Chinese Exercises & Massage

FOR HEALTH & LONGEVITY

Chinese Exercises & Massage

FOR HEALTH & LONGEVITY

by

DAHONG ZHUO, MD.
STAFF OF ANHUI MEDICAL SCHOOL
A.R. LADE
J. WONG

Hartley & Marks
PUBLISHERS

Published by

HARTLEY & MARKS PUBLISHERS INC.

P. O. Box 147 3661 West Broadway
Point Roberts, WA Vancouver, BC
98281 V6R 2B8

Printed in the U.S.A.

LIBRARY OF CONGRESS CATALOGING-IN-PUBLICATION DATA

Cho, Ta-hung.

Chinese exercises for health and longevity / by Dahong Zhuo.

p. cm.

Includes index.

ISBN 0-88179-158-X

1. Exercise therapy. 2. Health. 3. Medicine, Chinese.

I. Title. II. Title: Chinese exercises and massage for health and longevity

RM725.C45626 1998

615.8 2 DC21 97-49115

CIP

CONTENTS

PREFACE TO CHINESE EXERCISES 5
PREFACE TO CHINESE MASSAGE 9
HOW TO USE THIS BOOK 11

PART I
TRADITIONAL CHINESE EXERCISES

Introduction 17
1 *Tai Chi Chuan* 19
2 *Yi Jin Jing* — Muscle Strengthening Exercises 35
3 *Ba Duan Jin* — Eight Fine Exercises 49
4 *Shier Duan Jin* — Twelve Fine Exercises 59
5 *Chi Kung* — Invigorating Exercises 65
6 Other Traditional Chinese Exercises 77

PART II
CHINESE FITNESS EXERCISES

7 Fitness Exercises for Children 83
8 Fitness Exercises for the Sedentary 89
9 Fitness Exercises for the Elderly 97
10 Fitness Exercises for Pregnant Women 105
11 Fitness Exercises for Athletes 111

PART III
CHINESE THERAPEUTIC EXERCISES

12 Exercises for Hypertension 121
13 Exercises for Arteriosclerosis 131
14 Exercises for Coronary Heart Disease 135
15 Exercises for Gastrointestinal Problems 159
16 Exercises for Anxiety and Depression 167
17 Exercises for Insomnia 171
18 Exercises Following Brain Concussion 173
19 Exercises for Paralysis 174
20 Exercises for Sciatica and Lumbar Disk Problems 180

PART IV
PRINCIPLES &TECHNIQUES OF MASSAGE THERAPY

Introduction 186
21 Fundamental Techniques for Effective Massage 190
Section I: Commonly Used Techniques
1.Press Method 192
2.Rub Method 195
3. Push Method 197
4. Grasp Method 202
5. Roll Method 204
6. Dig Method 205
7. Pluck Method 207
8. Kneading Method 208
9. Vibrate Method 209
10. Drag Method 211
11. Chafe Method 212
12. Rub-roll Method 213
13. Pinch Method 215
14. Tweak Method 216

15. Flick Method 217
16. Knock Method 217
17. Pat Method 218
18. Hammer Method 219
19. Extension Method 221
20. Bend Method 223
21. Rotation Method 225
22. Shake Method 229
23. Stretch Method 230
24. Tread Method 236
Section II: Practicing Massage Techniques
1. Physical Training 237
2. Practicing the Techniques 240
22 Acupoints Commonly Used in Massage Therapy 245
23 How to Use Massage Therapy 256
Section I: Actual Practice
1. Amount of Massage 257
2. The Degree of Force to Use in Massage 257
3. Treat Each Case Individually 258
4. Important Considerations 259
Section II: Media Used in Massage 260
24 Clinical Applications of Massage Therapy 264
Section I: Actual Practice
1. Lumbar Strain 264
2. Chronic Lumbar Pain 266
3. Sprains 269
4. Bruise 273
5. Torn Muscles (*Muscular Lacerations*) 275
6. Flatfoot and Foot Strain 277
7. Frozen Shoulder (*Shoulder Periarthritis*) 279
8. Stiff Neck (*Torticollis*) 282
9. Bedsores (*Decubitus*) 284
10. Headache 286.

Section II: Common Ailments
11. Fatigue 288
12. Motion Sickness 290
13. Hemorrhoids 291
14. Insomnia 292
15. Indigestion 294
16. Anxiety and Nervousness 296
17. Menstrual Problems and Pain 297
18. General Chinese Massage Treatment 298

APPENDICES

1. Self-Massage for Strengthening the Body and Preventing Disease 300
2. Eye-Care Massage 302
3. Table of Weights and Measures 303
4. Table of Acupoints 304

INDEX

307

Preface to Chinese Exercises

In this modern age, the critical need for exercise therapy is especially felt when "life on wheels" and work with machines give us convenience and comfort at the cost of our health. The so-called diseases of civilization, or hypokinetic diseases, such as coronary heart disease and obesity, have become epidemic. In part, at least, their origin may be traced to lack of activity, and appropriate, regular exercise will do much to prevent them. In addition, with numerous new drugs appearing on the market each year, many patients and physicians tend to rely on medication, while fundamental recovery through therapeutic exercise is neglected. Clearly, the health and happiness of patients and their families will be enhanced by a knowledge of exercise therapy. A popular scientific book on this topic is a necessity today.

However, during my recent visit to North America, I was happy to find that, with the development of the holistic approach to health care in recent years, there has been a growing interest in Oriental preventive and therapeutic methods. Among those being brought to the attention of North Americans are programs of Chinese exercise therapy such as *Tai Chi Chuan* and *Chi Kung*, to mention only two of the most valuable.

Indeed, Chinese exercise methods are going to the West, and well deserve to do so. Chinese exercise carries a tradition of over 2,500 years. Numerous accounts found in medical classics and historical writings have shown its usefulness in maintaining health and promoting longevity. What is more important is that Chinese exercise therapy is now coming of age. The exercise programs which are widely used in China today represent a refinement of the ancient tradition. Over the past four decades Chinese clinical and experimental research has proved the effectiveness of Chinese therapeutic exercise and has revealed its underlying physiological mechanisms. Today the application of this kind of exercise therapy is guided by physiological and medical principles, thereby increasing the benefits to the patient. However, despite recent innovations, Chinese exercise programs still retain many unique traditional characteristics. It is this tradition which makes Chinese exercise therapy distinctive and gives it so much of its value.

Generally speaking, the Chinese systems of therapeutic exercise are characterized by slow and gentle movements with representative or symbolic implications, mental concentration during performance of the exercise, and the adjunctive application of self-administered massage. Physiologically and psychologically oriented, they have been found to be beneficial in chronic diseases, as well as where there are psychosomatic factors, and for preventive health in general. Most of the Chinese traditional exercise programs may be regarded as body/mind or body/image techniques, since both the body and the mind are trained during the practice. As a consequence, not only are the muscles, heart, and lungs strengthened, but the psychological and emotional states are also enhanced, promoting harmony and balance between body and mind. In this connection, I join many a physician of the West in suggesting that in today's world of hurried living and stress, these unique and ancient exercises may be a source of relaxation and peace of mind. They offer patients a means of relieving tension and shortening the recovery phase of long-term illness, particularly in diseases with a psychosomatic component, such as hypertension and peptic ulcer, as well as the psychoneuroses.

In addition, Chinese exercise therapy is effective in improving physical fitness and general well-being. It is well known that the middle-aged and elderly can benefit a great deal from the gentle movements of Chinese exercise. However, younger people—children as well as teenagers—will also find Chinese exercise interesting and of value, especially when they take up programs which demand strenuous effort to strengthen their muscles. Needless to say, the representative or symbolic aspects of many of the exercises will attract both young and old.

With these considerations in mind, I thought it worthwhile to write a book on Chinese exercise therapy for western readers, so that they might utilize this method of health care. As a physician trained in western medicine and with a research background in traditional Chinese medicine, I have been fortunate in being able to appreciate and evaluate traditional Chinese exercise therapy with an integrated point of view—from the standpoint of both western and Chinese medicine. The result is this practical guidebook on Chinese exercise therapy for the general reader and for people with chronic illness. In this book a number of traditional exercise programs are described in detail, and the application of these methods to a variety of diseases is dealt with in depth. Though Chinese methods are often used in conjunction with western methods in order to obtain the maximal therapeutic effect, this book emphasizes the Chinese methods.

The traditional system of Chinese exercise includes a strong preventive element for the promotion of general well-being and physical fitness. Regular and moderate exercise has long been considered valuable for health, fitness, and longevity. To reflect this tradition a number of well-known Chinese exercise programs are introduced in this book as examples of conditioning exercises. *Tai Chi, Yi Jin Jing,* and *Ba Duan Jin* all belong in this category. In addition, there are preventive health exercises specifically for sedentary people, the elderly, children, pregnant women, and athletes. In the sections for these programs, illustrations along with the description of the movements, as well as the benefits to be gained from the exercises, are presented. These exercises, many of which are characteristic of the traditional Chinese way, may be used to enhance physical strength, improve blood circulation, correct poor posture, increase flexibility and vigor, and to relax both body and mind. All will help promote the health of the exerciser.

The programs presented here are based on my own clinical experience and that of my colleagues in China. A substantial number of reports and presentations have demonstrated their usefulness and effectiveness in the management of disease. Chinese readers have shown much interest in these exercise programs, which I included in a Chinese text in 1976,* as have the many readers of the Japanese translation which followed. I shall be most happy if western readers also

*Zhuo Dahong: *Exercise Therapy in Chronic Diseases.* Beijing (Peking), People's Sports Press, 1976.

find this handbook useful in offering a simple and effective means to improve their health and fitness. It is also my sincere desire that this book will encourage the amalgamation of Chinese and western techniques of exercise therapy.

I am most indebted to my colleagues and associates at Zhongshan Medical College, Guangzhou (Canton), China, for their assistance in developing many of the programs presented in this book, to Dr. J. V. Basmajian of McMaster University and Dr. R. J. Shephard of the University of Toronto for their enthusiastic encouragement, to Dr. D. P. Barrett and Ms. S. W. Tauber for their valuable assistance in improving the style and language of the manuscript, to many other Canadian friends for their secretarial assistance, and to my publishers for their generous collaboration.

D. Zhuo
(Zhuo Dahong)
Guangzhou
The People's Republic of China

Preface to Chinese Massage

It has been my privilege to have worked on this text, translated from the original Chinese. My task was to check the accuracy of the medical terminologies used, especially to render them into the more current medical usage from the somewhat archaic terms obtained in the process of direct translation. I did this without changing the concepts and attitudes towards treatment of the original Chinese authors. I also reviewed the terminologies used in the sections pertaining to acupressure and, particularly, made some of the descriptions of point locations a little easier to follow. However, in this area especially, direct learning under supervision is the only really effective way to learn acupuncture point locations. This area of the text remains then, a guide to further study.

It is my feeling that the clinical work in massage therapy done in China is without equal in the world. The extremely effective work in this modality follows from the over three millennia of experience in traditional Chinese medicine in treating internal conditions of the body by manipulating, pressing, rubbing, heating, or needling surface areas of the body.

This text, then, supplies the western reader with an introductory perspective on the methods of and indications for Chinese massage therapy.

The overall basis of the text is for the treatment of a variety of pathological conditions from minor to severe. As such its primary audience will be health care professionals: massage therapists, physiotherapists, naturopaths, chiropractors, nurses, and physicians. Indeed, many of the conditions described require prior medical work-up and investigation while some require actual hospitalization; in this instance massage is just one of the many therapies utilized.

There is a still wider audience for this book, however. The general public has been over recent years demanding access to information in health areas formerly held exclusively by professionals. This includes information about effects of therapy, drugs, non-surgical alternatives, nutrition, methods of preventive medicine, and a whole host of related areas in health maintenance and general self-improvement.

Since massage applies itself very well as a general tool for relaxation and promotion of overall well-being, the interested and responsible layperson should find much useful information in this book about general methods of massage. Even the more clinically oriented sections will allow him or her to be aware of the therapeutic possibilities of the Chinese massage methods, inspiring the seeking out of practitioners who have a knowledge of such methods.

It is my hope that both my colleagues in western medicine and the interested lay reader will find this book a useful contribution to their store of knowledge.

Ronald Puhky, MD;
Bachelor of Acupuncture, College of Traditional Medicine, U.K.;
Diplomate, College of Traditional Chinese Medicine, Peking.
Peking, The People's Republic of China

HOW TO USE THIS BOOK

This book contains a great variety of exercise programs for individuals with different levels of health and physical fitness, and for all age groups. Each program is designed to produce specific effects, so that choosing the programs appropriate for one's needs will be a simple matter.

Benefits of the various exercises

- Relaxing the mind and body, calming oneself, and developing a sense of confidence: *Chi Kung* and/or *Tai Chi Chuan,* and *Shier Duan Jin.*
- Promoting basic fitness: a combination of one of the Chinese traditional exercise programs and a preventive health exercise program designed for one of the following groups: athletes, children, the elderly, pregnant women, or the sedentary.
- Improving the health of the heart, blood vessels, and lungs: one of the preventive health exercise programs designed for the various groups, combined with brisk walking or jogging.
- Improving muscle tone, posture, and stance: *Ba Duan Jin* and *Yi Jin Jing.*
- Maintaining or improving flexibility of the joints and spine, preventing back and neck pain: a combination of a preventive health exercise program, *Yi Jin Jing* or *Tai Chi Chuan,* and *Shier Duan Jin.*

Note: To help control weight, jogging or brisk walking are recommended.

For cure or better recovery from chronic disease, the third part of the book presents therapeutic exercise for particular diseases.

It is recommended that everyone using this book develop a daily exercise routine. Essential considerations in planning an exercise routine are the frequency, intensity, type, and time involved (FITT) in the exercises. If possible, the exercises should all be done in one or two daily sessions. Depending on individual needs, daily exercises should last at least ten minutes and may take up to half-an-hour. In most cases a moderate level of intensity is preferred. In terms of types of exercise, while the individual needs as described above should be considered, there is also room for personal preference.

For example, an exercise program for the average person is aimed at maintaining the health of the heart and lungs, increasing stamina, improving flexibility, and preventing mental stress. For these purposes, people in moderately good health may choose either of the following two programs.

(All exercises, except of course those for pregnant women, are suitable for both male and female exercisers.)

Example Program 1

Exercises for the sedentary, middle-aged, and those with mental stress
1. Preventive health exercise for the sedentary. 2. *Chi Kung for Fitness* (the Chinese way of meditation for mental and physical health). 3. *Shier Duan Jin* (which emphasizes self-massage or self-acupressure). *Note:* It is preferable to practice these three sets of exercises together in one program.

Example Program 2

Exercises for the elderly and those with poor cardiovascular health or poor posture
1. *Ba Duan Jin* and/or *Yi Jin Jing*. 2. *Chi Kung for Relaxation*. (A relaxation-meditation technique.) 3. Brisk walking. 4. Preventive health exercise for the elderly. *Note:* An elderly person should choose No. 4 (preventive health exercise for the elderly) instead of No. 1 (*Ba Duan Jin* and/or *Yi Jin Jing*).

Benefits of massage therapy

- Massage therapy is helpful for the treatment of numerous health problems, from minor to severe. It is generally suitable for both acute and chronic diseases.
- Massage treatments can help many conditions when used in conjunction with other primary treatments.
- Chinese massage is also used to promote harmony of body and mind as well as resistance to disease.
- Chinese massage will be of interest to health care professionals, such as massage therapists, physiotherapists, chiropractors, nurses and physicians, as well as anyone interested in health and alternative therapies.

It is recommended that anyone using these massage techniques pay attention to the specific needs of the patient and choose the massage techniques accordingly. Whether you are a professional massage therapist or a layperson, a positive relationship between the practitioner and the patient is essential. This book provides crucial information for those undertaking a long-term program of self-massage to assist in their own healing process.

PART I

Traditional Chinese Exercises

Introduction

Several basic exercise programs from the Chinese tradition are presented in this section. These popular and time-honored exercises are effective for both preventive and therapeutic purposes.

To obtain the maximum benefit from these exercises, one must try one's best to comply with certain requirements which are unique to the Chinese system of exercise.

In the first place, keep a peaceful mind and relaxed manner during the exercise. Focus your attention on the movement. You should be quite confident that you will benefit from doing the exercise.

Next, combine the movement with slow, gentle, and conscious breathing. This pattern of breathing will make you more relaxed and more aware of the movement.

Use your imagination when doing the exercise. Most of the traditional Chinese exercises, as indicated by their names, are representative or symbolic. Try to imagine what is suggested by the exercise, as if you were carrying out an imaginary task. For example, when doing the exercise "Shooting the eagle by drawing the bow with the hands," you should imagine there is an eagle in the sky and a bow in your hands. While watching the eagle attentively, you draw the bow to shoot the arrow at it.

Lastly, always combine exercise with self-administered massage. This is done either before exercise as a preparatory procedure, or following exercise to assist recovery and obtain benefits other than those directly resulting from the exercise. For example, massage on the face and neck produces tranquilizing effects and helps concentrate the mind on preparing for the exercises; massage on the joints following exercises induces a sense of relaxation and ease around the joints. In addition, massage on acupuncture points results in effects specific to those points as described in the following sections of this book.

For indications to a particular exercise, one may refer to the text of that section as well as the following sections dealing with particular diseases.

It is advisable to adhere to a set of programs which you find to suit you best. It is also acceptable to combine several programs at one time, or to alternate different programs from time to time.

CHAPTER I

Tai Chi Chuan

Translated literally the Chinese word *Tai* means great, *Chi* means origin, and *Chuan,* exercise with the hands. Hence *Tai Chi Chuan* is an exercise of great origin using the hands. It is so named because *Tai Chi* is regarded as the mother of *Yin* and *Yang,* while *Yin* and *Yang* are regarded as the parents of all things.* A good balance between *Yin* and *Yang* is essential to health, and *Tai Chi Chuan* is so valuable because it incorporates *Yin* and *Yang* in a balanced manner.

Tai Chi is a gentle and relaxing form of exercise. My research during my stay at the University of Toronto established that the average energy cost for the long form of *Tai Chi Chuan* is equal to walking at the speed of approximately 3½ miles per hour, putting it in the category of moderate exercise.

In my own experience and that of other Chinese physicians, *Tai Chi Chuan* produces remarkable effects in the treatment of a number of illnesses. It is also of great benefit to people in a variety of age groups, and with varying constitutions and levels of health. For those with emotional problems or prone to mental stress, *Tai Chi* brings relaxation and modification of the psychological profile, developing better concentration, attention, composure, self-confidence, and self-control.

For people with hypertension, it is a natural way to lower blood pressure. This effect occurs either immediately after a practice session or after a long-

* *Yin* and *Yang* are the two universal energies, which are polarized, and contain and complement each other. *Yang* is the creative initiator, and *Yin,* the cooperative, receptive energy.

term period of training. In turn, symptoms such as headache, dizziness, and insomnia are relieved.

For those with mild arthritis or rheumatism, practicing *Tai Chi* will increase the flexibility of the joints and prevent restriction of movement.

For people with atherosclerosis, it helps improve the circulation in the hands, legs, and feet. Symptoms such as numbness and weakness of the hands and feet will be relieved.

Derived from *Tao Yin* (the Way of Yin), *Tai Chi Chuan* has absorbed all the best qualities of Chinese traditional therapeutic exercises. As the movements are gentle and slow, they are particularly suitable for the middle-aged and elderly. Performance of *Tai Chi* requires relaxation of the muscles of the wrists, arms, shoulders, chest, abdomen, and back. The gentleness of the movement enables the performer to experience a feeling of relaxation, comfort, and ease. It may be said that *Tai Chi Chuan* brings peacefulness and rest to the mind. Meanwhile, relaxation of the muscles leads to relaxation of the arterioles, in turn reducing blood pressure. This is why a hypertensive patient may benefit from *Tai Chi*.

Tai Chi movements are directed by thought rather than by strength. While performing them, one must be relaxed and quiet, with the attention directed towards each movement of the exercise. Such concentration will bring relief in cases with emotional disorders, and provides an excellent exercise for the mind.

Tai Chi Chuan involves all the muscles and joints of the limbs and trunk. Each and every movement involves all muscles of the body. It is also a breathing exercise. During the practice of *Tai Chi,* breathing should be deep, steady, rhythmic, and gentle. Inhalation and exhalation should coincide with certain movements and in accordance with a set routine.

With the lumbar region as the axis of its movement, *Tai Chi Chuan* involves exercise of the trunk and facilitates the circulation of blood in the abdomen, thus improving digestion.

The intensity of *Tai Chi* is relatively low compared to jogging and other sports. Taking Simplified *Tai Chi Chuan* as an example, investigations have determined changes in physical functions during or immediately after the performance of these movements to be very slight (the heart rate measured at

105 beats per minute; blood pressure, 128/70 mmHg; pulmonary ventilation, 8.54 liters per minute; and energy cost, 2.3581 kcal per minute —only 11.92 kcal is expended if the exercise is completed in five minutes). The intensity of the older form of *Tai Chi* is a little higher than that of Simplified *Tai Chi Chuan,* but is still fairly low. Because of this low intensity, *Tai Chi* generally does not lead to fatigue or stress.

In addition to all its other benefits, and due to the complexity of its movements, *Tai Chi Chuan* helps improve coordination and balance.

Because of all this, *Tai Chi* has enjoyed much popularity among the Chinese people for over six hundred years, and is still highly valued today.

How to practice *Tai Chi* correctly

To obtain the maximum therapeutic effect of *Tai Chi Chuan,* one must practice it in accordance with certain principles:

- All movement should be gentle and soft, with the breath smooth and natural. *Tai Chi* should be performed gently, lightly, and in slow progression. Take your steps as lightly as a cat walks. Stretch your arms as gently as if you were pulling a thread of silk. It is desirable to move very slowly so that it takes 5–9 minutes to finish a set of Simplified *Tai Chi Chuan.*
- While performing *Tai Chi,* practice diaphragmatic breathing (abdominal breathing) naturally and rhythmically. Breathe in when doing raising or stretching movements; breathe out when doing lowering or bending movements. Never hold your breath during its performance.
- Relax the body and take an easy and comfortable stance. *Tai Chi Chuan* abhors straining and "grunting" motions. The stance should be easy and composed, and the body should be relaxed, especially the lower back and abdomen. It is inappropriate to strain the chest. Relax the muscles of the back so that the shoulders are dropped and relaxed. Your posture should follow these basic guidelines: Hold your chest in and straighten your back; drop your shoulders and lower your elbows. Then your stance will be easy and comfortable and your body will maintain good posture.
- Direct every movement with close attention, but do the exercises as effortlessly as possible. During the performance of *Tai Chi,* it is important to

allow your every movement to be directed consciously. You should have the image of the movement in your mind. Meditate over it quietly. "Draw" the image of the movement in your mind at the same time as you actually draw the image of the movement with your arms and legs.

- The strength of your muscles should be so controlled that you are making no visible effort, nor straining. Your limbs should move effortlessly, though actually you are using some strength to accomplish this.

It must be emphasized that *Tai Chi Chuan* is a very complicated exercise and cannot be self-taught. One must learn it from an experienced teacher. Fortunately, there are many *Tai Chi* centers in North America, and competent teachers are available in many cities. The following guidelines may be useful to those who are looking for a teacher of *Tai Chi*.

- Try to find a teacher who has been practicing *Tai Chi* for more than five years and has had experience in teaching it.
- If possible, select a teacher from among the active members of a well-established *Tai Chi* society.
- A *Tai Chi* teacher with a background of training in physical health education, or in health and life sciences, is preferred. Also, it is better to choose a health-oriented instructor than one oriented towards martial arts. However, proficiency in skill and knowledge should be the top criterion in making the choice.
- National origin is not important in selecting a *Tai Chi* teacher. Very often Caucasian teachers are as competent as their Chinese counterparts in teaching *Tai Chi*. For teachers of any nationality, an interest in and understanding of the Chinese philosophy of health and exercise is a definite asset to their teaching.

Simplified *Tai Chi Chuan*

Commencing form (1–4)

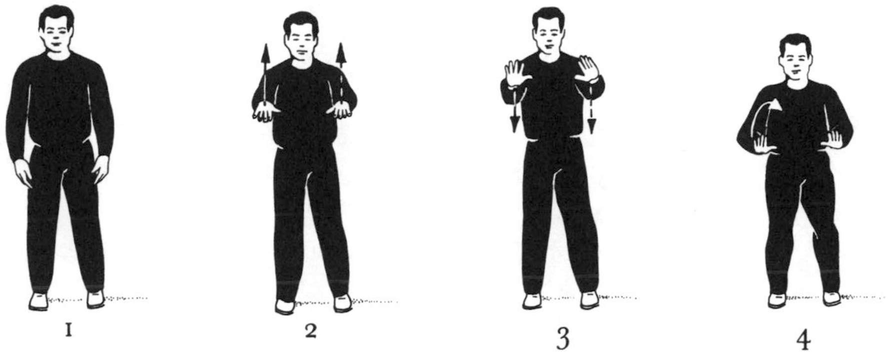

1 2 3 4

Parting the wild horse's mane on the left side (5–9)

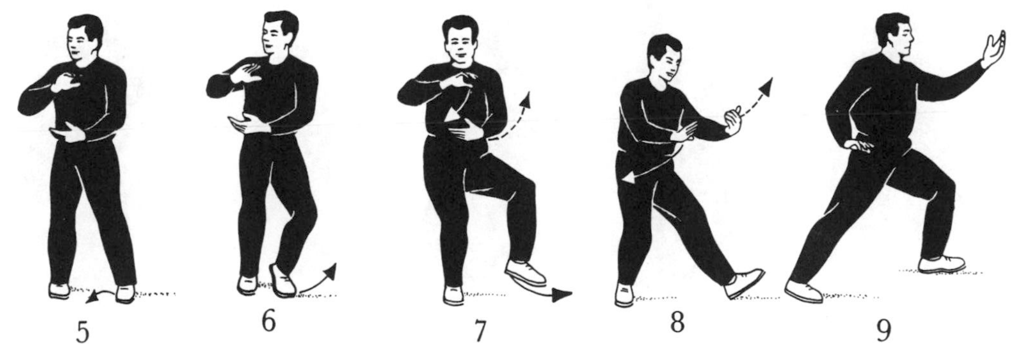

5 6 7 8 9

Parting the wild horse's mane on the right side (10–14)

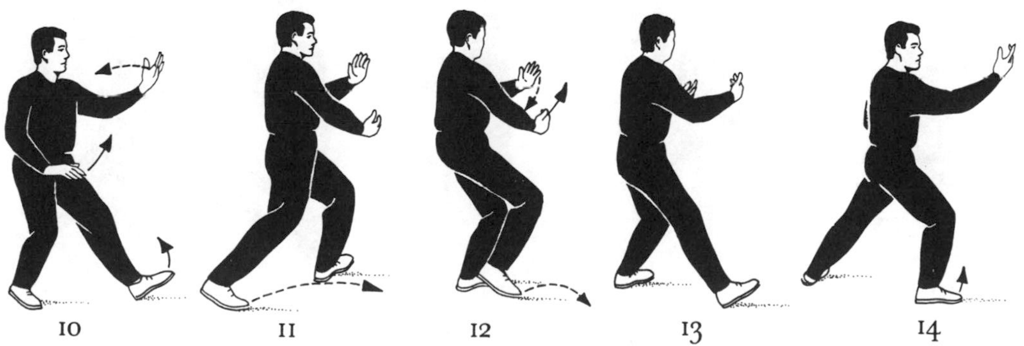

10 11 12 13 14

Parting the wild horse's mane on the left side (15–19)

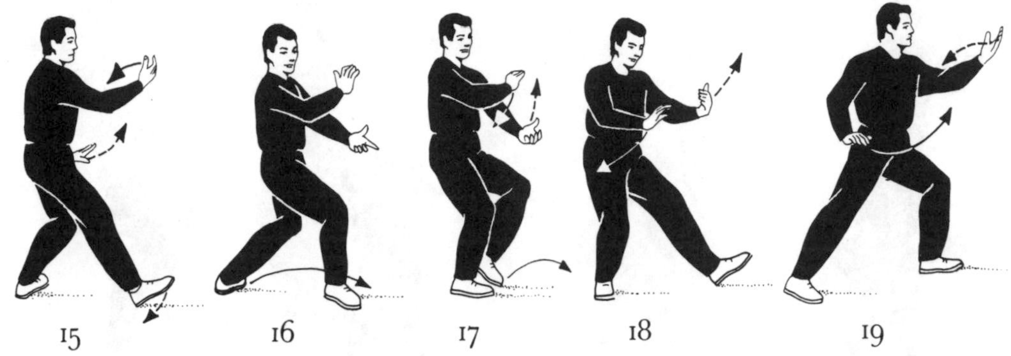

The white crane spreads its wings (20–22)

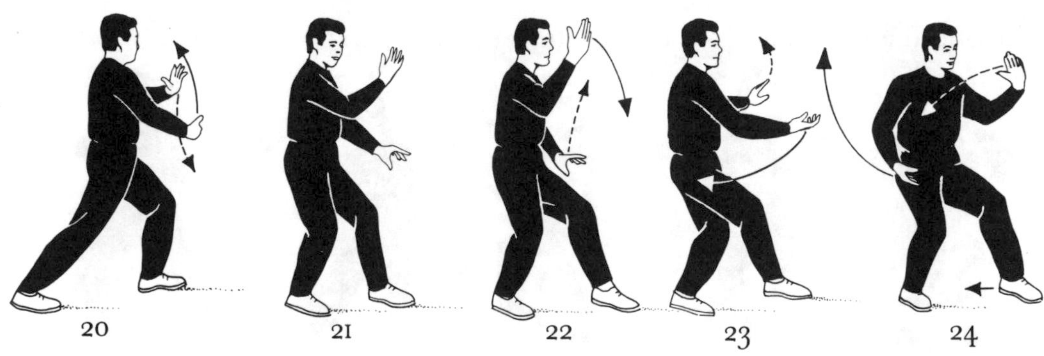

Brush knee and twist step on the left side (23–29)

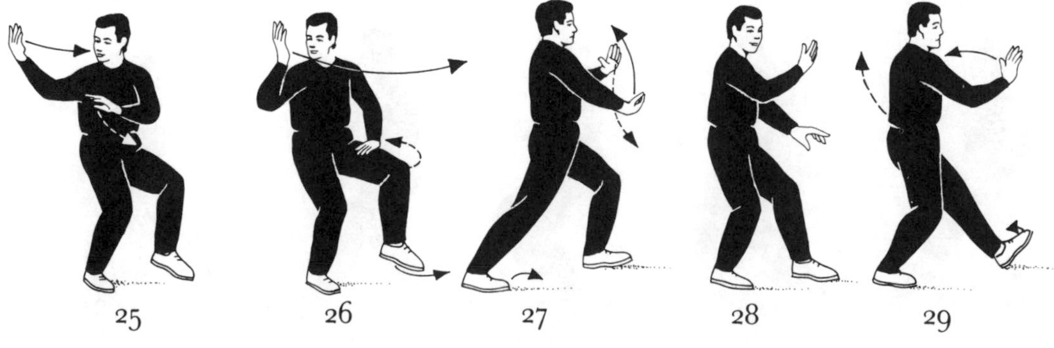

Brush knee and twist step on the right side (30–34)

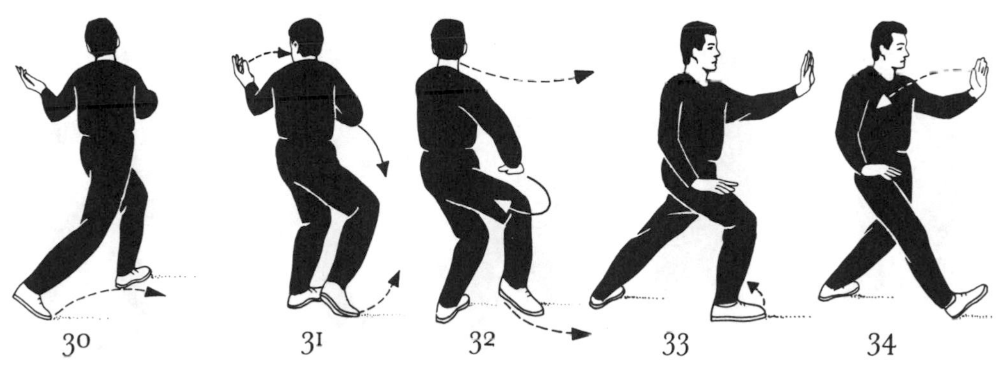

Brush knee and twist step on the left side (35–38)

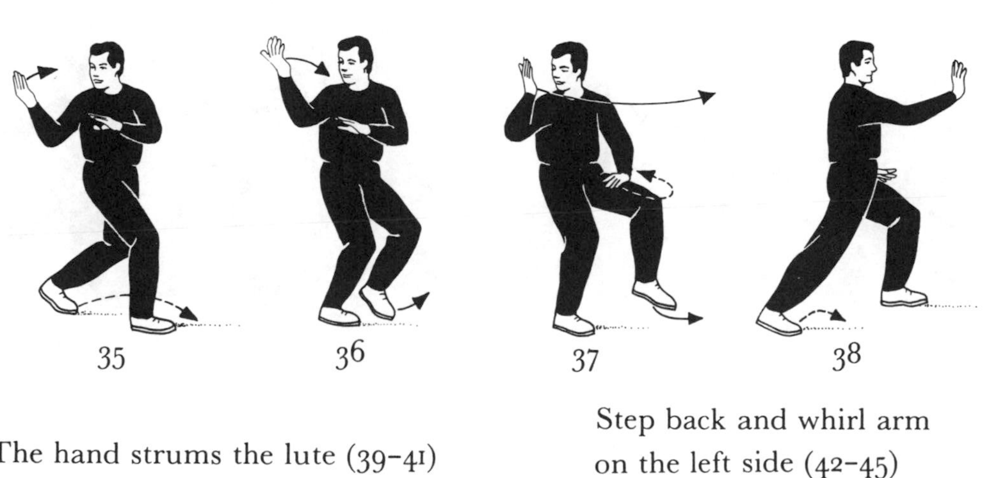

The hand strums the lute (39–41)

Step back and whirl arm on the left side (42–45)

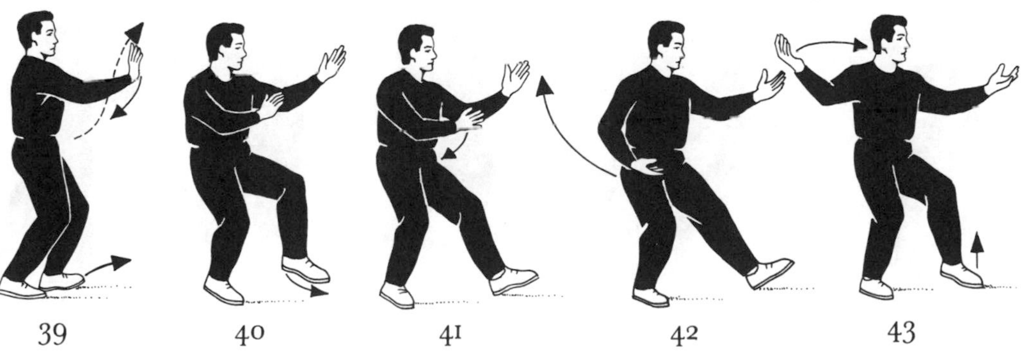

Step back and whirl arm on the right side (46–48)

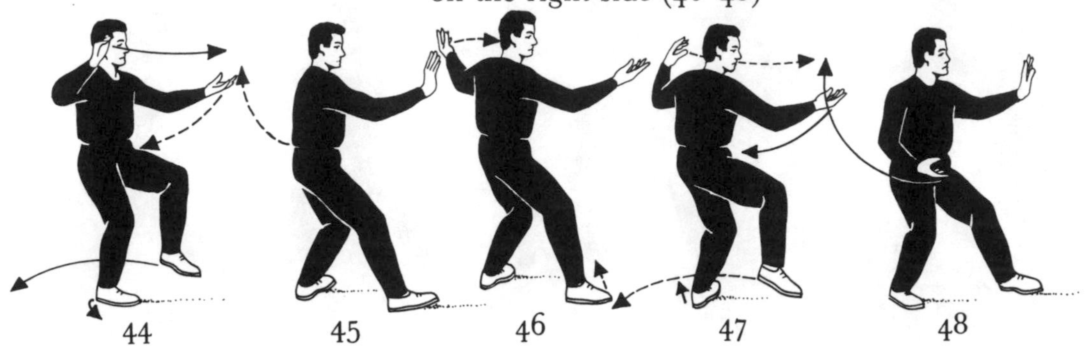

Step back and whirl arm on the left side (49–51)

Step back and whirl arm on the right side (52–54)

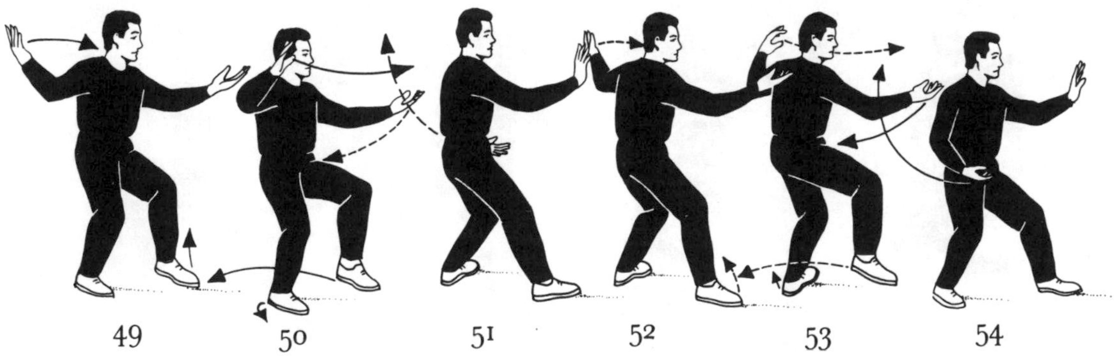

Grasp the bird's tail—left style (55–66)

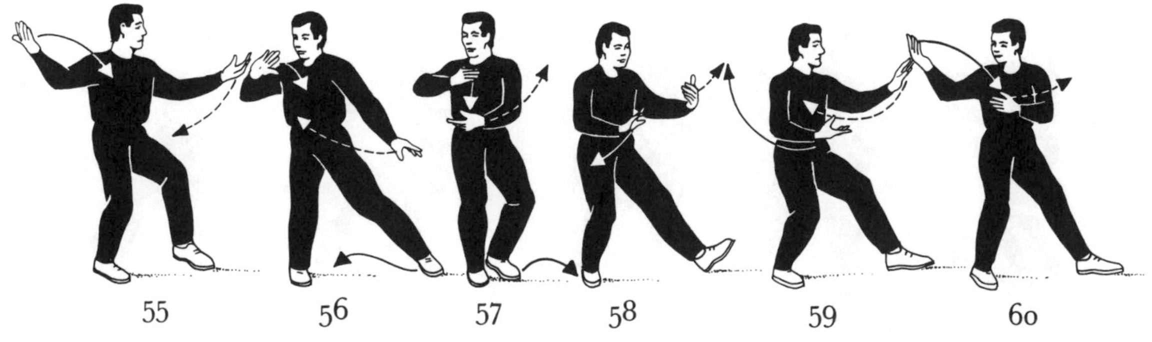

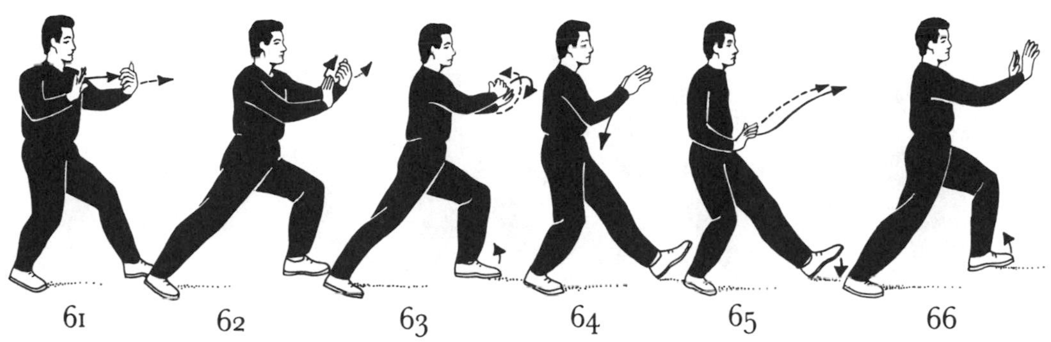

61 62 63 64 65 66

Grasp the bird's tail—right style (67–80)

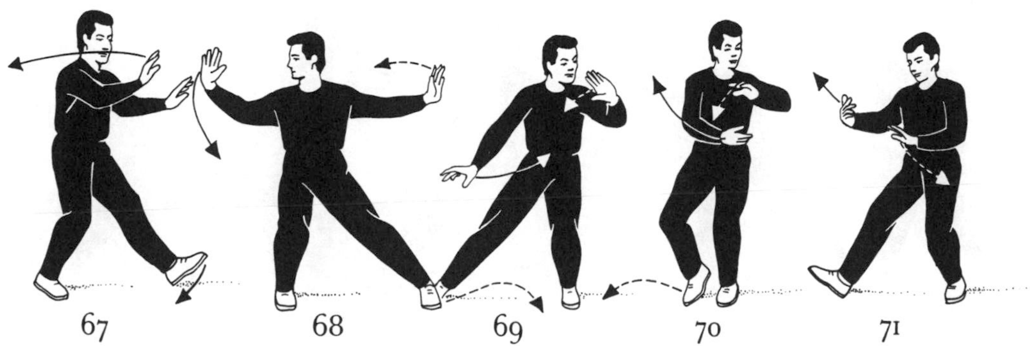

67 68 69 70 71

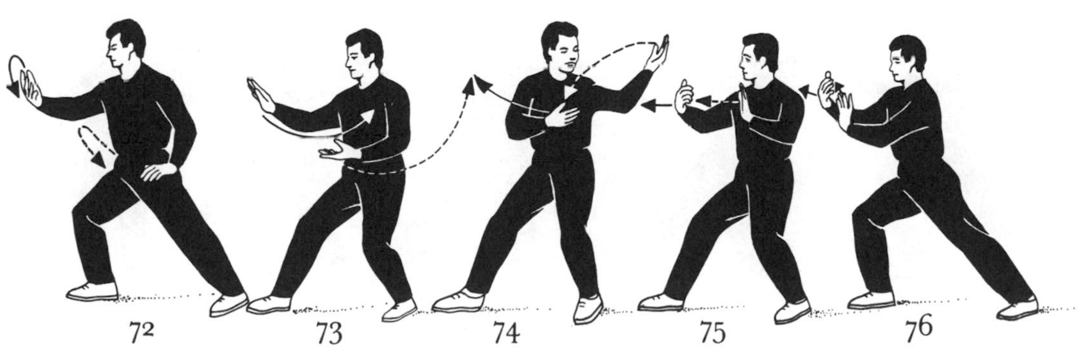

72 73 74 75 76

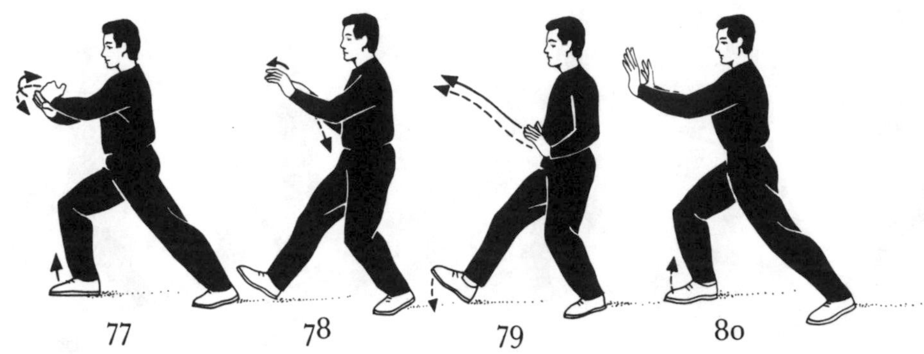

Single whip (81–86)

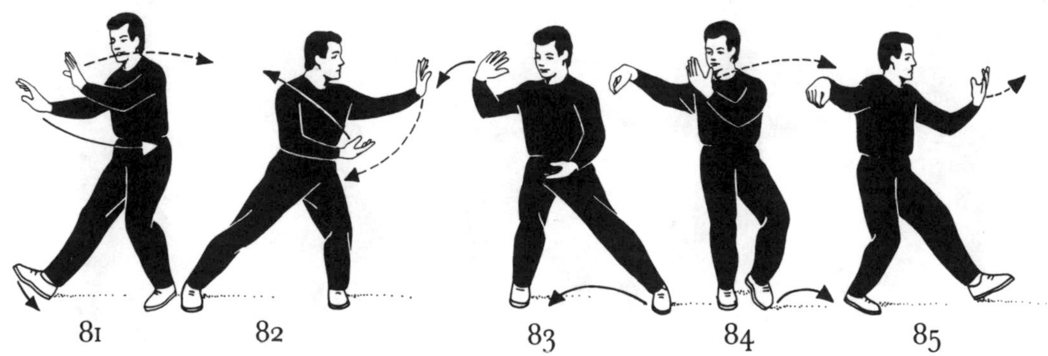

Wave the hands like clouds (87–100)

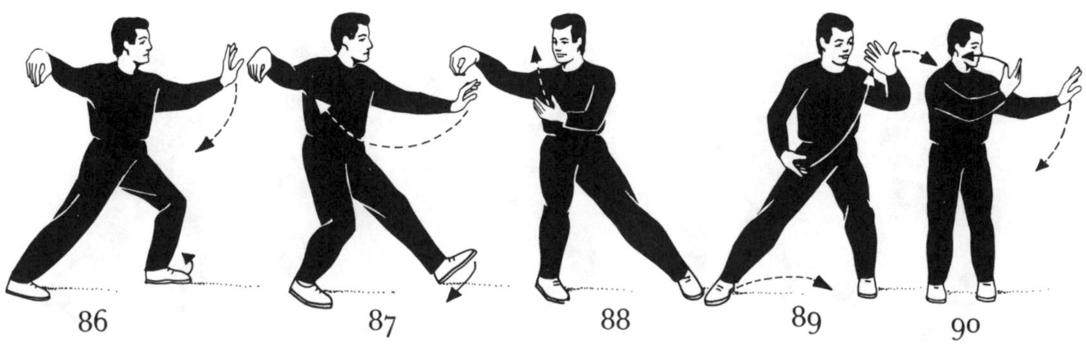

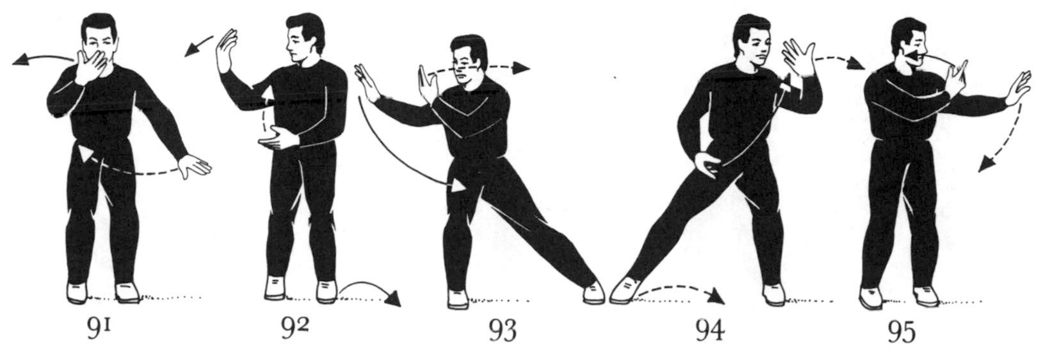

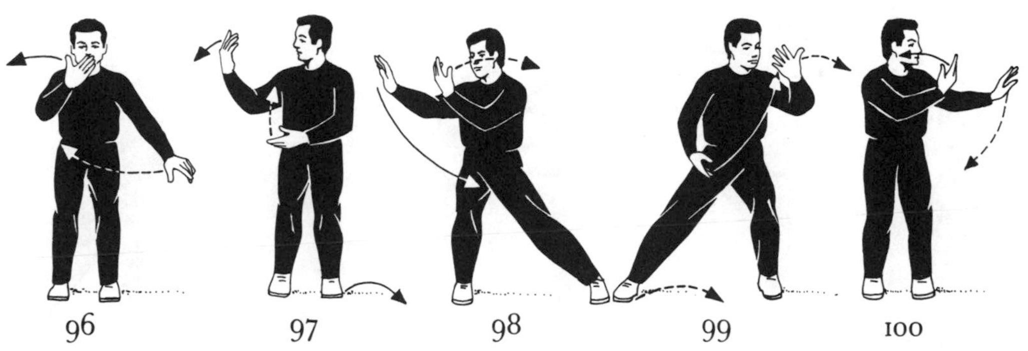

Single whip (101–5)

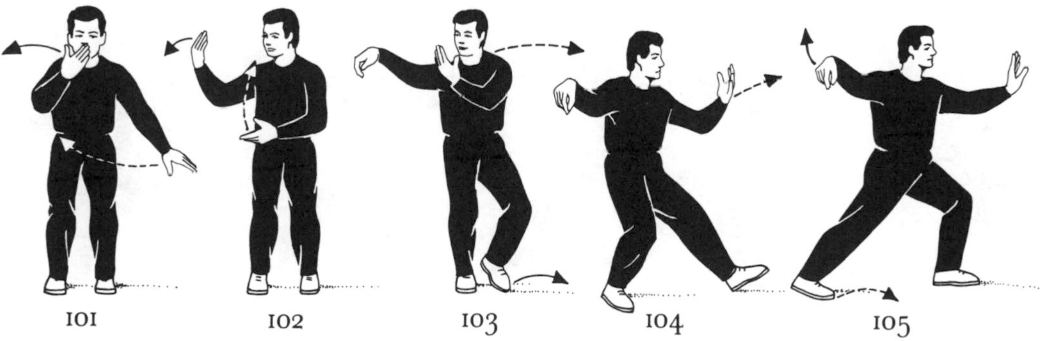

Pat the horse high (106–7)

Kick with the right heel (108–13)

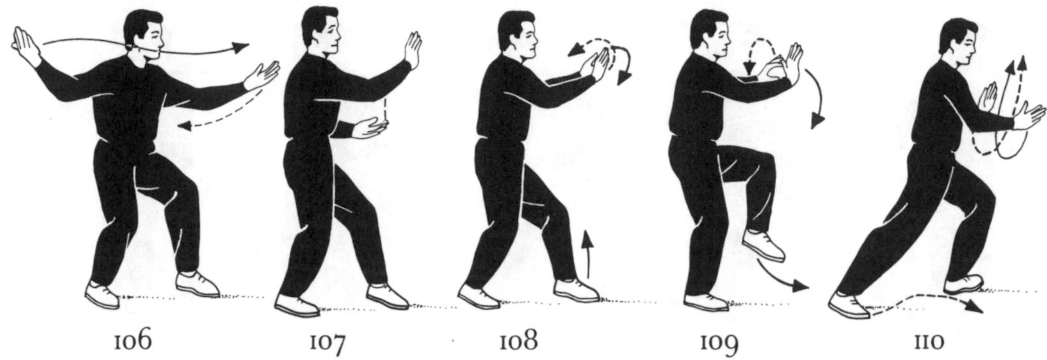

Strike opponent's ears with both fists (114–17)

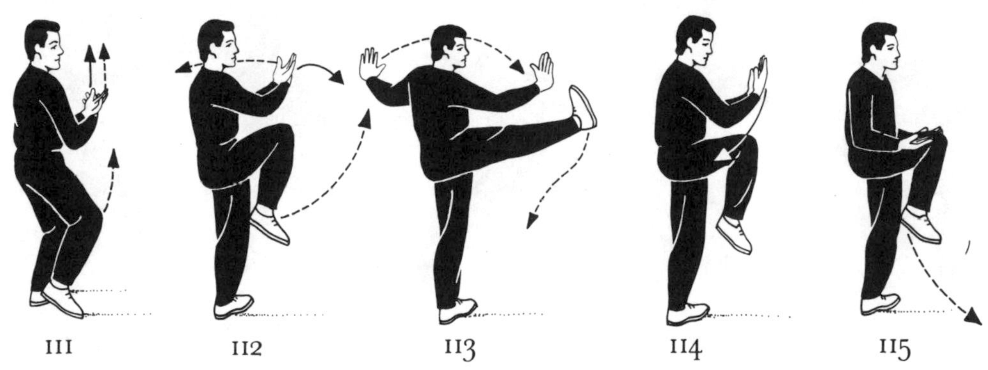

Turn and kick with the left heel (118–23)

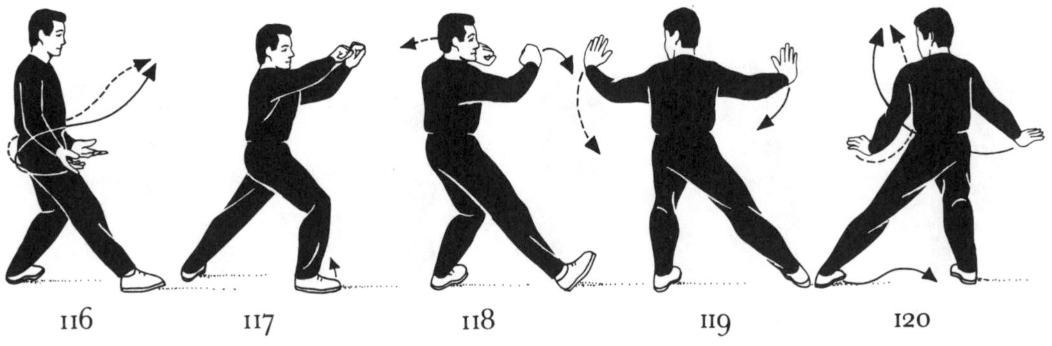

Push down and stand on one leg—left style (124–30)

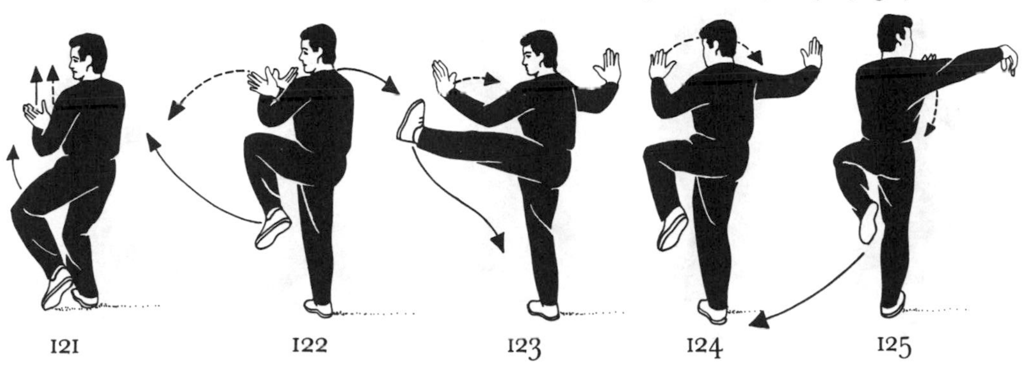

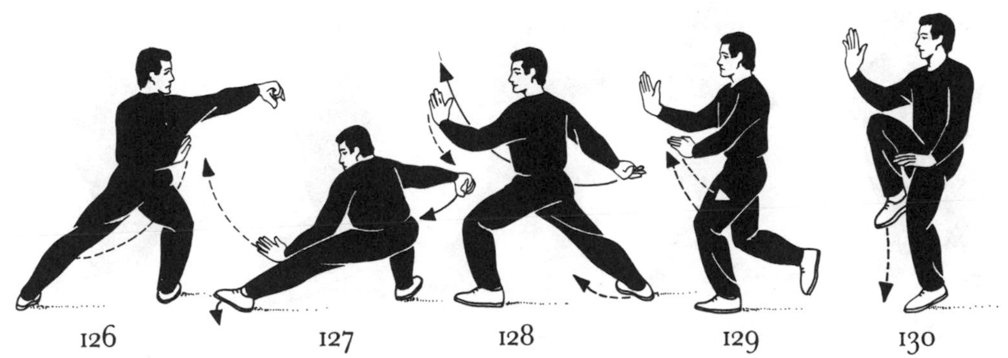

Push down and stand on one leg—right style (131–37)

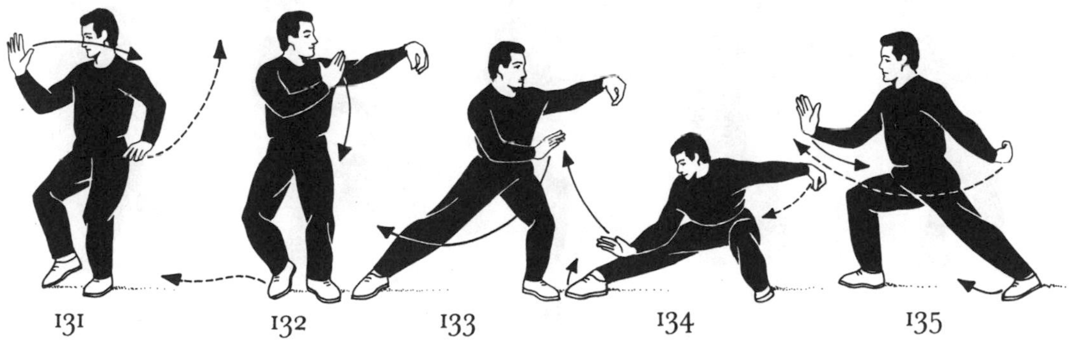

Work at shuttles—left style (138–42)

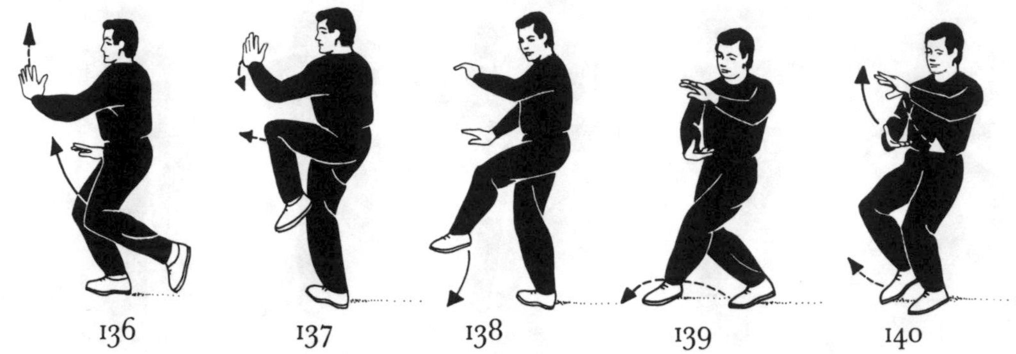

136 137 138 139 140

Work at shuttles—right style (143–48)

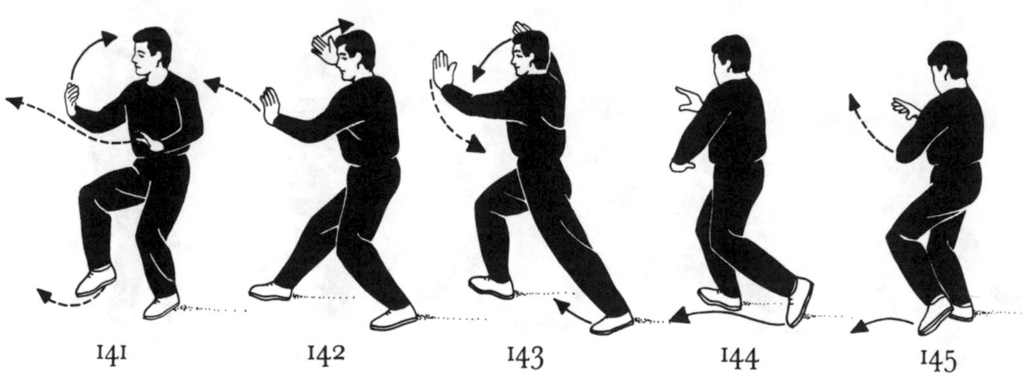

141 142 143 144 145

The needle at the bottom of the sea (149–50)

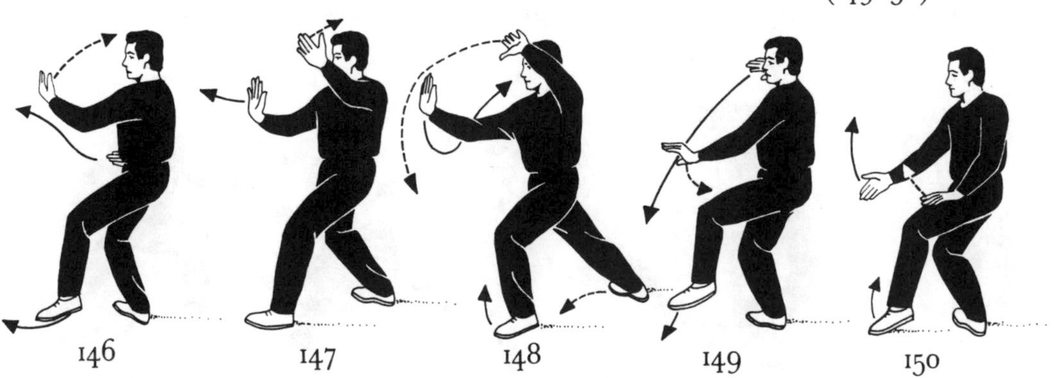

146 147 148 149 150

Flash the arm (151–53)

Turn, deflect downward, parry, and punch (154–60)

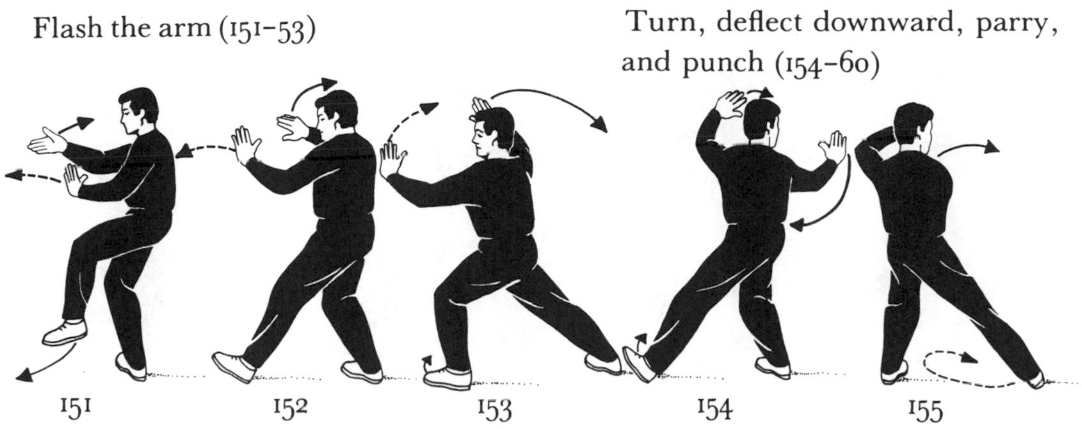

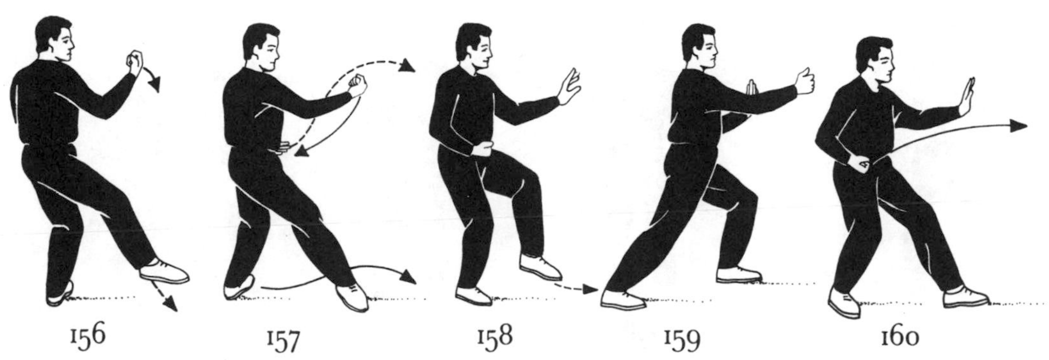

Apparent close-up (161–66)

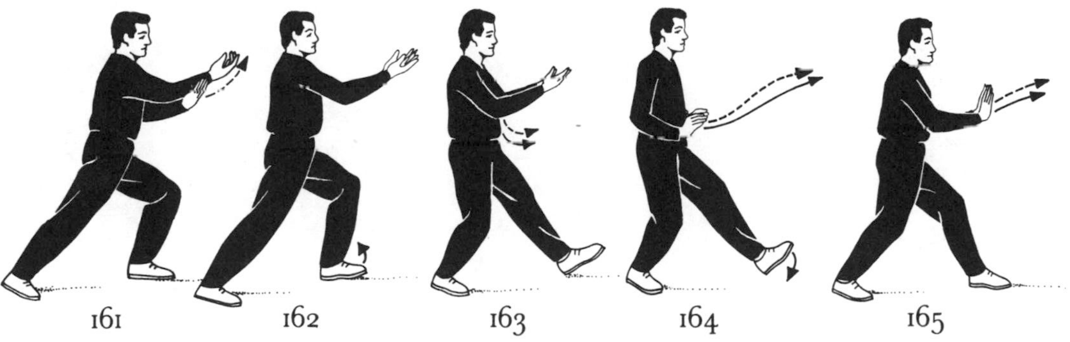

Cross hands (167–70)

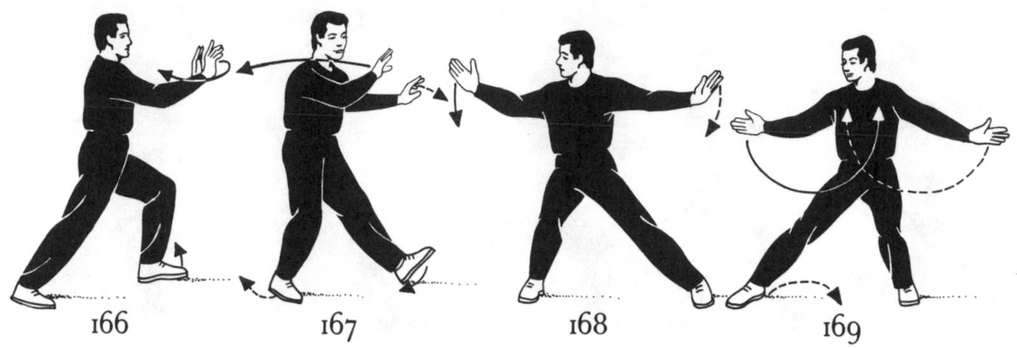

166 167 168 169

Closing form (171–73)

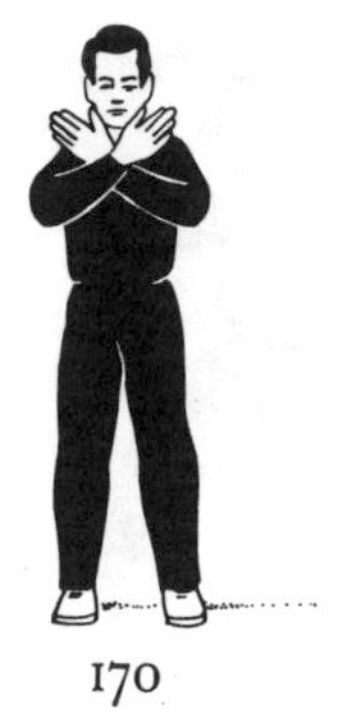

170

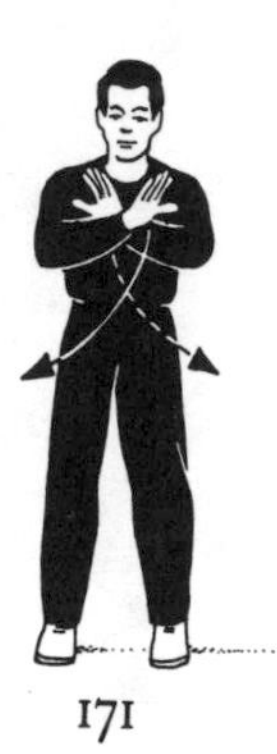

171

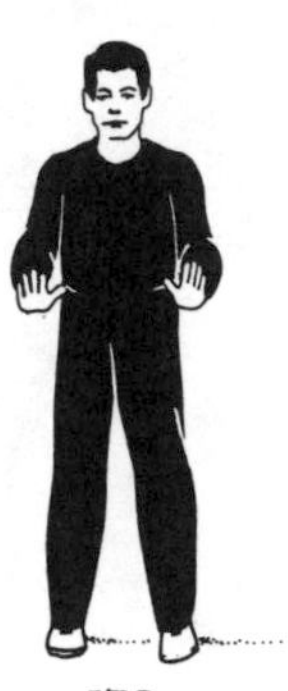

172

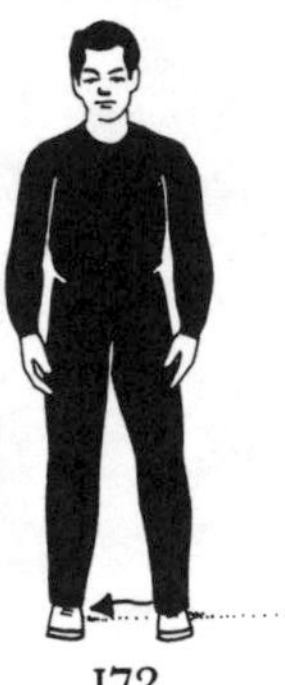

173

CHAPTER II

Yi Jin Jing—Muscle Strengthening Exercises

Yi Jin Jing is one of China's traditional forms of calisthenics. Its origin may be traced back over a thousand years. It consists of twelve exercises involving the head, arms, and trunk, and is performed in a standing position. Essentially, this program of exercise is isometric in nature. Unlike *Tai Chi Chuan, Yi Jin Jing* movements should be performed with significant vigor, though the motions are slow and appear gentle. Along with the vigorous movement, there should be relative stillness of mind, with the attention focusing on various parts of the body. As an exercise effective in strengthening muscles, it is still widely practiced today by Chinese masseurs and traditional bone surgeons, as well as by the average person wishing to maintain good muscle tone.

Yi Jin Jing can be done in full sequence or selectively. When done in full, as in the case of fitness training for younger people, one begins with Exercise 1 and proceeds in a smooth succession until the last exercise (Number 12) is completed. When done selectively, the exercises can be chosen in accordance with the needs of the exerciser. For example, those with neck pain will choose Exercise 4 (Reaching the stars) and Exercise 7 (Pulling the ear). To improve posture, Exercises 1, 2, and 3 can be chosen, while Exercise 8 is best for developing the knees and thighs. Individuals with hypertension should not do Exercises 10, 11, or 12, so as to prevent the risk of getting a headache or aggravating an already existing headache when lowering the head. The twelve exercises of *Yi Jin Jing* are as follows:

Exercises 1 thru 3 are stretching exercises, good for improving posture and expanding the chest. Like the other exercises (Numbers 4 thru 12) of *Yi Jin Jing,* they are called body/mind exercises, since attention and imagery are emphasized, helping to cultivate an alert mind. These three should be performed once each and in succession.

EXERCISE 1: *Making a gesture of respect with both hands facing the chest.*

STARTING POSITION: Standing, arms at sides, feet apart shoulder width, back erect, eyes straight ahead.

MOVEMENT: 1. Raise the arms slowly from the sides until they reach a horizontal position, palms downward, elbows straight. 2. Turn the palms inward, bend the elbows to let the hands approach the chest and stop at a distance of 6 inches (15 cm) in front of the chest.

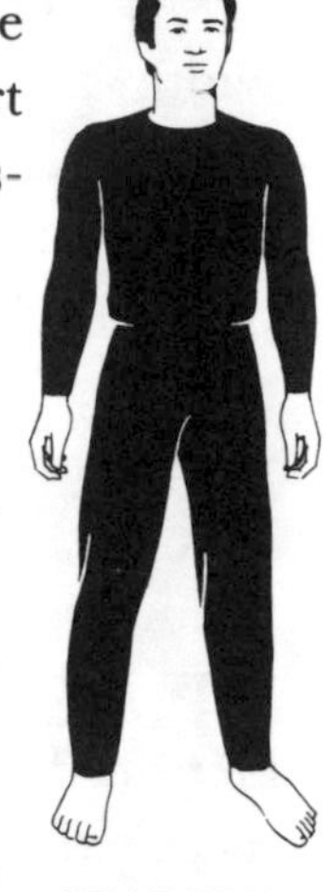

STARTING POSITION

Note: This exercise, as an initial and preparatory step, serves to adjust the body (relaxed and comfortable), adjust the mind (peaceful and concentrated), and adjust the breathing (smooth and natural).

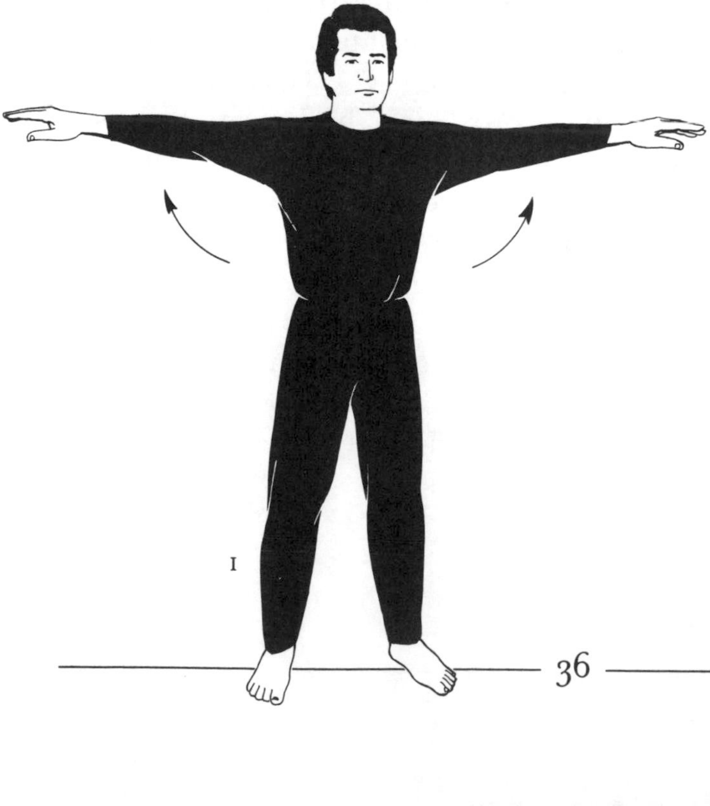

1

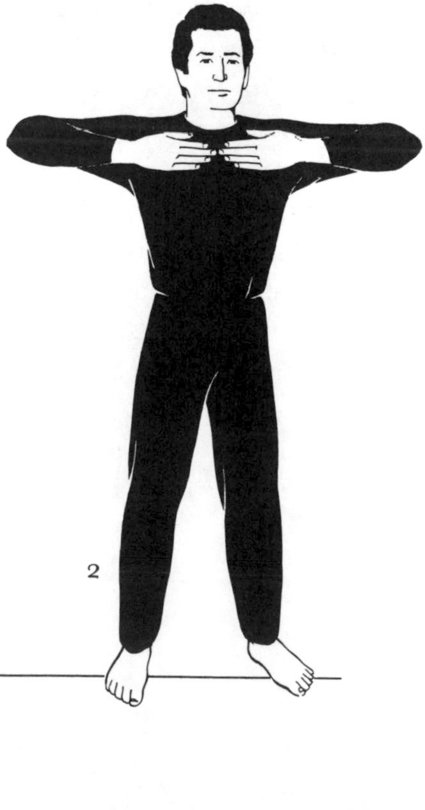

2

EXERCISE 2: *Heaving.*

STARTING POSITION: Standing, feet apart shoulder width, arms at sides, back erect, eyes straight ahead.
MOVEMENT: 1. Toes firmly touching the ground, turn the palms upward. 2. Raise the heels slightly about one inch (2–3 cm). Toes touching the ground, extend the arms horizontally, palms upward, and hold. Attention is focused on palms and toes. Breathe naturally.

Note: Movements of hands and feet should be performed simultaneously.

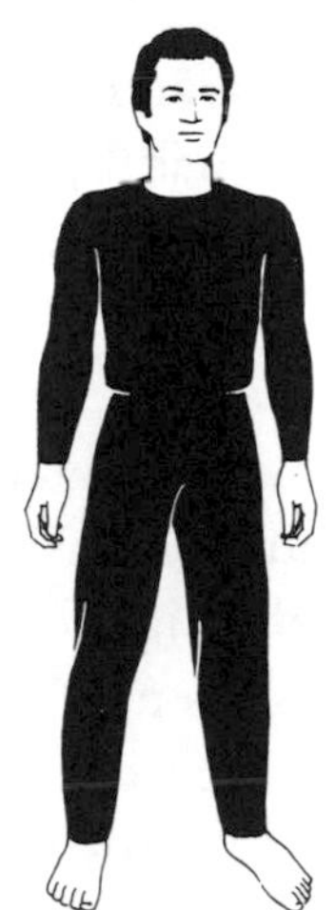

STARTING POSITION

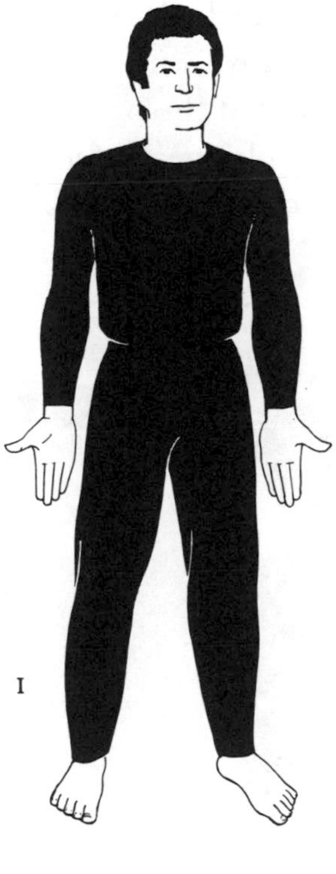

1

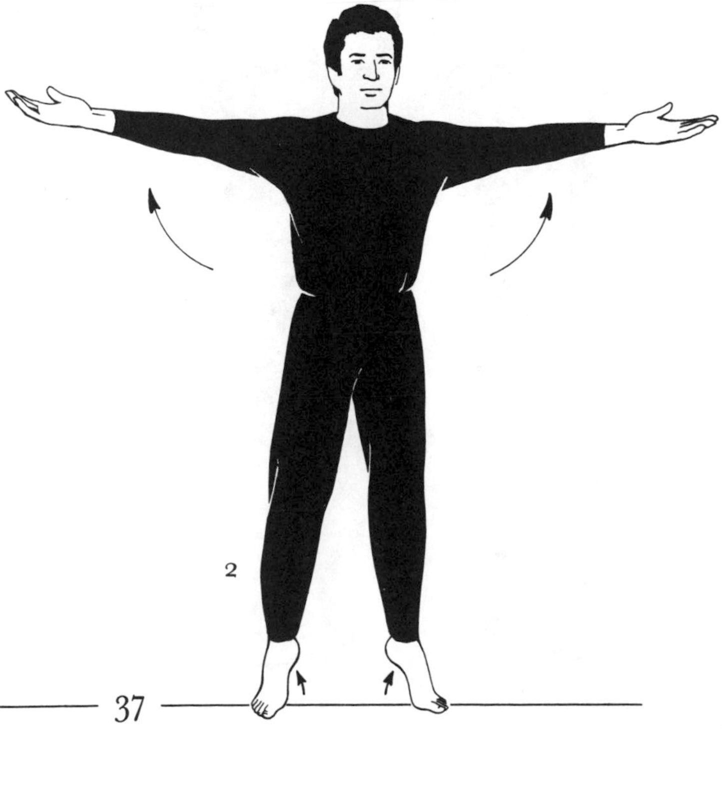

2

EXERCISE 3: *Pushing towards the sky.*

STARTING POSITION: Standing, feet apart shoulder width, arms extended horizontally, palms upward.

STARTING POSITION

MOVEMENT: 1. Raise the arms slowly from the side, as if drawing an arc, until they reach a vertical position. 2. Then turn palms upward, fingers pointing inward as though the hands are pushing up towards the sky. Meanwhile raise the heels higher than in Exercise 2, toes touching the ground. Clench the jaw and place the tip of the tongue against the roof of the mouth, breathing smoothly and deeply. Attention is focused on both palms (watching the palms from the mind). 3. Clench the fists and slowly lower the arms to the "heaving" position (arms extended horizontally out to the sides, with the palms open and upward). Heels down.

Note: "Watching the palms from the mind" does not mean looking at the palms with the eyes. It simply means focusing your attention on the palms.

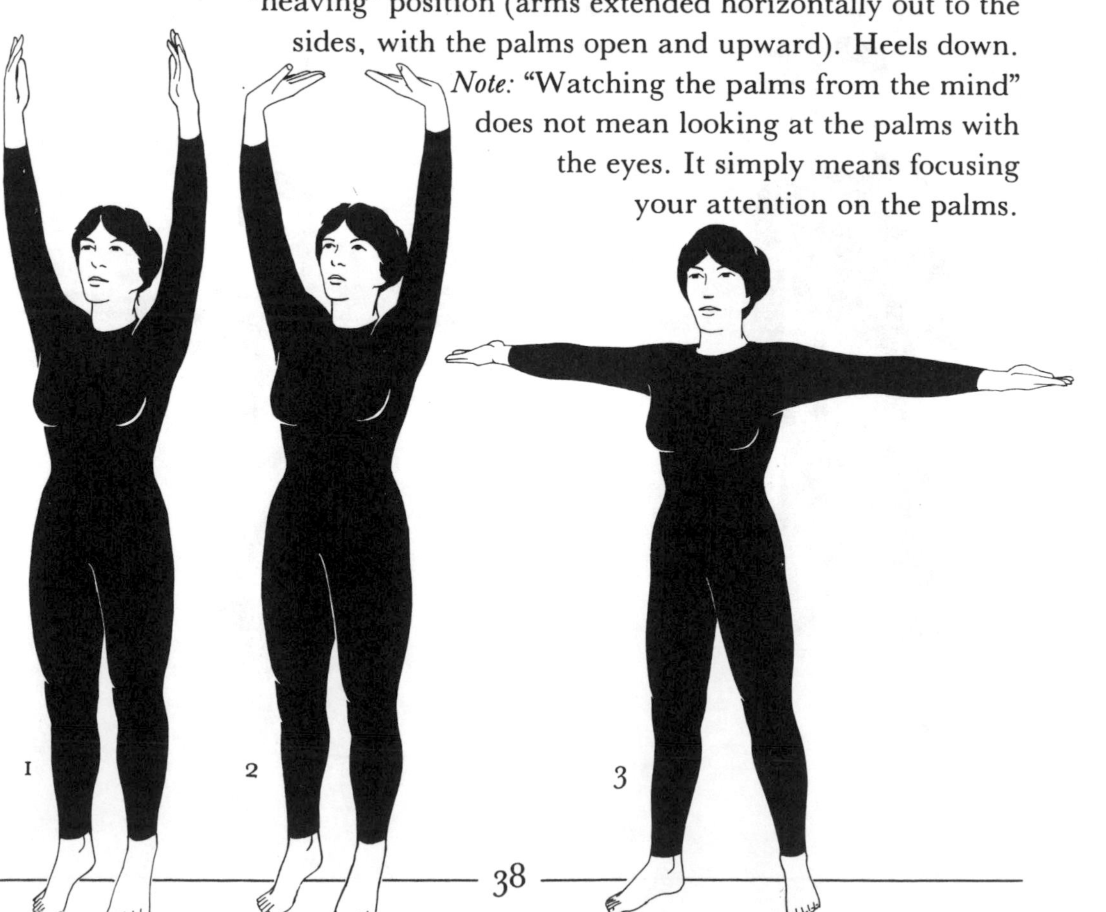

EXERCISE 4: *Reaching the stars.*

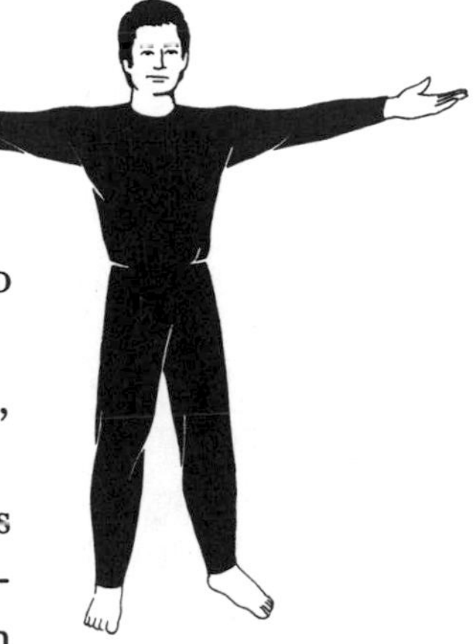

STARTING POSITION

This exercise develops flexibility of the shoulder joints and the upper spine. It helps to prevent the frozen shoulders and stiff neck common among the middle-aged and elderly. Since the exercise involves static contraction of the arm muscles while holding the reaching position, it is also good for strengthening the arms.

STARTING POSITION: Standing, feet apart shoulder width, arms extended horizontally, palms open and upward.

MOVEMENT: 1. Raise the right arm slowly until it reaches a vertical position. Turn the palm downward, fingers together pointing inward. Raise the head upward and turn right, with the eyes looking at the right palm. Meanwhile, bring the left arm down and turn the left palm with the back of the hand touching the back. Hold this position for a while. Take 3–5 breaths. 2. Raise the left arm (as in step 1 for the right arm). Raise the head and turn left with the eyes looking at the left palm. Bring the right arm down and touch the back with the back of the right hand. Hold. Take 3–5 breaths.

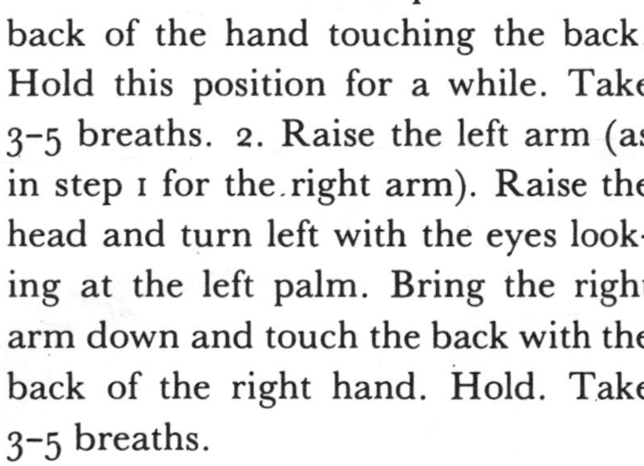

1

Repeat this exercise 3–5 times.

Note: While looking at the upper hand, attention is focused on the back, which is being touched by the other hand. When breathing in, press the back lightly with the hand. When breathing out, relax. Breathing should be rythmic, smooth, and slow.

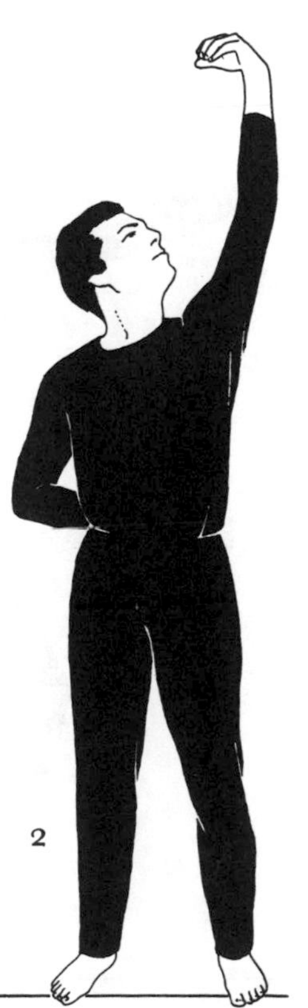

2

EXERCISE 5: *Pulling the tails of nine oxen.*

This is an isometric exercise which involves contracting the arm muscles as tightly as possible for the required length of time, thus helping develop strength in the arms.

STARTING POSITION: Standing, feet apart shoulder width, left arm raised upward, the head turned up with eyes looking at the left palm, the right arm flexed backward with the back of the right hand touching the lower back.

MOVEMENT: 1. Remove the right hand from the back. Bring it forward and stretch the arm until the hand is raised to the shoulder level, elbow slightly bent, fingers together and slightly bent. Meanwhile, the right foot takes a step forward with the knee bent and the left leg stretching straight behind. Bring the left arm down and stretch it behind, fingers together and slightly bent, palms upward. Breathe in, and focus attention on the right hand which is pulling with effort, as if pulling the tails of oxen. Breathe out, and focus attention on the left hand which is now pulling with similar

STARTING POSITION

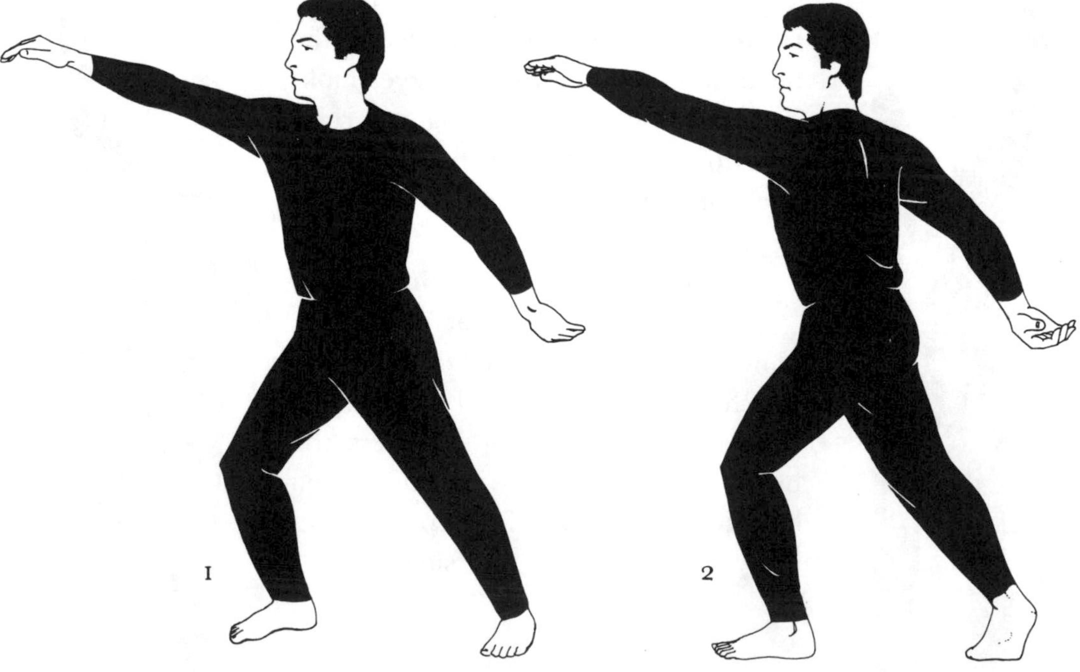

effort from behind, as if pulling the tails of oxen. Repeat several times. As a result of straining, the legs, trunk, shoulders and elbows will tremble slightly when pulling. 2. The left foot takes a step forward with the knee bent and the right leg stretching straight behind. Turn the left wrist and stretch the left arm forward. Bring the right arm down and stretch it behind (same position as step 1, only reversed). Breathe in, and focus attention on the left hand. Breathe out, focusing attention on the right hand. The requirements for the pulling movement are the same as in step 2.

Repeat this exercise 3–5 times.

Note: Breathe naturally with the abdomen relaxed. The pulling should be somewhat strained.

EXERCISE 6: *Pushing the mountain.*

This exercise strengthens the arms and helps correct a rounded upper back.

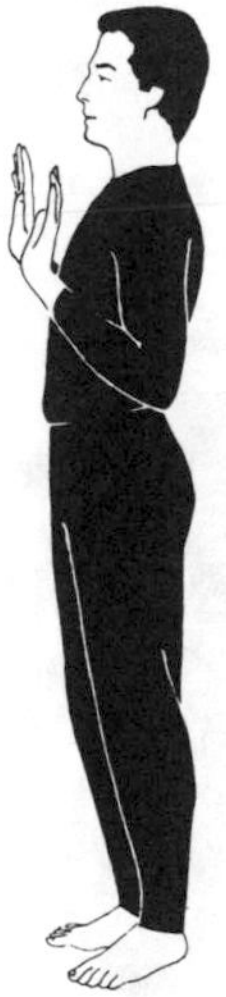

STARTING POSITION

STARTING POSITION: Standing, feet together, elbows bent at sides with fingers spread and pointing upward, palms forward.

MOVEMENT: Hands erect and form a right angle at the wrists, palms outward ("mountain pushing hands"). Push hands slowly forward, increasing the effort gradually until the elbows are fully extended. Meanwhile keep the body straight, eyes straight forward. Then bring the hands back to the starting position alongside the chest.

Repeat this exercise 3–5 times.

Note: At the end of the pushing, effort is exerted to the maximum, as if you are pushing a mountain. Breathe out while pushing. Breathe in when relaxing.

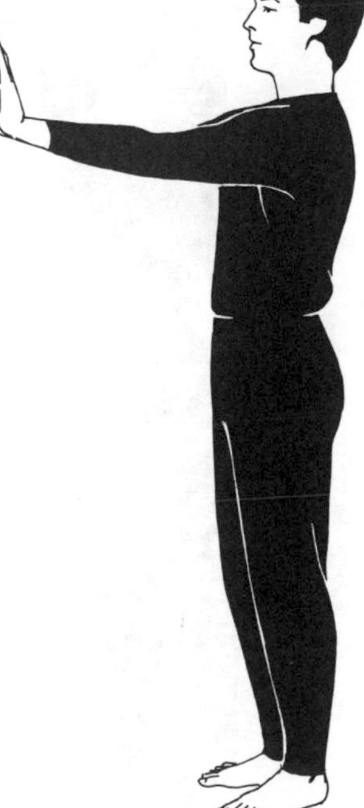

EXERCISE 7: *Pulling the ear.*

The benefits gained from this exercise are much the same as those in Exercise 4 (Reaching the stars), though to a lesser extent.

STARTING POSITION: Reach standing: Standing, feet together, arms fully extended forward horizontally, palms facing forward.

STARTING POSITION

MOVEMENT: 1. Raise the right hand to the back of the head. Press the head with the palm, and pull and press the left ear with fingers. The right shoulder is fully extended. Meanwhile, turn the head to the left and place the left hand on the back with the back of the hand touching the space between the shoulder blades. Breathe in, pulling and pressing the left ear with the right hand. At this time, there will be a sense of strain at the head and right elbow. Attention is focused on the right elbow. Breathe out and relax. Repeat the above breathing 3–5 times. 2. Bring the right hand down and put it on the back with the back of the hand touching the space between the shoulder blades. Raise the left hand to the back of the head. Press the head with the palm, pull and press the right ear with the fingers, lightly. The left shoulder is fully extended. Meanwhile, turn the head to the right. Breathe in, pulling and pressing the right ear with the left hand. At this time, the head and elbow again experience a sense of strain. Attention is focused on the left elbow. Breathe out and relax. Repeat this 3–5 times.

Repeat the entire exercise 3–5 times.

Note: Keep the body straight and the breathing smooth.

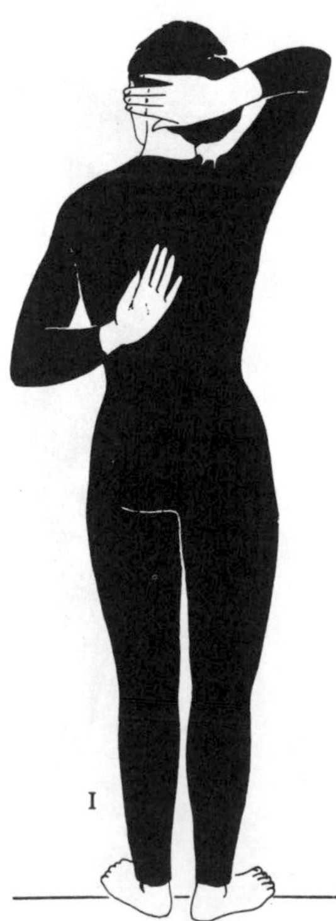

1

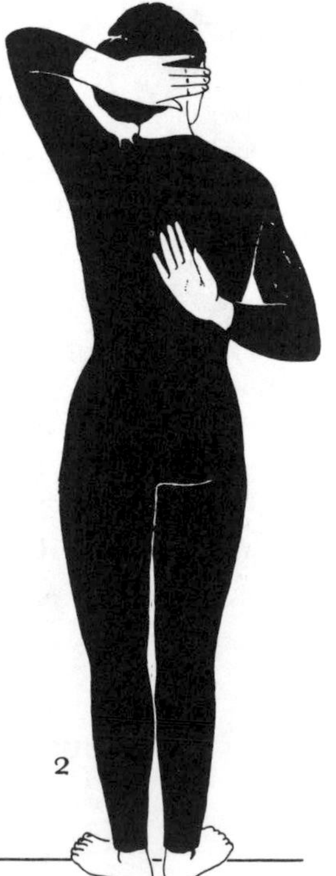

2

EXERCISE 8: *Lifting the plates.*

This is a good exercise for strengthening the thighs and knees. It is recommended for both prevention and treatment of weak and painful knees resulting from the degeneration of their cartilage.

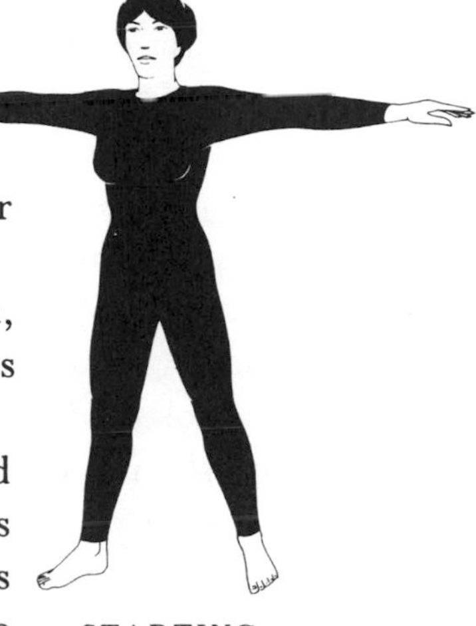

STARTING POSITION

STARTING POSITION: Standing, feet apart shoulder width, arms extended sidewards at shoulder level, palms downward.

MOVEMENT: 1. Bend the knees (ride standing), head and back remaining straight. Bend the elbows and press the hands downward with increasing effort as the knees continue gradually to bend, fingers apart with the thumbs pointing inward. Press the hands down to about 6–8 inches (15–20 cm) above the knees. 2. Turn the palms upward. Raise the hands slowly as if you were lifting heavy objects weighing a thousand pounds, and begin straightening the knees gradually to a standing position.

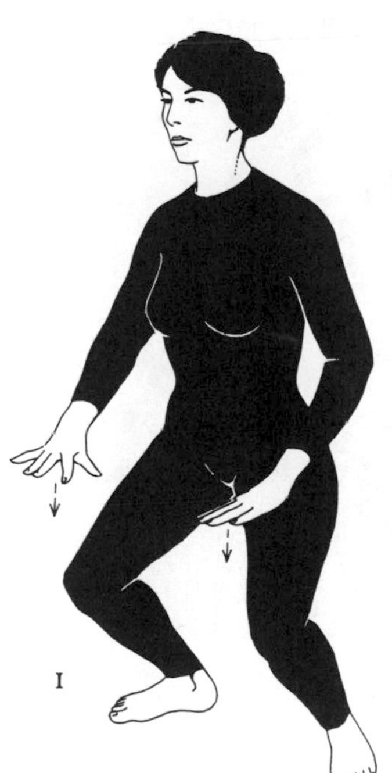

1

Repeat this exercise 3–5 times.

Note: The movement should be slow. Strenuous effort must be made in doing the "lifting." During the exercise, close the mouth and place the tip of the tongue against the roof of the mouth, eyes wide open and straight ahead. Breathe out as the hands press down, breathe in as they lift up.

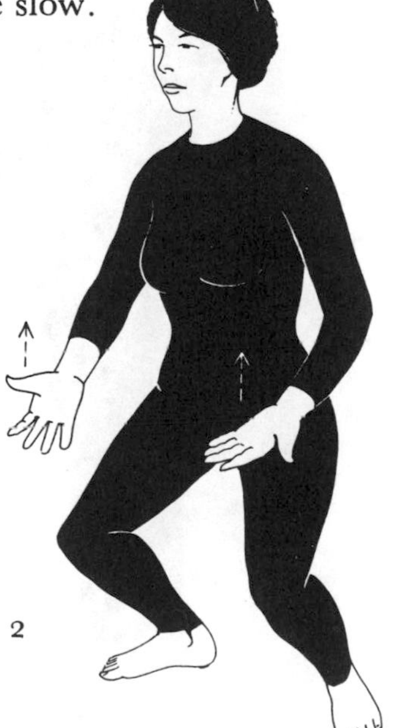

2

EXERCISE 9: *Stretching the arms.*

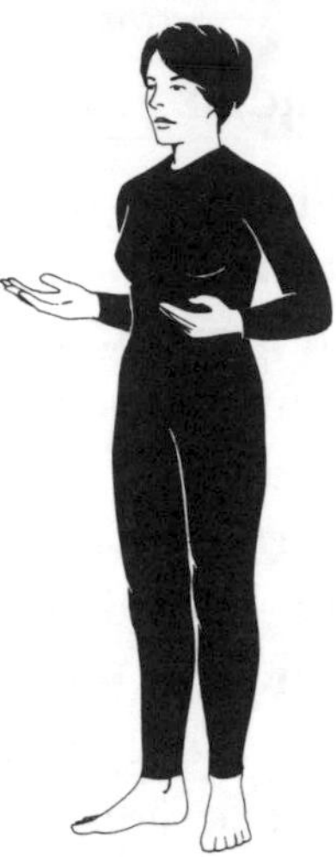
STARTING POSITION

This exercise develops the arms.

STARTING POSITION: Standing, feet slightly apart, arms bent at sides of chest, palms up.

MOVEMENT: 1. Turn the left hand with the palm downward and make a loose fist. Bring the left hand close to the hip. Meanwhile, turn the right hand with the palm downward and make a loose fist. Stretch the right arm forward towards the left. Turn the head and the trunk slightly to the left at the same time. 2. Bring the right fist close to the right hip. Meanwhile stretch the left arm forward towards the right (to the reverse of position 1). Repeat 3–5 times.

Note: Breathe in through the nose when stretching the arm. Breathe out through the mouth when the stretching is completed.

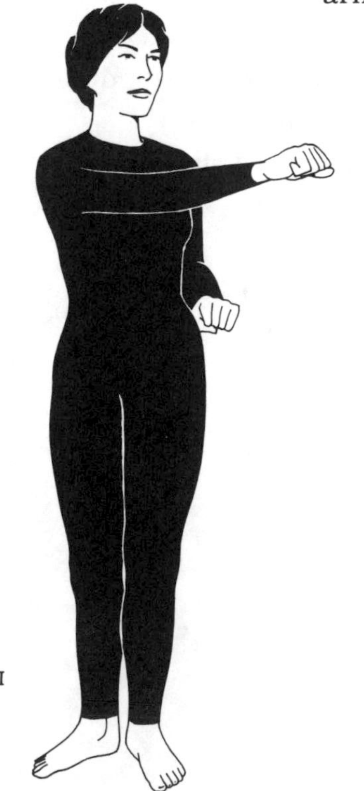
1

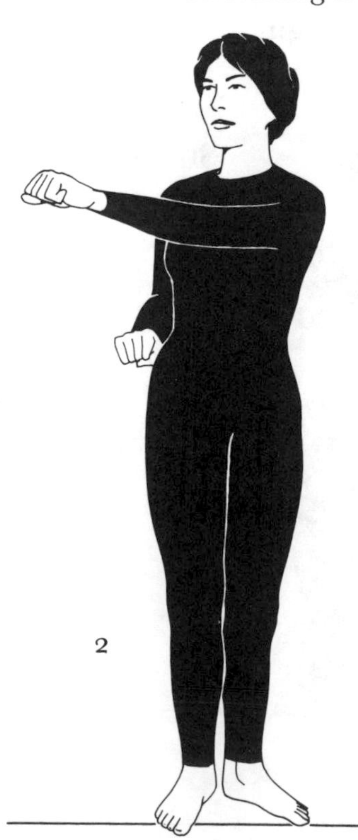
2

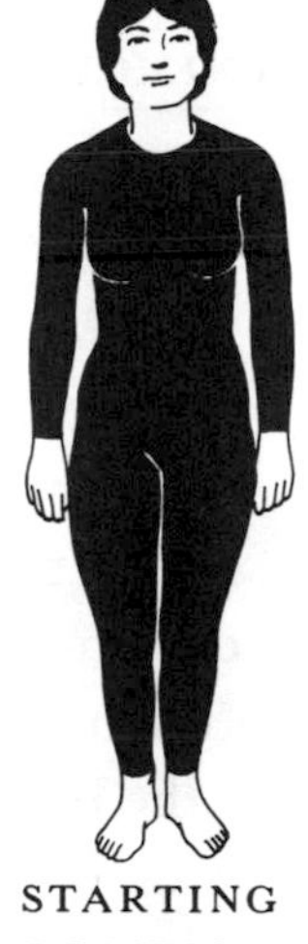
STARTING POSITION

EXERCISE 10: *The hungry tiger jumping towards the food.*

This exercise strengthens the hands, arms and neck. It also develops flexibility of the hip and knee joints.

Caution: Those with hypertension are not permitted to do this exercise.

STARTING POSITION: Standing, feet together, arms at sides.

MOVEMENT: 1. Take a step forward with the right foot. Bend the right knee, while the left leg is stretched behind with the knee kept straight. Meanwhile, lean the body forward. Press the fingers to the ground. Raise the head a little, keeping the eyes wide open looking sternly straight ahead. 2. Slowly and slightly bend, then extend, both elbows simultaneously. When bending the elbows, the trunk falls and the head and chest move forward little, just like a tiger moving towards its food. When extending the elbows, the trunk rises again, and the head and chest move backward a little. Repeat 3–5 times, then stand up. Take a step back with the right foot, and return to the starting position.

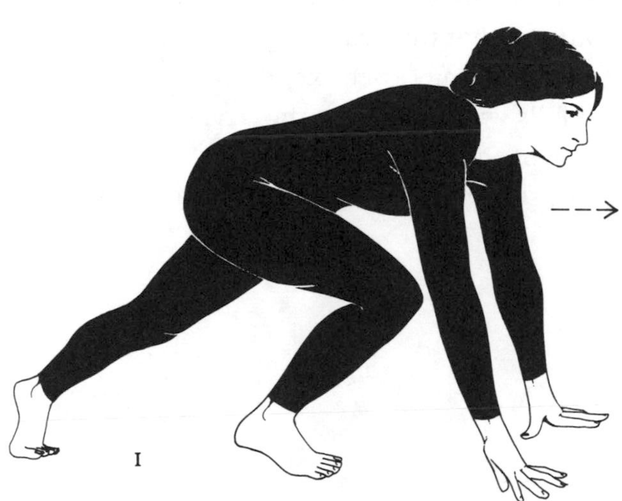
1

Repeat the above two movements, this time stepping forward with the left foot. This exercise is to be done only once.

Note: Breathe in as the head and chest move backward. As they move forward, breathe out.

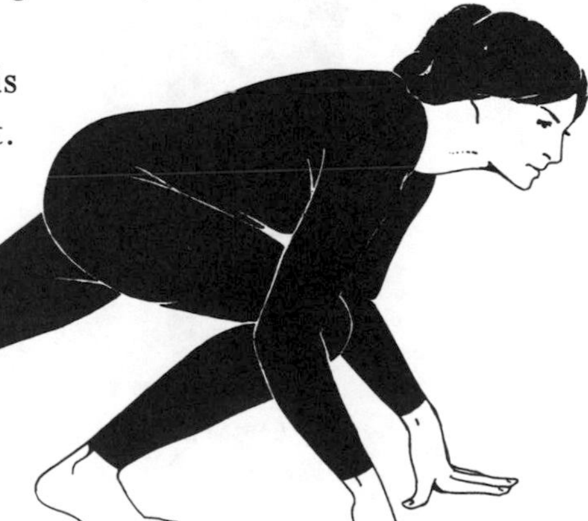
2

EXERCISE II: *Bowing.*

This exercise develops flexibility of the spine and hip joints. It also helps prevent dizziness.

Caution: Avoid overstraining. Those with hypertension are not permitted to do this exercise.

STARTING POSITION: Standing, feet together, arms at sides.

MOVEMENT: 1. Place the hands at the back of the head, palms covering the ears. Extend the shoulders so that the elbows point outward. 2. Bend the trunk forward so that the head falls to the point in front of the knees, just as in bowing (knees kept straight). The degree to which the head falls will depend on the individual. In this position, tap the back of the head with the index fingers 10–20 times. Then stand up, slowly straightening the trunk, and return hands to sides.

STARTING POSITION

Repeat this exercise 2–5 times.

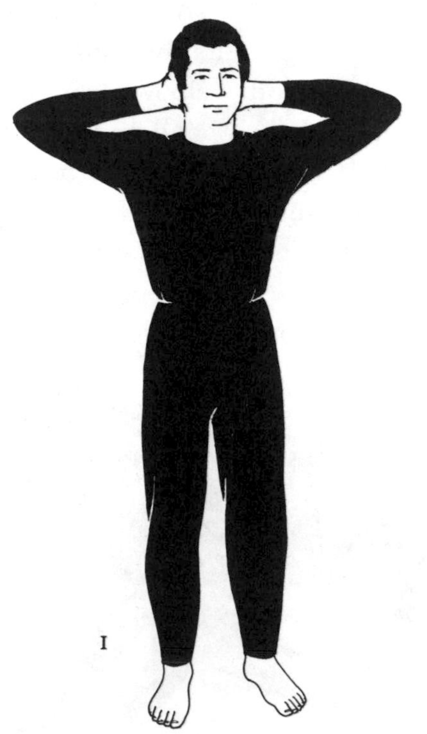

1

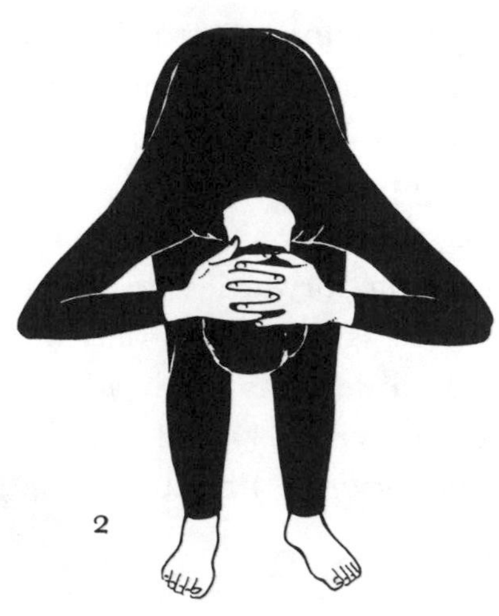

2

ıg forward.

elops flexibility of the spine and hip joints.
ɜrstraining. Those with hypertension are not
exercise.

Standing, feet slightly apart, arms at sides.

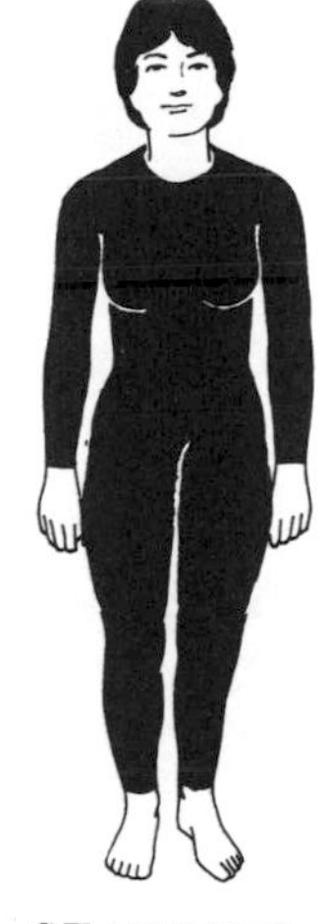

STARTING POSITION

…VEMENT: 1. Raise the hands and push forward until the elbows are fully extended, palms forward. 2. Cross the hands, palms downward, while the arms are fully extended. Then bring the hands back in front of the chest. Uncross the hands. 3. The trunk bends forward and the hands push downward as much as possible. Raise the head, eyes straight ahead. Keep the knees straight. 4. Raise the trunk and stand up. Bend and extend the elbows seven times. 5. Finally, jump in place seven times with the arms hanging naturally.

This completes the whole program of *Yi Jin Jing*.

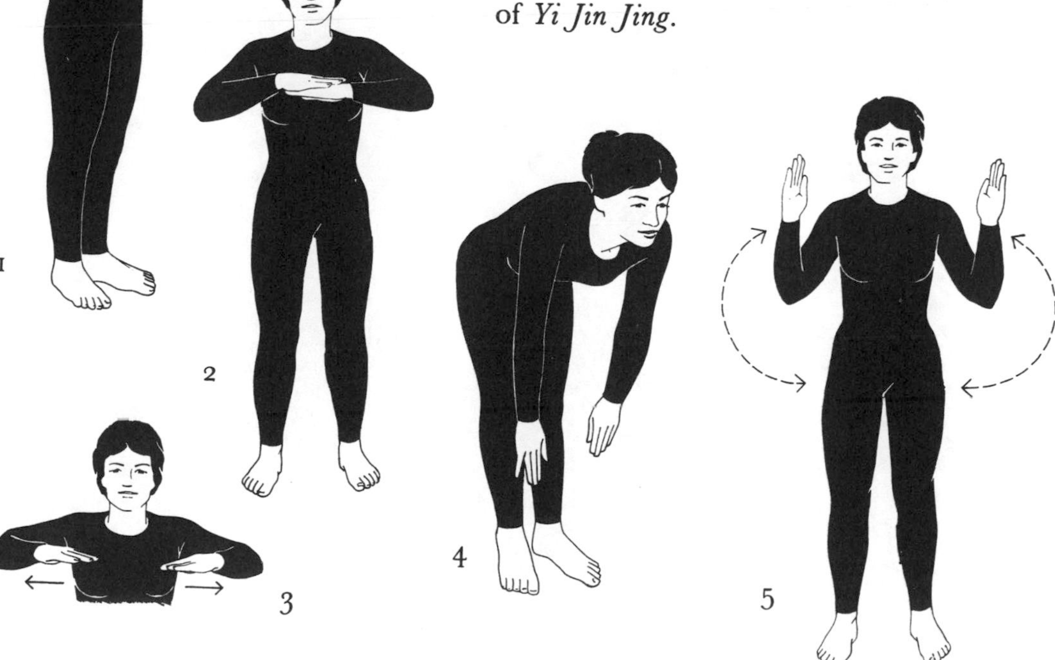

CHAPTER III

Ba Duan Jin—Eight Fine Exercises

Ba Duan Jin is a form of calisthenics which has been practiced in China for more than eight hundred years. It comprises eight exercises performed while standing. The traditional name of each exercise describes its movement and its effect on the body. Interestingly enough, the effects which are referred to coincide in part with modern concepts of exercise physiology.

Traditionally, *Ba Duan Jin* is performed with some effort or strain. However, the effort must be internal and not shown outwardly. Jerking movements and overstraining should be avoided. The advantage of *Ba Duan Jin* is that it is very effective in strengthening the arm and leg muscles, and in helping to develop the muscles of the chest, thus promoting good posture and helping to correct the defect of a rounded back. Because of this, it may be recommended for the youngster with weak muscles or defective posture. Modified *Ba Duan Jin* which is to be practiced gently without any effort or strain is suitable for the chronically ill and the elderly in poor physical condition. The traditional exercises of *Ba Duan Jin* are as follows:

EXERCISE 1: *Regulating the internal organs by raising both hands to the sky.*

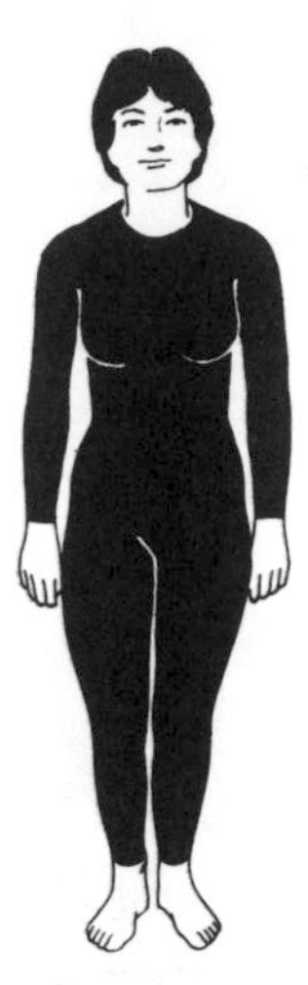
STARTING POSITION

This stretching exercise is good for improving posture. In addition, the movement of raising the arms is known to extend the range of vertical motion of the diaphragm, thus promoting deeper respiration, and providing soft "massage" to the stomach and intestines.

STARTING POSITION: Standing, heels together, arms at sides, eyes straight forward.

MOVEMENT: 1. Raise the arms from the sides slowly. Interlace the hands, and raise the heels about 2 inches (5 cm). 2. Turn the palms upward, and straighten out the elbows with effort. Raise the heels one inch higher. Hold this position for a while. 3. Unclasp the hands. Bring the arms down slowly. Keep heels raised. 4. Lower heels slowly. Repeat this exercise 8–16 times.

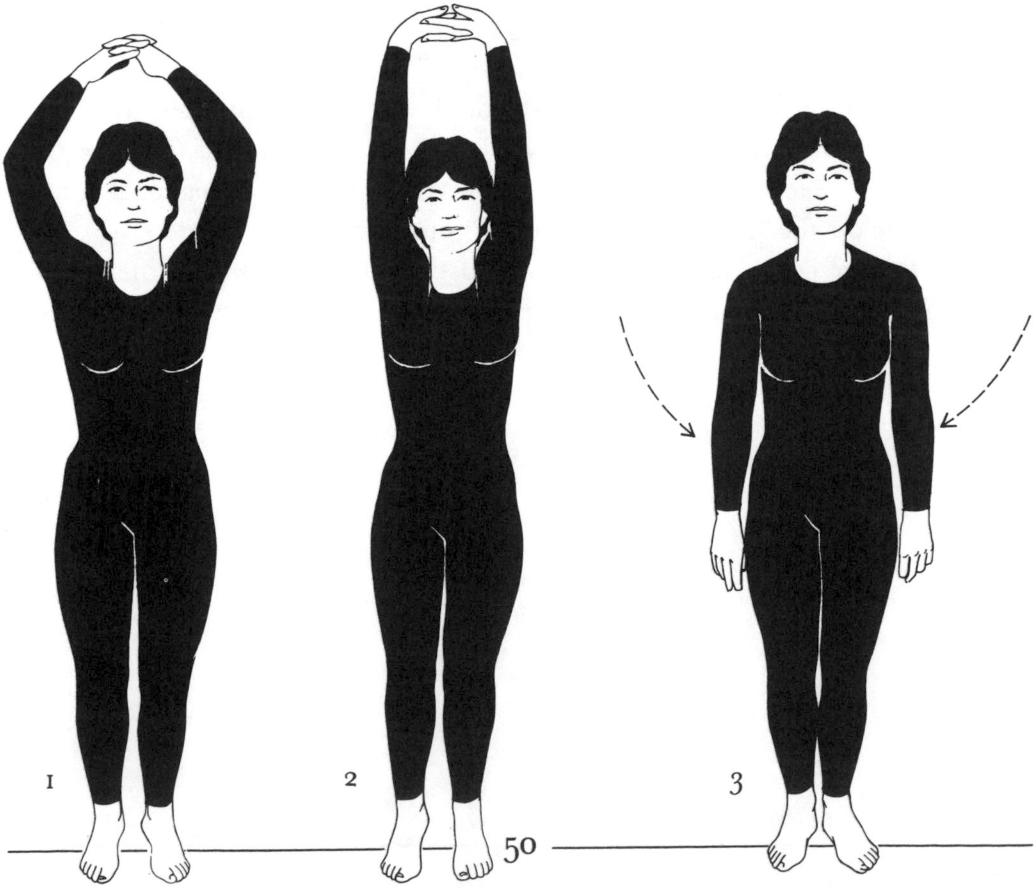

EXERCISE 2: *Shooting the eagle by drawing the bow with the hands.*

This exercise develops the muscles of the shoulder girdle and the sides of the chest. It is also good for strengthening the thighs.

STARTING POSITION: Standing, toes together.

MOVEMENT: 1. Take a step to the left with the left foot, keeping heels down, toes pointing forward. Bend the knees until the thighs are parallel to the ground, trunk erect. Cross the arms in front of the chest with the right arm outside the left, fingers spread. Turn the head to the left and look at the right hand. 2. Clench the left fist with the index finger pointing upward and the thumb pointing outward, palm facing left. Stretch the left arm slowly to the left until the elbow is fully extended. Meanwhile clench the right fist. Move the right arm slowly to

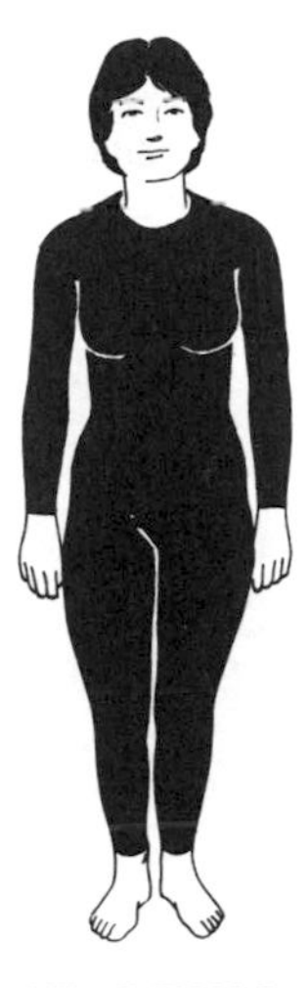

STARTING POSITION

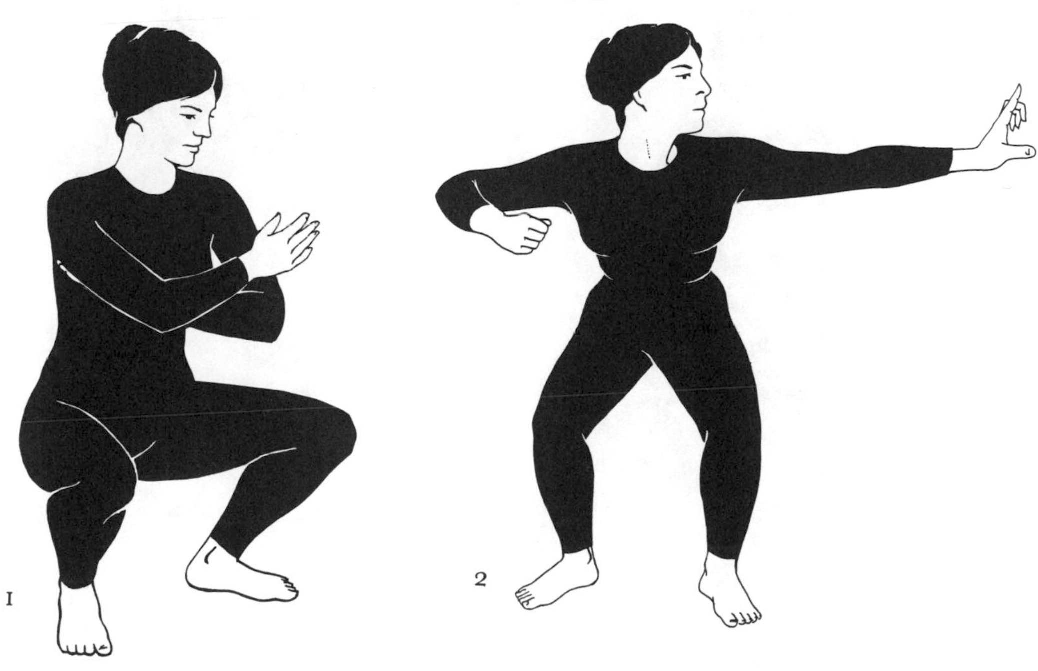

the right as if drawing a bow, the right elbow pointing outward. Look at the left index finger. 3. Relax the arms and return them to the crossed position in front of the chest, with the left arm outside the right. Turn the head to the right, looking at the left hand. 4. Clench the right fist with the index finger pointing upward and the thumb pointing outward. Stretch the right arm slowly to the right until the elbow is fully extended. Meanwhile, clench the left fist. Move the left arm slowly to the left, and let the left elbow point outward. Look at the right index finger.

Repeat this exercise 8–16 times.

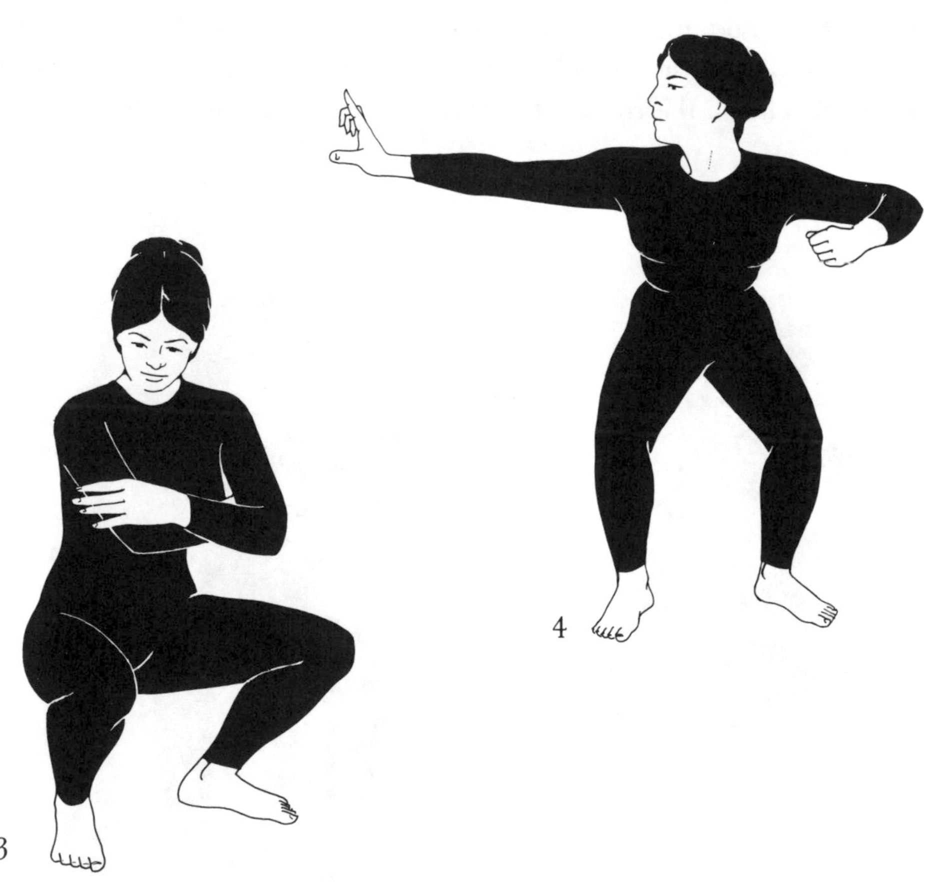

EXERCISE 3: *Regulating the spleen and stomach by raising the hand upward.*

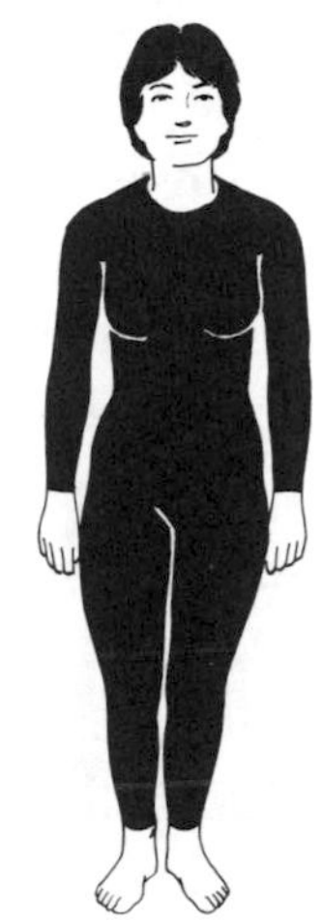
STARTING POSITION

As in Exercise 1, this exercise increases the range of vertical motion of the diaphragm and helps regulate the digestion. It also develops the upper back, shoulders, and the back of the upper arms.

STARTING POSITION: Standing, arms at sides.

MOVEMENT: 1. Turn the left hand and raise it up from the side with the palm upward, fingers together and pointing to the right, elbow fully extended. Meanwhile, the right hand pushes downward with effort, palm down, fingers pointing forward. 2. Bring the left arm down to the starting position. The left hand pushes downward with effort, fingers pointing forward. Meanwhile, turn the right hand and raise it up from the side with the palm upward, fingers together and pointing to the left, elbow fully extended.

Repeat this exercise 8–16 times.

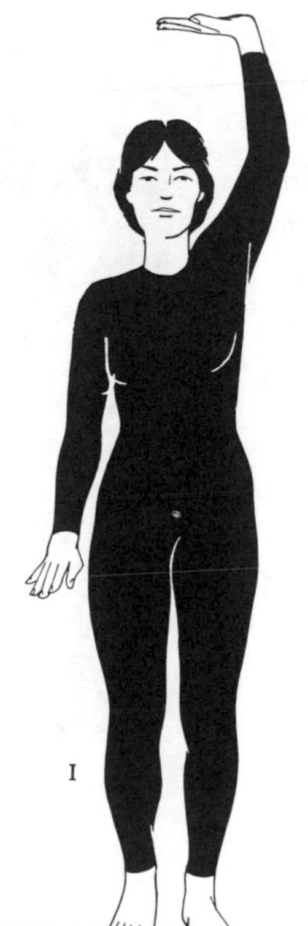
1

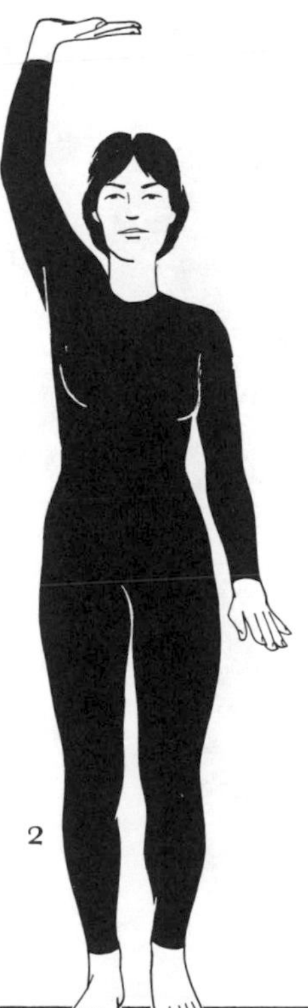
2

EXERCISE 4: *Curing the five troubles and seven disorders* by turning the head backward and gazing sternly.*

This exercise is good for developing the neck. It is recommended for the prevention and treatment of neck pain or stiff neck due to rheumatism or degenerative disorders. It also helps relieve dizziness in patients with hypertension.

STARTING POSITION: Standing, head upright, arms at sides, palms pressing the thighs.

STARTING POSITION

MOVEMENT: 1. Turn the head to the left slowly with the eyes looking sternly backward. Expand the chest with the shoulders slightly extended. Then return to the starting position, eyes straight ahead. 2. Turn the head to the right slowly with the eyes looking sternly backward. Expand the chest with the shoulders slightly extended. Again, return to the starting position, eyes straight ahead.

Repeat this exercise 8–16 times.

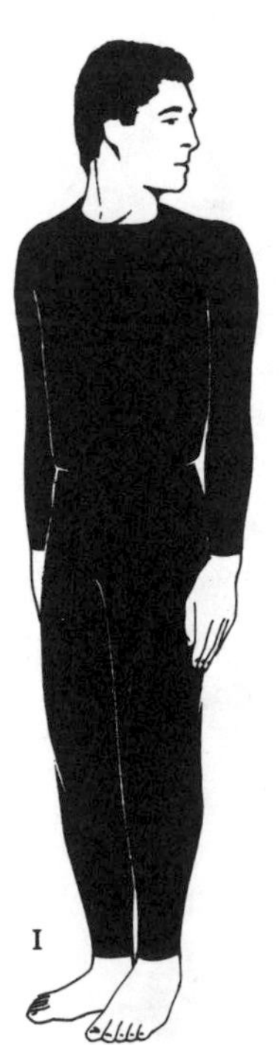

1

**Note:* The five troubles are troubles of the five organs: the heart, liver, spleen, lungs, and kidneys. The seven disorders are disorders arising from overeating, anger, overexertion, chilliness, extreme climate, anxiety, and apprehension. This exercise is said to cure these disorders because it promotes a sense of wellbeing.

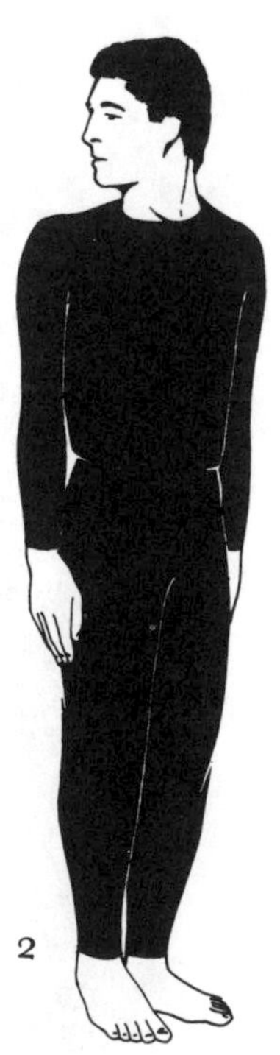

2

EXERCISE 5: *Tranquilizing the fiery heart* by turning the head around and swinging the hips.*

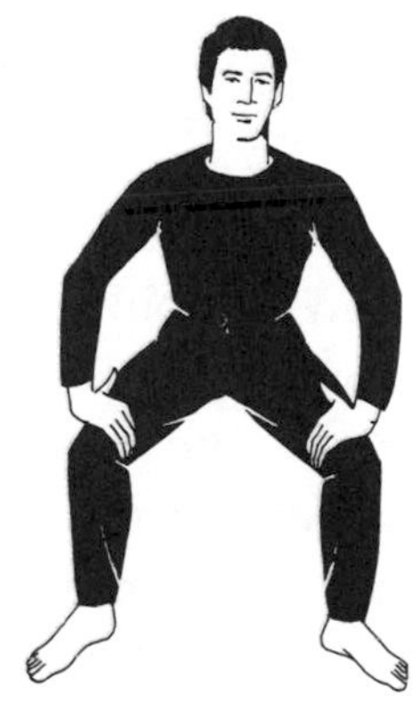

STARTING POSITION

This exercise strengthens the thighs and develops the flexibility of the spine.

STARTING POSITION: Stride standing (feet wide apart), knees bent, assume a horse-riding posture. Palms on the knees and thumbs pointing towards the body. Trunk erect.

MOVEMENT: 1. Bend the trunk and head low to the right, and then rotate the head in a small circle. Meanwhile, the hips swing slightly. Return to the starting position. 2. Extend the trunk and the head to the left, and rotate the head in a small circle, then return to the starting position. Repeat the above two movements, rotating the head in the opposite direction.

Repeat the entire exercise 8–16 times.

**Note:* The term "fiery heart" refers to a group of symptoms arising from mental agitation, such as sleeplessness and restlessness. This exercise, like other moderate exercises, has the effect of regulating the psychological state, or "tranquilizing the fiery heart."

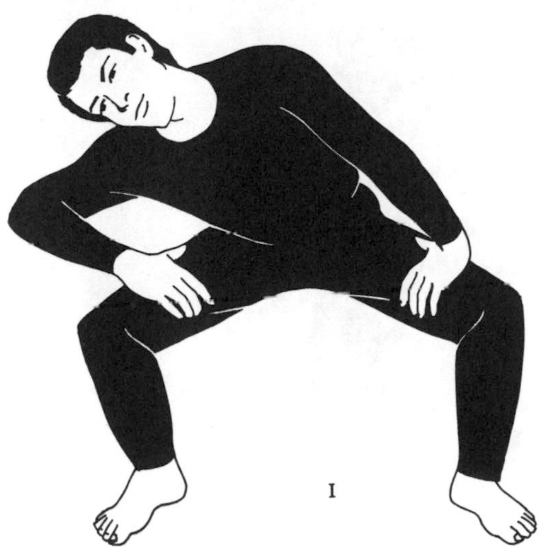

1

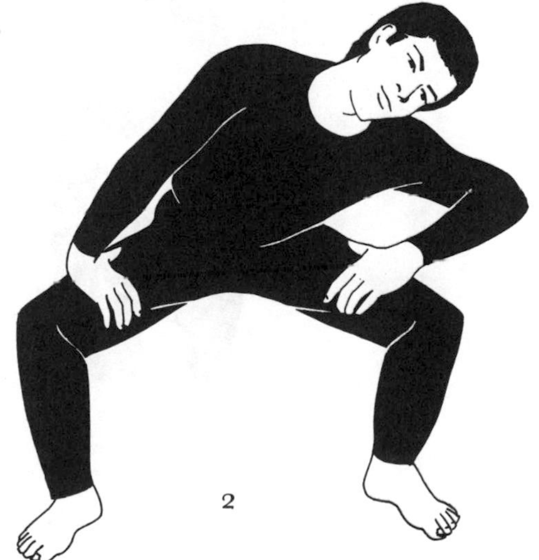

2

EXERCISE 6: *Strengthening the loins and kidneys by bending forward with hands touching the feet.*

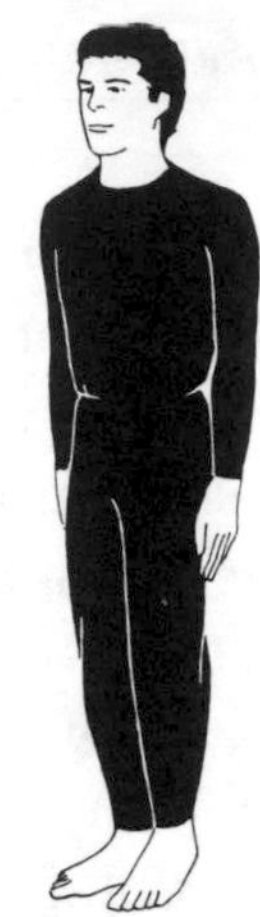
STARTING POSITION

This exercise develops the flexibility of the lumbar spine and hip joints. It helps in preventing backache. Those with lower back problems should not do this exercise.

STARTING POSITION: Standing.

MOVEMENT: 1. Bend the trunk forward slowly and as low as possible, knees kept straight. Meanwhile, stretch the arms downward with the hands touching or grasping the toes or ankles. Then raise the head slightly. Hold this position for a few seconds, then return to the starting position. 2. Extend the trunk backward with both hands placed on the lower back. Then return to the starting position.

Repeat this exercise 8–16 times.

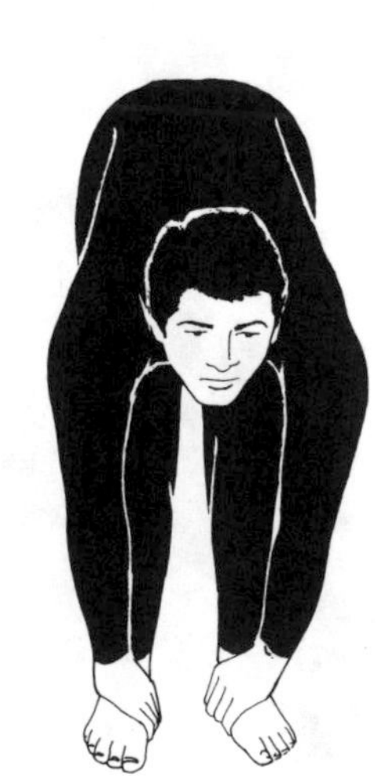
1

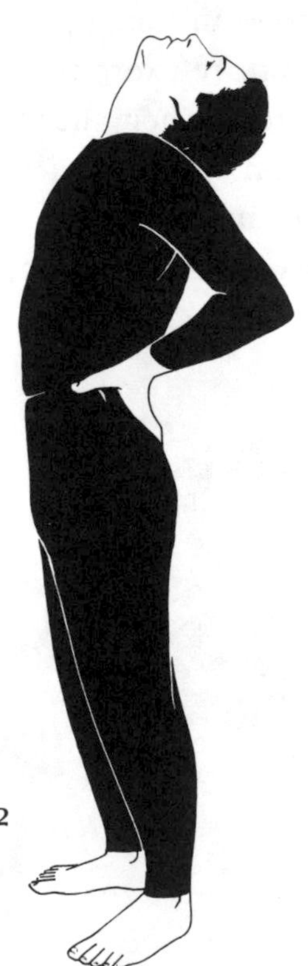
2

EXERCISE 7: *Increasing the vital energy by tightening the fists and gazing sternly.*

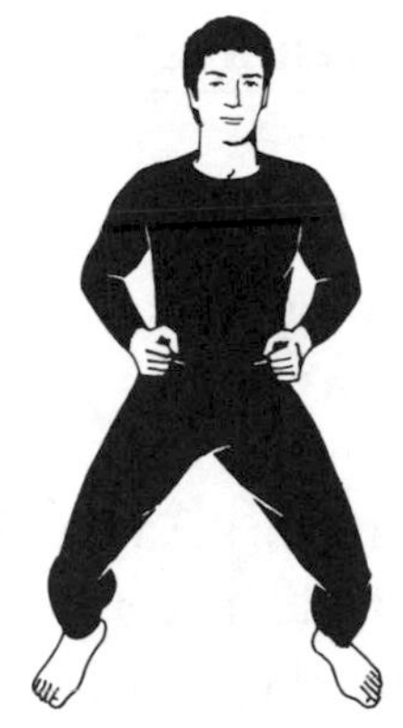
STARTING POSITION

This exercise develops the arms. Opening the eyes wide and gazing sternly are methods used traditionally to increase effort during the exercise.

STARTING POSITION: Stride standing (feet separated shoulder width), knees bent, hands forming fists alongside the waist.

MOVEMENT: 1. Stretch the left arm forward as far as possible, fist tightened as if hitting a target, elbow fully extended. Meanwhile, clench the right fist with the elbow pointing backward. Eyes are kept wide open and gazing ahead sternly. 2. Bring the left fist back to the side of the waist, and stretch the right arm forward as far as possible, fist tightened as if hitting a target, elbow fully extended. Meanwhile, clench the left fist at the side of the waist with the elbow pointing backward. Eyes kept wide open and gazing ahead sternly. Then bring the right fist back to the side of the waist.

Repeat this exercise 8–16 times.

1

2

EXERCISE 8: *Keeping all diseases away by raising the heels seven times.*

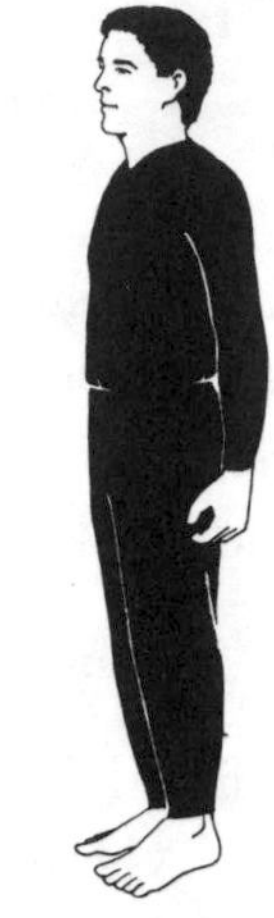
STARTING POSITION

This exercise is good for improving posture and developing the calf muscles.

STARTING POSITION: Standing, toes together, palms on thighs.

MOVEMENT: 1. Expand the chest, keeping the knees straight. Raise the heels as high as possible and push the head upward with effort. 2. Lower the heels, returning to the starting position.

Repeat this exercise 8–16 times.

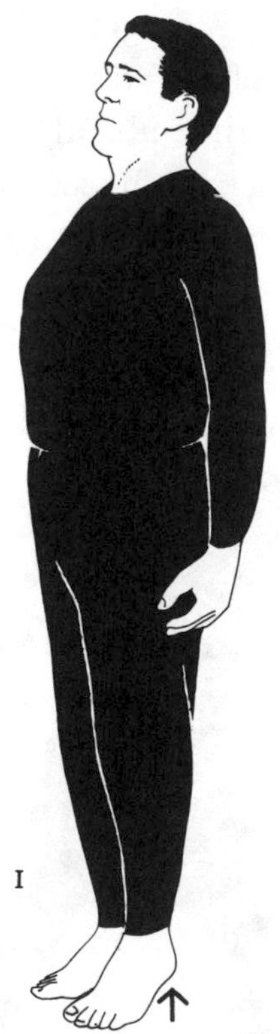
1

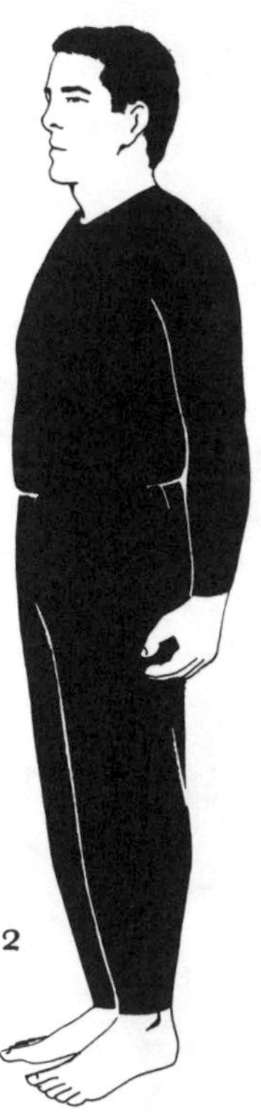
2

CHAPTER IV

Shier Duan Jin — Twelve Fine Exercises

Shier Duan Jin (Twelve Fine Exercises) is a traditional Chinese therapeutic exercise derived from the ancient *Tao Yin* (the Way of *Yin*). This program of exercise is a combination of bodily movements and self-administered massage. Usually the exercises are performed while sitting cross-legged on the floor or on a bed. Simple and effective, this program, through its invaluable therapeutic effects on the general well-being, is particularly suitable for the elderly and the chronically ill.

EXERCISE 1: *Biting the teeth.*

Close the mouth. Let the upper and lower teeth bite against each other. When doing this movement, open and close the jaw alternately. Repeat 20–30 times. It is said that this exercise prevents the teeth from becoming loose and is helpful in the treatment of periodontitis.

EXERCISE 2: *Moving the tongue around.*

Close the mouth. Move the tongue around, touching the gums and massaging the insides of the cheeks. This can stimulate the secretion of saliva and is said to have some therapeutic effect on gum inflammation and periodontitis.

EXERCISE 3: *"Washing" the face.*

Rub the hands together to warm the palms. Then "wash" the face by stroking it with the palms 20–30 times. It is said that this massage helps improve the circulation of blood to the skin, and maintain its elasticity and tone.

EXERCISE 4: *Beating the "drum of heaven."*

1. Put the hands on the back of the head, and cover your ears with the palms. Place the index fingers on the middle fingers. 2. Then slap the index fingers down to tap the back of the head (near the acupuncture point *feng chi*) 20–30 times. You may hear a sound of drumming. It is said that this massage may relieve headache and dizziness. According to traditional Chinese medicine, acupuncture on the *feng chi* point may cure headache and dizziness. Massage (percussion) on this point is expected to have a similar effect.

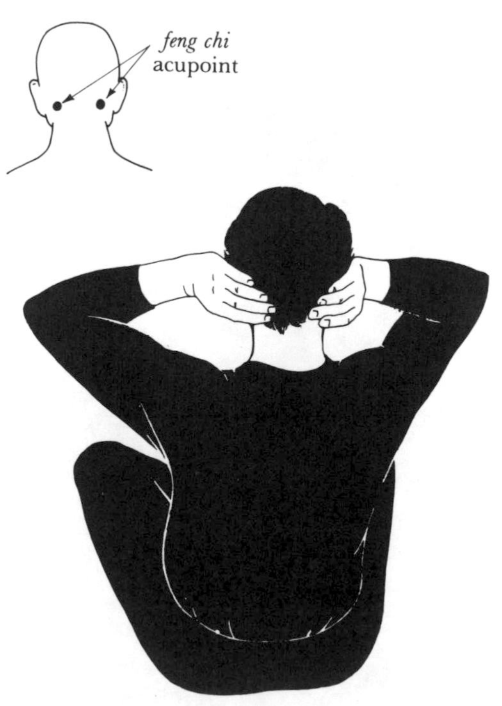

EXERCISE 5: *Winding the pulley.*

1. Starting with the elbows bent at a right angle beside the chest, and the forearms forward, clench the fists, palms downward. 2. Stretch the arms forward and upward, and then draw them downward and backward in a circular pattern, as in winding a wheel or a pulley. This circular movement of the shoulders is helpful for the prevention and treatment of periarthritis of the shoulder joints.

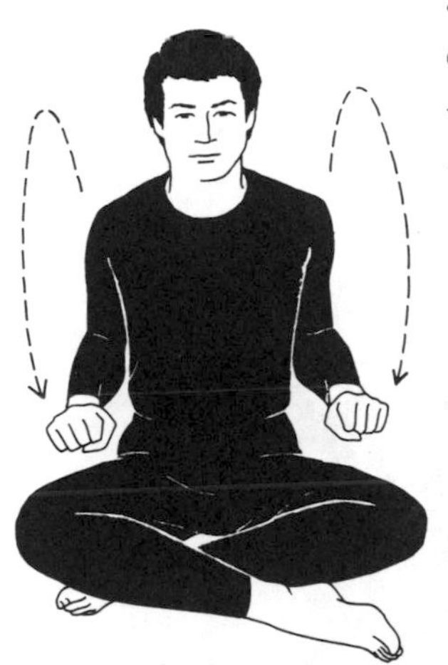

1

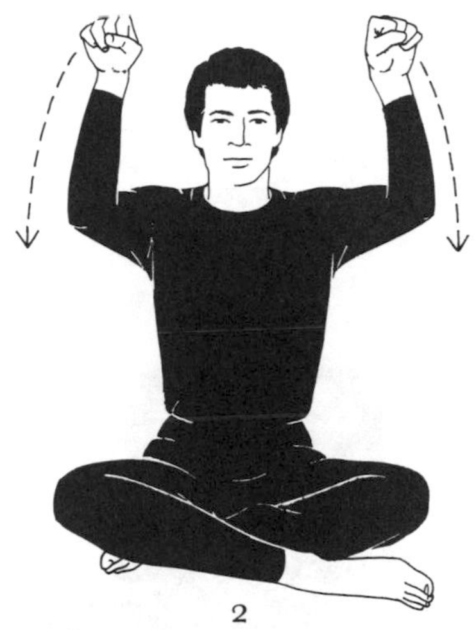

2

EXERCISE 6: *Pushing towards the sky.*

1. Interlace the hands in front of the abdomen, palms upward. 2. Raise the hands up above the head and turn the palms upward, making an effort to stretch the arms as if pushing towards the sky, elbows fully extended. Repeat 10–20 times. This is good for expanding the chest and strengthening the shoulder joints.

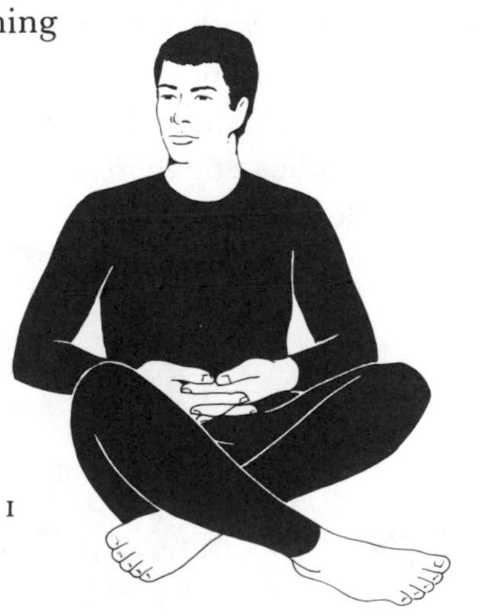

1

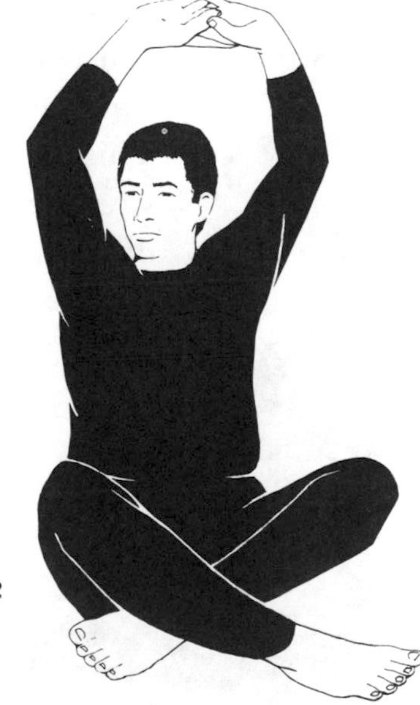

2

EXERCISE 7: *Drawing a bow.*

1. Cross the arms in front of the chest with the right arm outside the left, fingers spread. Turn the head to the left and look at the right hand. 2. Clench the left fist with the index finger pointing upward and the thumb pointing outward, palm facing left. Stretch the left arm slowly to the left until the elbow is fully extended. Meanwhile clench the right fist. Move the right arm slowly to the right as in drawing a bow. Repeat this movement 10–20 times. The effects on the body are similar to those of Exercise 6.

1 2

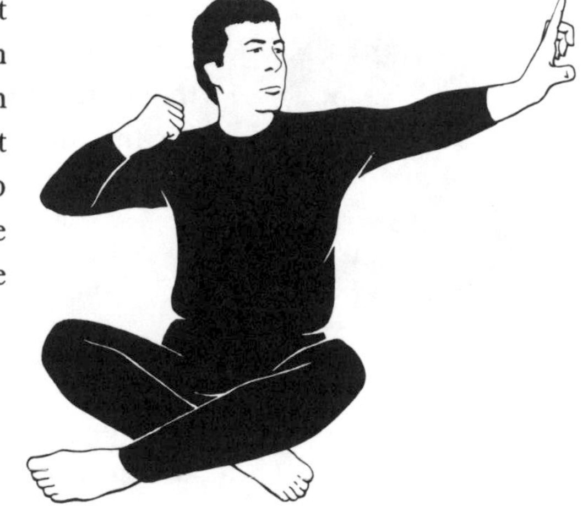

EXERCISE 8: *Bending the trunk with the hands touching the feet.*

1. Sit on the floor with legs kept straight (long sitting). 2. Bend the trunk forward and touch the feet with the hands. Repeat 10–20 times. This is good for maintaining the mobility of the spine and stretching the back muscles and hamstrings. However, sitting in this way is contraindicated where there is a back problem.

1 2

EXERCISE 9: *Stroking the* dan tian* *(field of pills).*

Dan tian is a traditional acupoint located about 2 inches below the umbilicus. In practice, stroking the *dan tian* is almost the same as stroking the lower abdomen. The massage is performed with three fingers of the right hand. Acupuncture on this point is indicated in cases of indigestion, lower abdominal pain, and excessive nocturnal emissions, and massage over this point is expected, and has been observed, to relieve the aforementioned symptoms. Massage for five minutes.

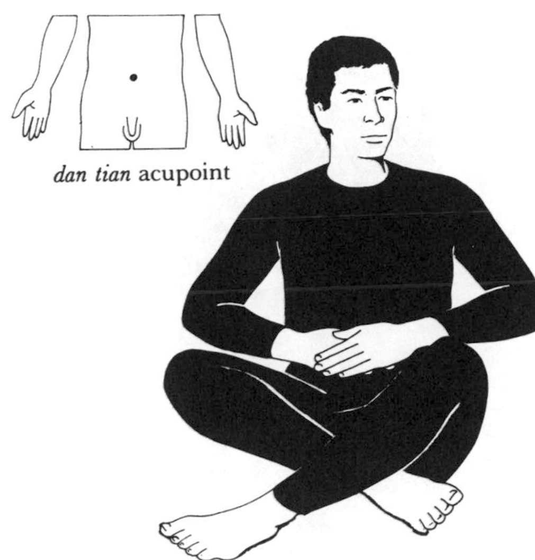
dan tian acupoint

**Note:* In Chinese, the word *dan* means pill, and *tian* means field. The ancient Chinese scholars noted that when one meditates, focusing the awareness on the center of the lower abdomen, one can sense a "warm pool" forming in that area. This small pool of warmth is said to be a valuable "pill." And so *dan tian* is called the "field of pills."

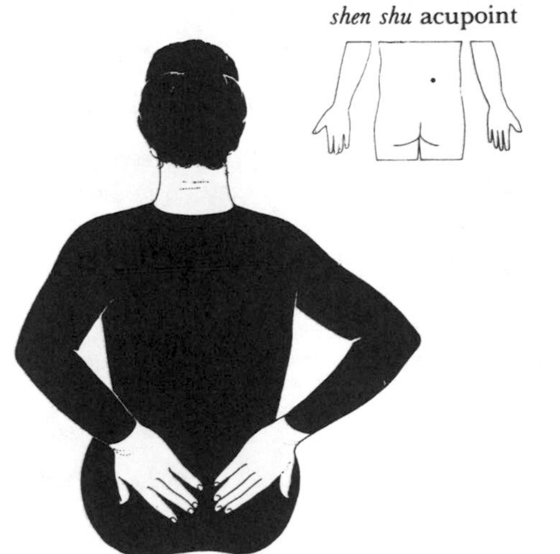
shen shu acupoint

EXERCISE 10: *Stroking the* shen shu *(kidney point).*

Rub the hands together to warm the palms. Then stroke the lower back with both hands for five minutes. The point *shen shu* is located on the lower back. Acupuncture or massage on this point has a preventive and therapeutic effect for backache caused by straining the back muscles.

EXERCISE 11: *Stroking the* yung chuan.

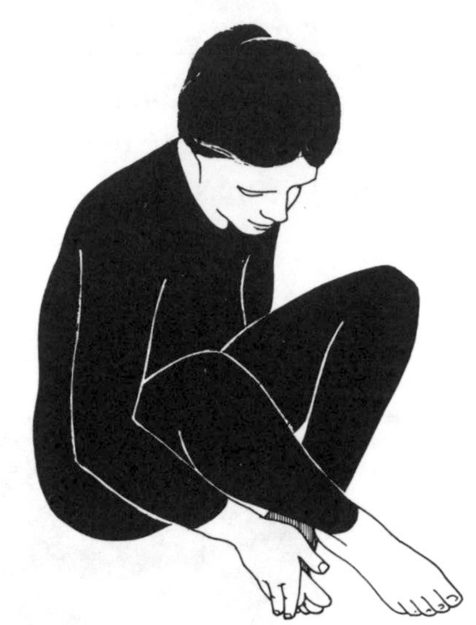

Rub the hands together to warm the fingers. Then stroke the left sole with three fingers of the right hand until there is a feeling of warmth in the sole. Then, stroke the right sole with the left hand. The acupoint *yung chuan* is on the sole of the foot. Massage on this point is helpful in the treatment of insomnia and palpitation, and is good for strengthening the feet as well.

yung chuan
acupoint

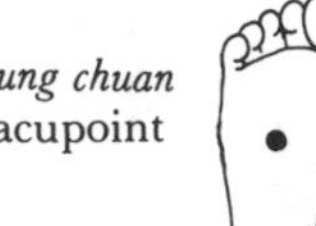

EXERCISE 12: *Stretching the legs.*

Stand. Taking a step backward, stretch the left leg. Then return to the starting position. Do the same with the right leg. Repeat this exercise 10–20 times. This exercise improves the blood circulation in the legs and helps relax the muscles.

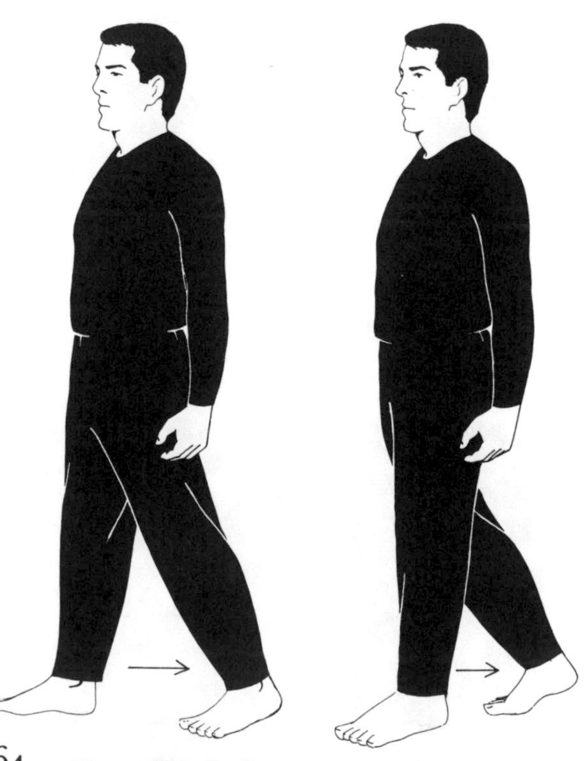

The above exercises and massage may be practiced in the morning after getting up and/or in the evening before going to sleep. They may be practiced in the complete series or selectively, that is, only some of them per session. One may establish one's own priority according to symptoms, as well as vary the number of repetitions or time allotted each exercise in a given routine.

CHAPTER V

Chi Kung—Invigorating Exercises

Chi Kung is a special form of traditional Chinese exercise. The Chinese term *Chi* means the air one breathes in and out. It also refers to the vitality or energy in the body. The term *Kung* means exercise, skill, or training. Translated literally, then, *Chi Kung* is a breath-training or invigorating exercise. Essentially, *Chi Kung* is an exercise which combines breathing with meditation and relaxation.

Technically, the practice of *Chi Kung* has three aspects: adjusting the posture, adjusting the breathing, and adjusting the mind. These three elements are closely associated with each other, and mastering *Chi Kung* means learning and mastering the techniques of these "three adjustments."

In China, *Chi Kung* is used widely to treat a number of diseases and to promote longevity. Scientific studies have shown that *Chi Kung* is quite effective in preserving the energy of the body. It may be called an "energy-saving" exercise. *Chi Kung* is also renowned for its remarkable capacity for bringing relaxation to both mind and body. It is thus a good remedy for many of the stress-related diseases. In addition, through the mechanical action of the *Chi Kung* breathing exercises, the internal organs benefit greatly since the exercises provide an "internal massage."

In China, many kinds of *Chi Kung* are practiced. Today the most popular forms are *Chi Kung for Relaxation, Chi Kung for Fitness,* and *Chi Kung for the Internal Organs.* The methods and applications of these three are described in this section.

How to practice *Chi Kung* correctly

In order to benefit from *Chi Kung* the following principles must be observed.

- *Relaxation, quiet, and ease:* During the practice, relax both body and mind. First of all, loosen the belt and clothing. Relax the body; drop the shoulders, keeping the chest in. This posture is maintained without any effort. If uncomfortable, continue to readjust the posture until the muscles of the entire body, especially those of the abdomen, are relaxed. Then relax the mind, letting it dwell on pleasant and peaceful things. All anxiety and unhappiness should be kept out. Focus attention on the practice, and then adjust your breathing. Smooth and easy breathing will help the body to relax better. A sense of relaxation during exhalation may be experienced.

  Quietness and stillness require concentration of the mind. Attention is focused on the practice of *Chi Kung* without other thoughts interfering. When entering the state of quietness and stillness, one will feel a sense of emptiness in the mind. Sensations resulting from external stimulation (sound, light) become weaker. Sometimes the limbs seem to no longer exist or to not be where they are.

  At the initial stage, a beginner may find it hard to concentrate. Irrelevant and random thoughts emerge now and then, and make him or her vexed and uneasy. If this happens, relax and quiet yourself with auto-suggestion such as "My thoughts are turned inward and I am at ease." After a period of training, you will gradually succeed in calming down and entering a state of inward quietness, feeling serene and still.

- *Integrating breath with concentration:* During the practice of *Chi Kung,* the training of concentration and regulation of respiration should be combined. Breathing is directed by thought which controls its rhythm, depth, and speed, constantly directing it in and out.

  The essence of training one's concentration consists of turning towards an inward quietness. Regulation of the breathing aims at developing a pattern of smooth, deep, slow, and rhythmic breathing, done easily and without hoarseness. Breath-training is especially emphasized in *Chi Kung for the Internal Organs,* while *Chi Kung for Fitness* and *Chi Kung for Relaxation* emphasize the training of concentration.

- *Alternating stillness with activity: Chi Kung* is a form of physical training requiring little motion of the body, so it is advisable, if possible, to also participate in other therapeutic exercises and sports. Generally, active exercises are scheduled to follow *Chi Kung.*
- *Gradual progress: Chi Kung* is an art and skill. A long time is required to master its special method. Only patience and gradual progression will lead to success. The introduction to quietness and the training of breath should begin with simple methods and then gradually proceed to more demanding and complex methods. The length of a *Chi Kung* session usually begins with fifteen to twenty minutes, gradually increasing to between thirty and forty-five minutes.

Apart from the aformentioned principles, there are some maxims which a *Chi Kung* participant should follow:

Stop all reading and recreational activities between ten and fifteen minutes before a session, so as to bring the body and mind to a quieter state. This is important if one is to experience a successful *Chi Kung* session.

The duration of each session is best determined by the participant. When it is felt that the session should come to an end, open the eyes slowly, rub the face with the hands, and then stand up and do some stretching exercises.

Because it would be difficult to concentrate, *Chi Kung* should not be practiced when feeling hungry, nor after a full meal. The same is true in cases of fever, bad colds, diarrhea, and the like.

The possible side effects of *Chi Kung*

It is quite safe to practice *Chi Kung for Relaxation, Chi Kung for Fitness,* and *Chi Kung for the Internal Organs,* because if practiced correctly, these three kinds of *Chi Kung* will not cause any undue side effects. Beginners, however, may find it difficult to get used to the particular position, breathing, and concentration demanded by *Chi Kung.* In addition, lack of proficiency in the skill of

Chi Kung will sometimes cause abnormal responses in the body during the performance. Unfavorable reactions such as the following may be prevented or overcome by taking suitable measures.

- Backache after prolonged sitting. This is the result of malposition in sitting. For those who have had back problems, it is advisable to begin the practice in a lying position, and gradually shift to a sitting one. The length of each session may be cut down by those who feel discomfort in the back.
- Numbness of the legs when sitting cross-legged. This may be prevented by bending and stretching the legs immediately before assuming the cross-legged sitting position. If numbness occurs in the course of sitting, it is advisable to massage the legs or adjust the position to make the legs feel at ease, or to stand up and stretch the legs. If the numbness disappears, the participant may return to the original sitting position.
- Discomfort and shortness of breath. This may be seen in beginners, when they try to do very deep breathing. Malposition and poor motivation also may produce discomfort and difficulty in concentrating. Appropriate adjustment of respiration and position will help produce a state of calm and make breathing easier.
- A suffocating feeling in the chest, and pain over the lower costal (rib) region. This may be caused by inappropriate respiration—holding the breath in the throat or chest. If this occurs, the participant should change the breathing pattern by not holding the breath.
- Drowsiness and even falling asleep. This may come about when in a lying position. If so, a sitting position should be taken instead, with the eyes open, focused gently on the tip of the nose. A cup of hot tea or a short walk around the room will also help one keep alert.
- Strange sensations. Sometimes, during profound *Chi Kung* relaxation, one may experience a sensation of numbness, scorching, itching, or a flow of warmth in the skin or in the muscles of certain parts of the body. There is no cause for alarm when this occurs. The strange sensation will disappear or be reduced if one focuses attention on the lower abdomen.
- Palpitation. This may arise from hyperventilation or prolonged breath

holding, or emotional tension. If one strives to find the cause one can then remove it.

- Headache and fainting. These may be caused by strained breathing or emotional upset. Again, it is necessary to find the cause in order to remove it.
- Discomfort in the head due to pulsation of the temporal artery. This occurs sometimes when practicing *Chi Kung* while lying on one's side. The discomfort will be removed by adjusting the position of the head so that the temporal region is not pressed firmly.

Chi Kung for Relaxation: Method and Application

Chi Kung for Relaxation is relatively simple to perform. It is indicated for chronic diseases in general.

POSITION: Lying on the back, with high pillows under the head. The shoulders and upper back are supported by towels or soft pads. The head is kept straight in line with the body. Arms are at the sides and relaxed. Legs are kept straight. Eyes, slightly closed. The mouth is shut with the upper and lower teeth touching, and the tip of the tongue placed against the roof of the mouth.

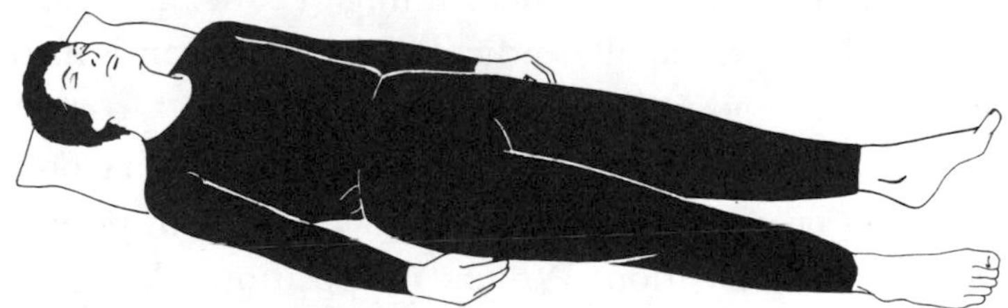

RESPIRATION: Breathe naturally through the nose. Regulate the breathing and let it be fine (not hoarse), rhythmic in speed and depth, and steady (without jerking or blocking).

RELAXATION: Use a cue word to induce the relaxation response. The participant is to mentally repeat, first the word "quiet" with each inhalation, then the word "relaxed" with each exhalation. Thinking about the word "relaxed," deliberately relax a part of the body at the same time. Thus, for each breath a part of the body is to be relaxed. The procedure begins with the head. After the head is relaxed, relax in turn, the arms, hands, chest, abdomen, upper back, lower back, hips and buttocks, legs, and finally the feet. After that, scan over the whole body to see whether there are any specific regions which may still be tense. If there are, make some adjustment to allow that region to be relaxed. After all muscles are relaxed, focus on the blood vessels, then the nerves, and finally, the internal organs (especially the affected organs), imagining each of these being relaxed. Such a use of imagery has been found to bring about a sense of relaxation in the areas where the attention is focused.

FREQUENCY AND LENGTH OF TRAINING: These depend on the individual. Generally speaking, hospitalized patients are required to practice three or four 30-minute sessions daily. Others who do not have sufficient time to do this are advised to practice one or two 30-minute sessions daily. The course of *Chi Kung* therapy varies. Generally, it takes 3–4 months to obtain significant therapeutic results.

Chi Kung for Fitness: Method and Application

Chi Kung for Fitness emphasizes the training of concentration to attain an inward quietness. It is principally indicated for hypertension, the psychoneuroses, heart disease, and pulmonary emphysema.

POSITION: The position commonly adopted is sitting on a stool. It may also be performed sitting cross-legged or standing. Patients in poor physical condition may take a lying position. Whichever position is chosen, keep the eyes slightly closed, the mouth shut with the upper and lower teeth touching, and the tip of the tongue placed against the hard palate.

1. *Sitting on a stool.* Sit on a big stool, feet apart and touching the floor. The knees are bent at a right angle. The trunk remains straight. The thighs are parallel to the floor with the hips bent at a right angle. The palms are placed on the thighs comfortably, with the elbows bent slightly. The head is kept straight. Drop the shoulders and hold in the chest.

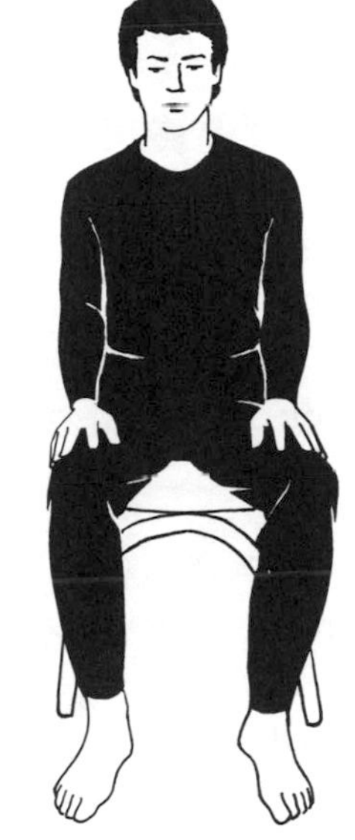

2. *Sitting cross-legged.* Sit on a cushion with the legs crossed comfortably and the feet under the thighs. Interlace or clasp the hands and place them on the lower abdomen below the navel, palms upward, thumbs crossed.

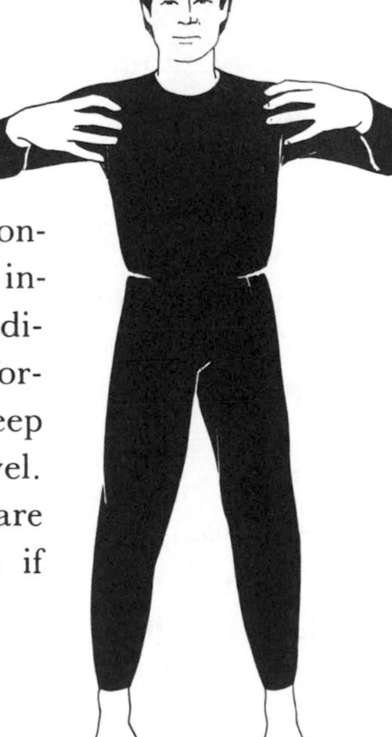

3. *Standing.* Since the position of standing consumes more energy and requires more effort, it is indicated only for patients in moderately good condition. Stand on the floor, feet apart, toes pointing forward and slightly inward, knees slightly bent. Keep the trunk straight. Raise the arms to shoulder level. Bend and drop the elbow slightly as if the arms are circling a big tree. Flex the fingers slightly as if holding a ball in the hand.

RESPIRATION: Use either diaphragmatic breathing or chest-abdominal breathing.

1. *Diaphragmatic breathing.* When breathing in, expand and protrude the abdomen; when breathing out, contract the abdomen, pressing it down. The breathing gradually becomes deeper and deeper until a rate of six to eight breaths per minute is attained. Breathe comfortably and easily, without any strain.

2. *Chest-abdominal breathing.* As in *Chi Kung for Relaxation,* breathe naturally through the nose. Regulate the breathing and let it be fine (not hoarse), rhythmic in speed and depth, and steady (without jerking or blocking).

QUIETNESS TRAINING: To induce the state of inward quietness, the basic method is to focus attention on the lower abdomen. As a preparatory or introductory procedure, one may begin by counting breaths, then following the breath with one's attention. After two or three weeks of training, one may change the method to focusing attention on the lower abdomen.

Counting the breaths. One begins by counting one's breaths. Each breath includes inhalation and exhalation. Counting begins with number one (the first breath counted), and proceeds to number ten. The counting is repeated again from one to ten, until one can concentrate fully, and gradually enters a state of inward quietness. If the counting is interrupted by irrelevant drifting thoughts, one should draw one's attention back and focus it on counting again from the very beginning.

Following the breath. Let your attention follow the descent of the inhaled air from the nose down into the lung, and then the ascent of the exhaled air from the lung up to the nose. This method is more natural than counting breaths. Yet it may still be interrupted and one's thoughts may be attracted outward, drifting far off. If this occurs, one should draw the attention inward again and focus it on the movement of the inhaled and exhaled air.

Focusing the attention on the lower abdomen. Thought is lightly and gently focused on the lower abdomen about two inches below the navel. The "attachment" of one's thought should be loose and done without any reluctance or stress. If this "attachment" is broken by the interference of drifting thoughts, draw the attention inward and again "attach" it to the lower abdomen.

FREQUENCY AND LENGTH OF TRAINING: As in *Chi Kung for Relaxation,* these depend on the individual. Generally speaking, hospitalized patients are required to practice for 30 minutes, 3–4 times daily. Others who do not have time for 3 or 4 sessions, should practice once or twice daily, for 30 minutes each.

The following table outlines the program used in teaching patients in the *Chi Kung for Fitness* class at Zhong Shan Medical College Hospital.

Table 1. Program for the Practice of *Chi Kung for Fitness*

Stage	First Stage (1st week)	Second Stage (2nd–4th week)	Third Stage (5th week)
Position:	Lying or sitting.	Sitting on stool or sitting cross-legged.	Sitting or standing.
Respiration:	Natural, deep breathing.	Diaphragmatic breathing (deep).	Diaphragmatic breathing (deep).
Inducing quietness:	Counting breaths and following the breath.	Following the breath. Focusing attention on the lower abdomen.	Focusing attention on the lower abdomen.
Frequency and length:	3–4 sessions/day, 15–20 mins. per session.	3–4 sessions/day, 30 mins. per session.	3–4 sessions/day, 30–45 mins. per session.
Require-ments:	1. Correct posture. 2. Smooth, rhythmic, and steady breathing. 3. Focusing attention on the breath.	1. Correct posture. 2. Smooth, rhythmic, deep, and steady breathing. 3. Inward quietness.	1. Correct posture. 2. Smooth, deep, rhythmic, slow, steady, and relaxed breathing. 3. Profound inward quietness. 4. Relief of symptoms. 5. Interest in *Chi Kung.*

Chi Kung for the Internal Organs: Method and Application

The method of *Chi Kung for the Internal Organs* emphasizes training of the breath. It is indicated in the treatment of peptic ulcer, viral hepatitis, chronic constipation, and gastroptosis (downward displacement of the stomach).

POSITION: Preferably lying on the side or sitting on a stool.

1. *Lying on the side.* In general, lying on the right side is preferable, with the head slightly bent forward, the right hand placed on a pillow about three inches from the head, palm upward. The left arm is extended comfortably with the hand placed on the left hip, palm downward. Both legs are bent comfortably. The left leg is placed on the right leg. The mouth is shut with the upper and lower teeth touching, the tip of the tongue placed against the hard palate. Keep the eyes slightly closed.

Note: Those who feel a pulsation of the artery on the side of the head, while practicing *Chi Kung* in this position, may instead adopt the position of lying on the back: Lying on the back, with high pillows under the head, keep the shoulders and upper back supported by towels or soft pads. The head is kept straight in line with the body. Arms are at the sides and relaxed. Legs are kept straight. The eyes, mouth, and tongue are the same as above.

2. *Sitting on a stool.* Sit on a big stool, feet apart and touching the floor. The knees are bent at a right angle. The trunk remains straight. The thighs are parallel to the floor with the hips bent at a right angle. The palms are placed on the thighs comfortably with the elbows bent slightly. The head is kept straight, with the shoulders dropped and the chest held in. The eyes, mouth, and tongue are the same as in Position 1, above.

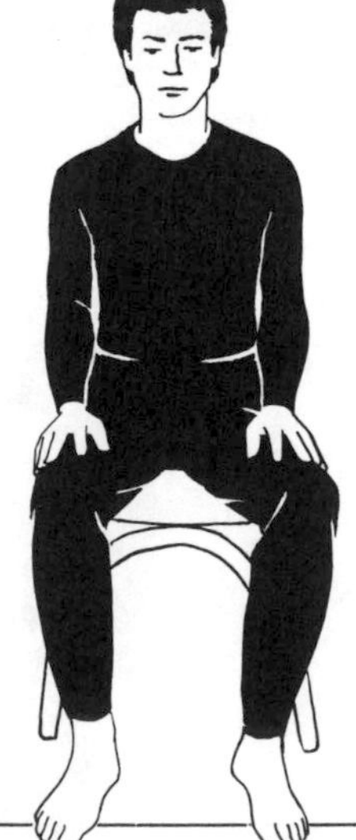

RESPIRATION: Utilizing the pattern of interval respiration, the patient is asked to pause and hold between each breath. The breathing is diaphragmatic and through the nose. The pattern of breathing is as follows:

Inhale - exhale - pause. Hold the breath, raise the tongue, and concentrate on some words in the mind. Lower the tongue - inhale. . . and so on.

While holding the breath, interrupt the respiratory movement for a while and focus the attention on the lower abdomen. Never strenuously, close off the air at the throat or at the upper abdomen. With continued practice the time of the interval between each breath will gradually lengthen. This may be helped by reciting a phrase silently, usually one word per second. In general, it is advisable to recite 3–7 words during each interval, since the length of holding the breath will be 3–7 seconds. The content of the phrase should be self-chosen and should have a positive impact. For example, at the initial stage, one may recite "Quietness is fine," that is, three words for holding the breath for three seconds. Later, "Quietness and relaxation are wonderful" (five words, when holding the breath for five seconds), and then, "Quietness and relaxation give me perfect health" (seven words, when holding the breath for seven seconds). The psychological effects of interrupted respiration are not yet clearly understood. It is possible that interrupted breathing induces regular changes in abdominal pressure, which then can stimulate the blood circulation in the abdominal cavity and improve the movement of the bowels.

QUIETNESS TRAINING: By reciting phrases mentally, in order to focus attention on the breath, one becomes relaxed in both mind and body, enabling one to expel any irrelevant thoughts and to gradually enter a state of inward quietness.

CHAPTER VI

Other Traditional Chinese Exercises

Breathing exercise

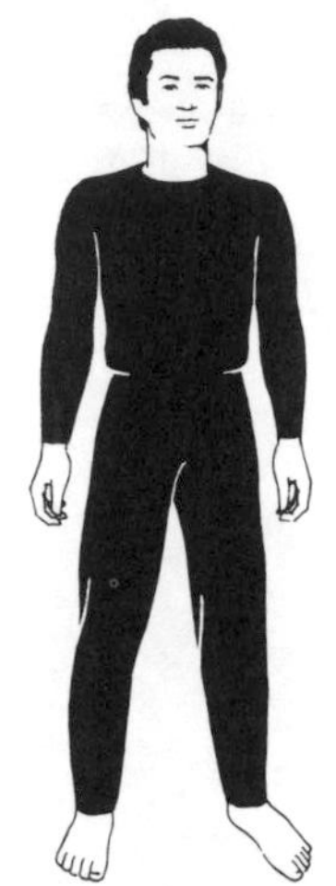

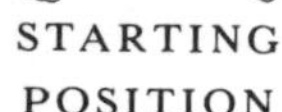
STARTING POSITION

This dynamic breathing exercise is done with large-ranging movements of the limbs and trunk. As a type of calisthenics, it has been observed to have a beneficial effect on general physical well-being, and to be helpful in the treatment of some chronic diseases, such as hypertension.

STARTING POSITION: Standing, relaxed, feet apart, arms at sides.

MOVEMENT: 1. Raise the arms forward and upward slowly until they reach a vertical position, with fingers extended. Breathe in. 2. Squat with the knees bent and bring the arms slowly down to the sides, and breathe out. Return to the position in step 1, breathing in. Then squat again, breathing out.

Repeat this exercise 10–20 times.

For the advanced practitioner, the exercise of twisting the body may be added to the above movements. (See Exercise 22, page 152.)

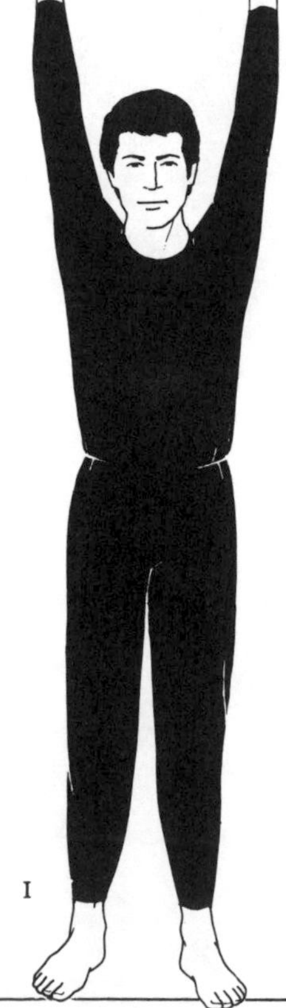
1

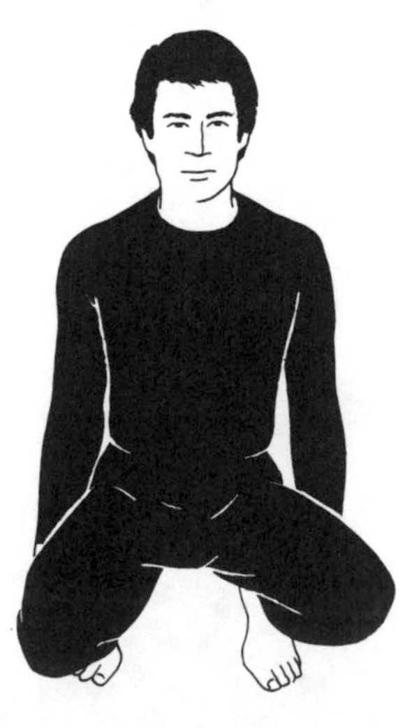
2

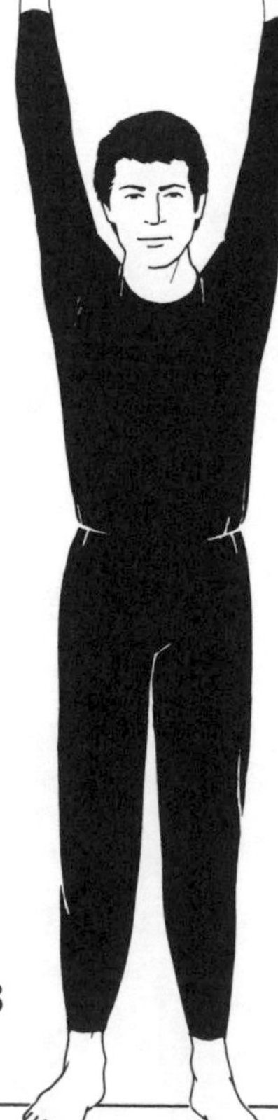
3

Exercise with the *Tai Chi* Stick

The *Tai Chi* Stick exercise is one of China's most ancient calisthenics. Like *Tai Chi Chuan,* it is gentle in nature, demanding that the participant be relaxed, quiet, and composed throughout the exercise. It may be used in the treatment of the psychoneuroses, peptic ulcer, and other chronic diseases.

EXERCISE 1: *Circling at a resting position.*

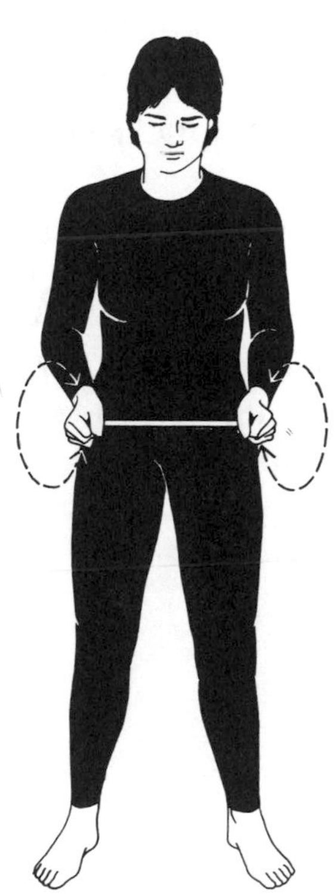

STARTING POSITION: Standing (feet apart), sitting on a stool, or lying on one's back. Elbows bent, fingers slightly flexed, palms holding a stick about 14 inches (35 cm) long at both ends, body relaxed, eyes partly closed. Focus attention on the lower abdomen. Breathe in and out smoothly.
MOVEMENT: With the stick held between the two palms, draw a circle in front of the abdomen, like a wheel rolling incessantly, at the rate of 40–50 cycles per minute.

EXERCISE 2: *Circling while moving the legs up and down.*

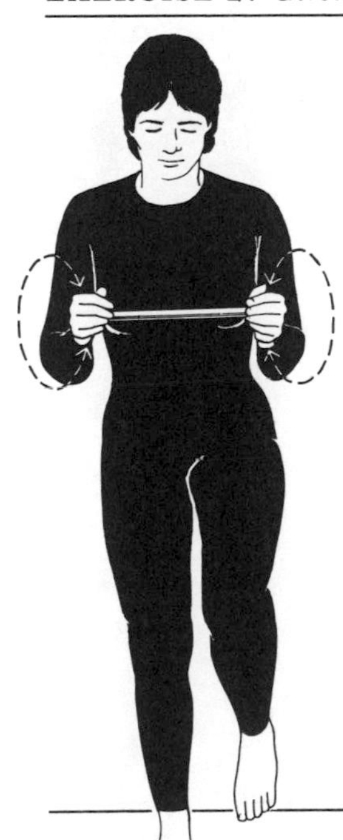

STARTING POSITION: Standing.
MOVEMENT: Bend the left leg upward and, at the same time, draw a circle with the stick held between the two palms. Lower the left foot and draw a circle with the stick. Bend the right leg upward and, at the same time, draw a circle. Lower the right foot and, at the same time, draw a circle.

EXERCISE 3: *Circling while walking.*

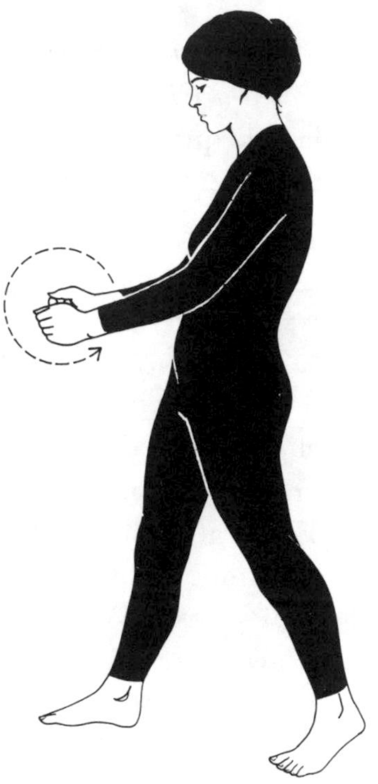

STARTING POSITION: Standing.
MOVEMENT: Step forward, and circle with both hands at the same time, the stick held between the palms. The rate is one circle for each step.

There may be various responses of the bodily function during the practice of the *Tai Chi* Stick, such as sweating, a sensation of warmth on the fingers, and sometimes twitching of the muscles.

Precaution: Progress gradually. For a beginner, each session should last about 2–5 minutes. After a training period of 3–4 weeks, the length of each session may be increased to 5–10 minutes. After a month or two, 10–20 minutes for each session is suitable.

PART II

Chinese Fitness Exercises

CHAPTER VII

Fitness Exercises for Children

This program is good for children (age 7–15), to develop cardiorespiratory fitness, flexibility, and good posture.

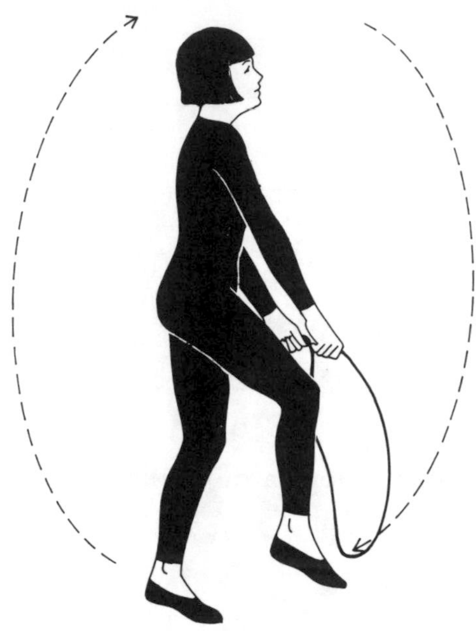

EXERCISE 1: *Rope jumping.*

PURPOSE: To develop the heart and lungs.
STARTING POSITION: Standing with a rope held in the hands.
MOVEMENT: 1. Free skipping with a rope 25–50 times. 2. Skipping the rope on the spot 25–50 times with jogging steps. 3. Skipping the rope on the spot 25–50 times, feet together.

Rest one minute between each of the above.

This sequence may be repeated three times.

EXERCISE 2: *Hitting the bean bag.*

PURPOSE: To develop strength in the upper arms.
STARTING POSITION: Standing before a bean bag, fists clenched.
MOVEMENT: Stretch out the arms and punch the bean bag with the left and right fists alternately.

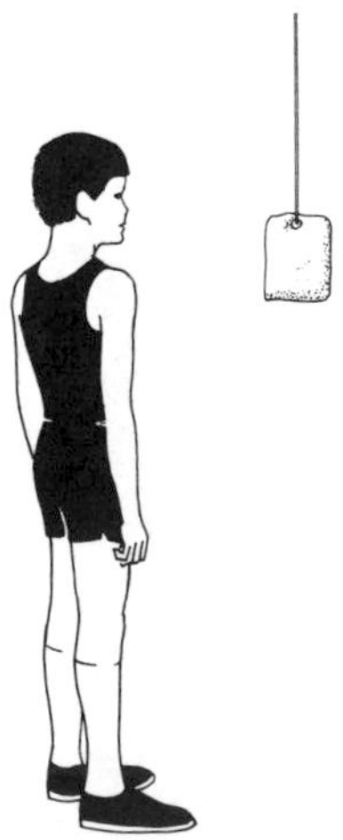

STARTING POSITION

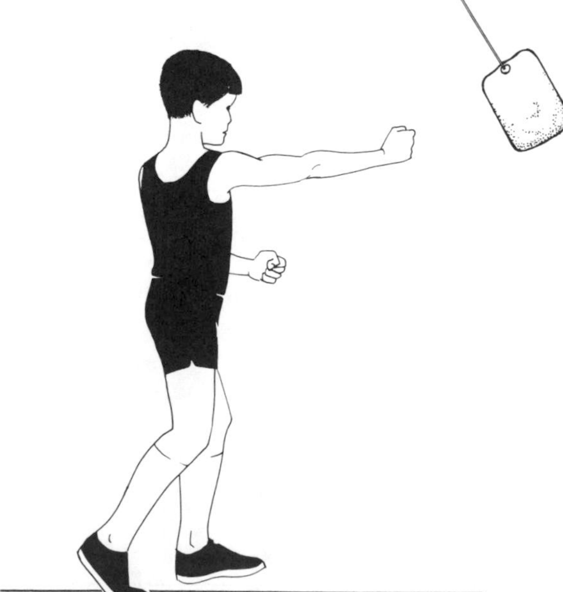

EXERCISE 3: *Monkey play.*

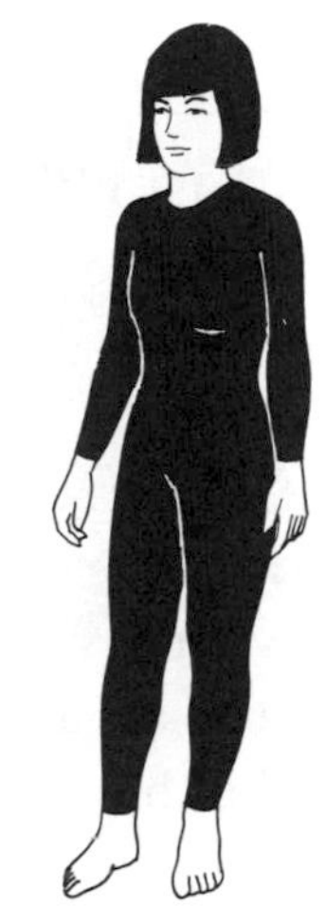

STARTING POSITION

PURPOSE: To develop agility.

STARTING POSITION: Standing, feet apart, arms hanging naturally at the sides.

MOVEMENT: 1. Jump forward with the left foot landing on the ground, while the right foot remains suspended in the air with the knee slightly bent. At the same time, reach forward with the left hand, fingers firmly held together, to imitate the picking movement of a monkey. The right arm is slightly bent at the side. Then jump backward and return to the starting position. 2. Jump forward with the right foot landing on the ground, while the left foot remains suspended with the knee slightly bent. At the same time, reach forward with the right hand, fingers firmly held together, to imitate the picking movement of a monkey. The left arm is slightly bent at the side. Then jump backward and return to the starting position.

Repeat this exercise 8–10 times.

Note: This exercise should be performed in a swift and lively manner, just as a monkey might do it.

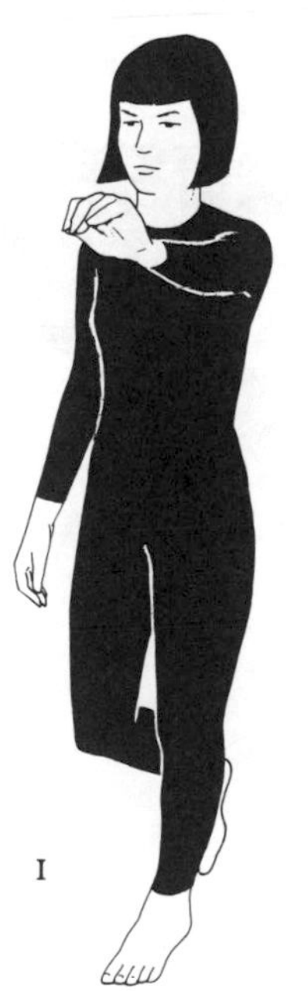

1

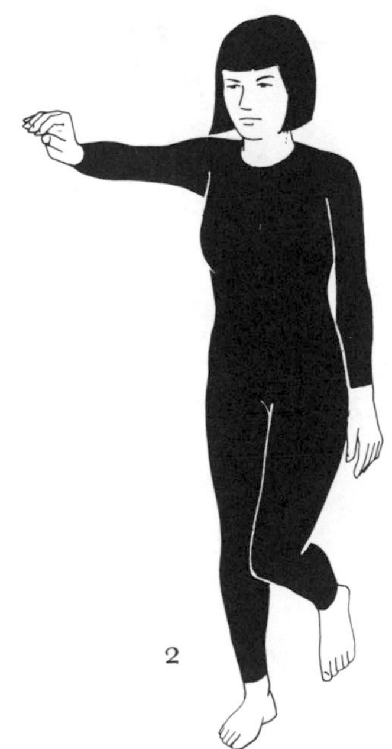

2

EXERCISE 4: *Tiger walking.*

PURPOSE: To develop the flexibility of the lumbar spine and hip joints.

Caution: This exercise is not suitable for children with back injuries.

STARTING POSITION: Standing with feet separated shoulder width.

MOVEMENT: 1. Bend the trunk forward, bending the knees so the back is almost parallel to the floor. Grasp the left ankle with the left hand, and the right ankle with the right hand. 2. Take a step forward with the right foot, while turning the head to the right. 3. Then take a step forward with the left foot, while turning the head to the left. Walk 8 steps in this manner. Then raise the trunk and return to the starting position. Breathe naturally in a rhythmic manner 8–10 times.

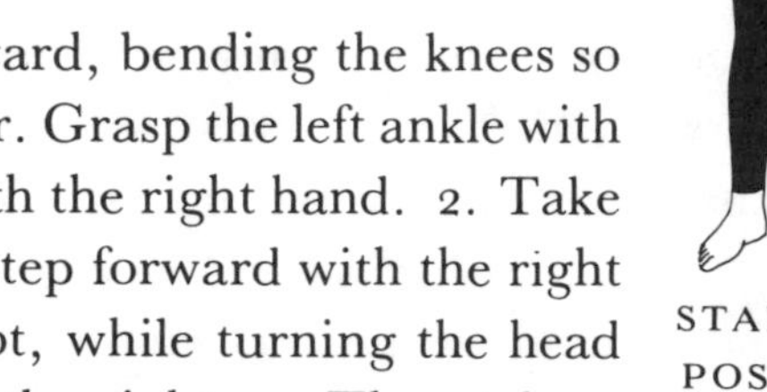

STARTING POSITION

Repeat this exercise 2–4 times.

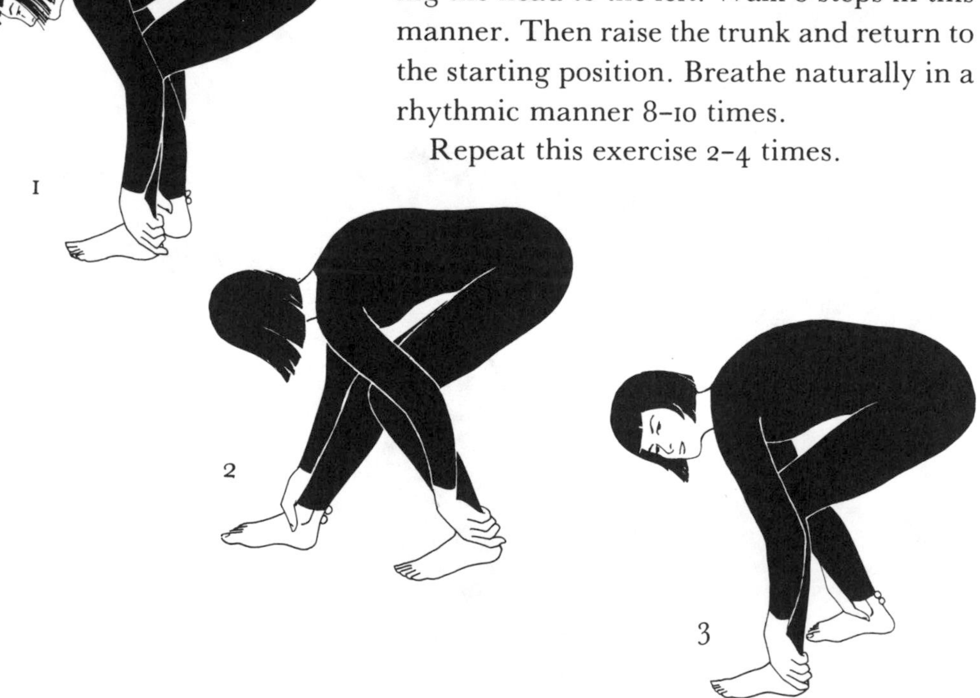

EXERCISE 5: *Worm wriggling.*

STARTING POSITION

PURPOSE: To develop the muscles of the back and to prevent scoliosis.
STARTING POSITION: Lying on the back, arms at sides, feet together.
MOVEMENT: Move the body along the floor in the direction of the head by shrugging the shoulders for 2–3 minutes.

Note: The movement of the body looks like the wriggling of a worm. Do not use the hands to assist the movement.

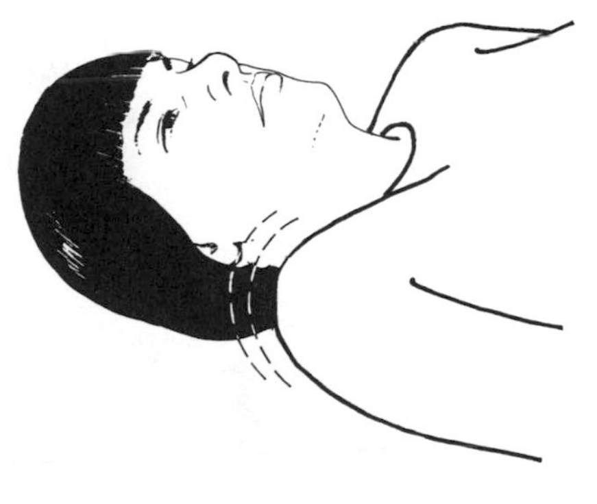

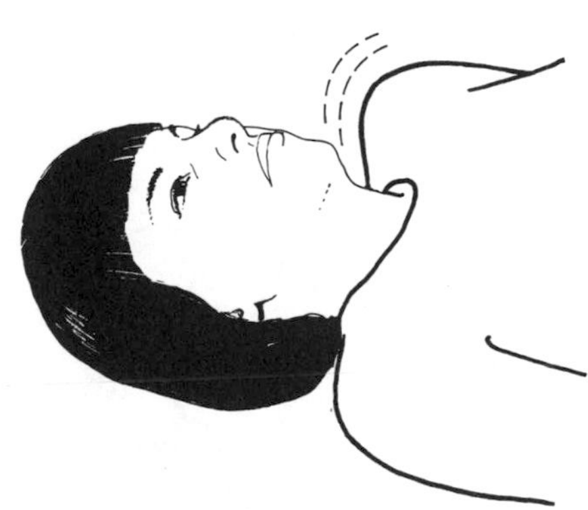

EXERCISE 6: *Tip-toe walking.*

PURPOSE: To strengthen the feet and calf muscles, and develop good posture.
STARTING POSITION: Standing, shoes off.
MOVEMENT: Raise the heels off the floor and walk on the tips of the toes. Walk 100 steps.

Note: Keep the heels raised as high as possible.

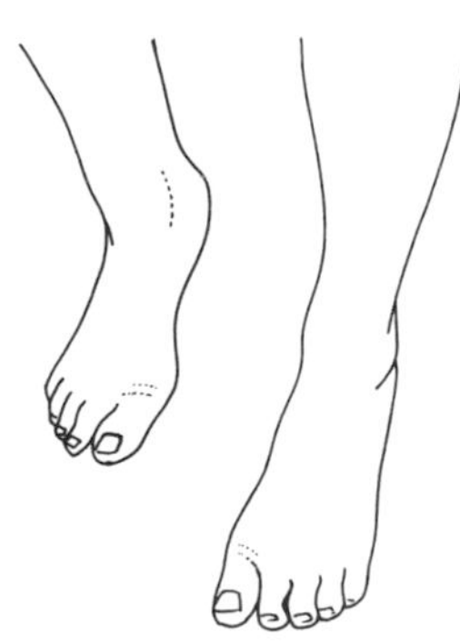

EXERCISE 7: *Edge walking.*

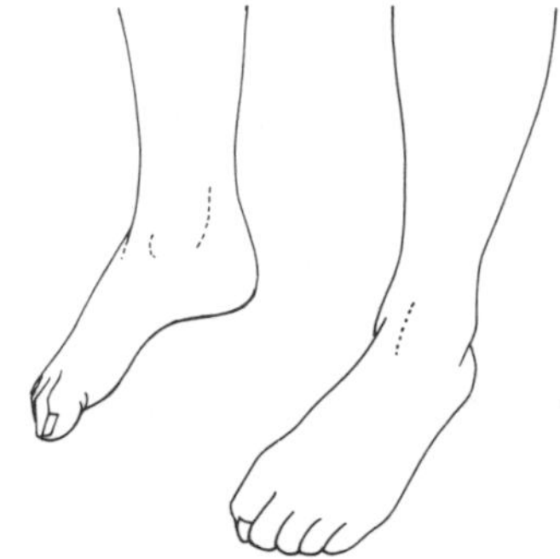

PURPOSE: To prevent flat feet, and strengthen the ankle joints.

Caution: This exercise is not suitable for children with ankle problems resulting from injuries to the lateral ligament.

STARTING POSITION: Standing, shoes off.

MOVEMENT: Walk with the feet pointing forward, but with the insides of the feet off the floor (walking on the "edge"). All body weight is supported by the outsides of the feet. Walk 100 steps.

EXERCISE 8: *Eye massage.*

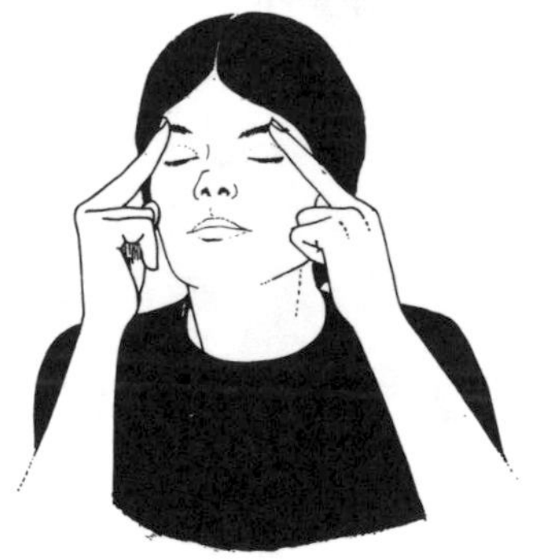

PURPOSE: To relieve eye strain and promote good eyesight.

STARTING POSITION: Sitting with eyes closed.

MOVEMENT: Stroke and press the region around the eyes in a circular motion with the index and middle fingers of both hands, left hand for the left eye and right hand for the right eye.

Note: Do this massage with clean hands.

CHAPTER VIII

Fitness Exercises for the Sedentary

Sedentary people should take an exercise break at least once a day in order to keep fit and avoid degenerative conditions such as coronary heart disease and degenerative musculoskeletal problems. The following program is designed to meet such a need. It may be done during an exercise break at work or at home.

EXERCISE 1: *Swinging the arms.*

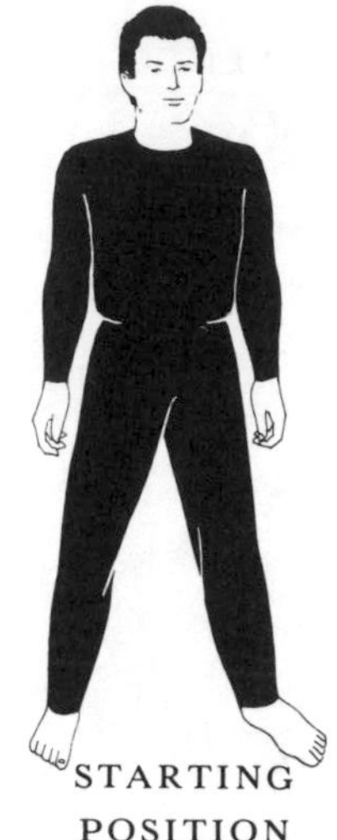
STARTING POSITION

PURPOSE: To improve digestion, blood circulation, and general well-being, and to keep the shoulder joints in good shape and prevent "frozen shoulders."

STARTING POSITION: Standing with the feet shoulder width apart. The trunk is straight, head erect but relaxed, mouth closed naturally, the tip of the tongue placed against the hard palate, eyes looking forward. Arms hang naturally at the sides. Fingers spread naturally.

MOVEMENT: Swing both arms forward and upward as high as the navel. Then swing them downward and backward naturally. With the continuing, rhythmic swinging of both arms, the lumbar region and the pelvis sway forward and backward with the same rhythm. Repeat this swinging motion 100–200 times (about 2–4 minutes), initially. Later, as the level of fitness improves, the number of swinging motions may be increased to 300–500.

Note: 1. Relax the entire body as much as possible during the exercise. 2. The swinging motion should be light, rhythmic, and effortless, performed at an easy and comfortable rate, about 50 swings per minute. 3. Continue to breathe naturally during the exercise.

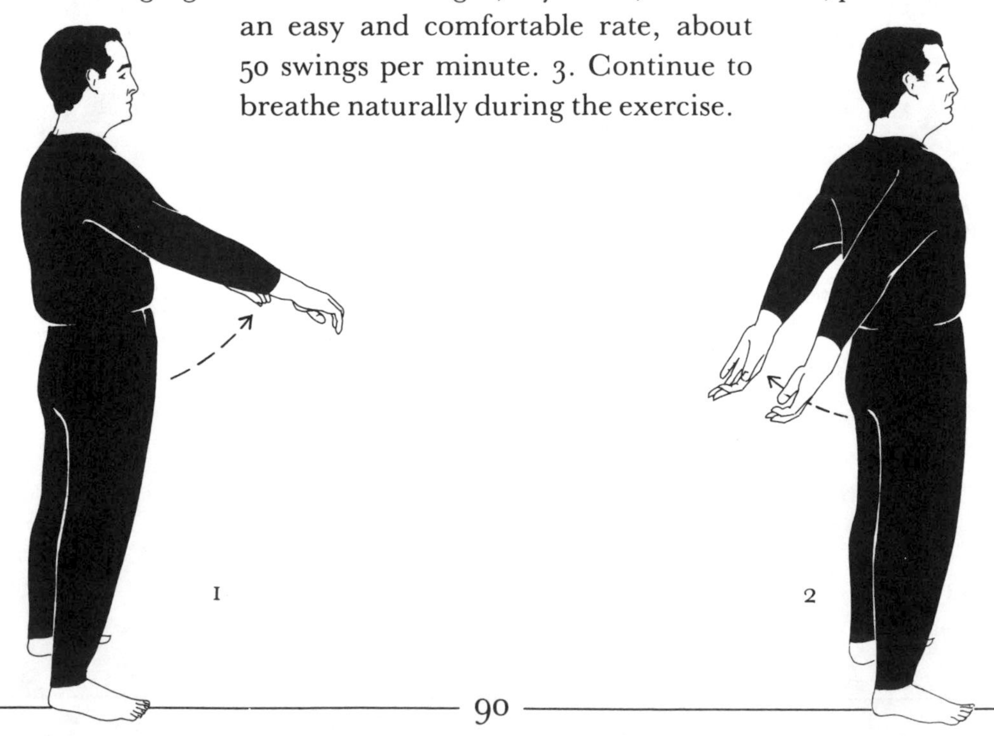

EXERCISE 2: *Twisting the trunk and looking backward.*

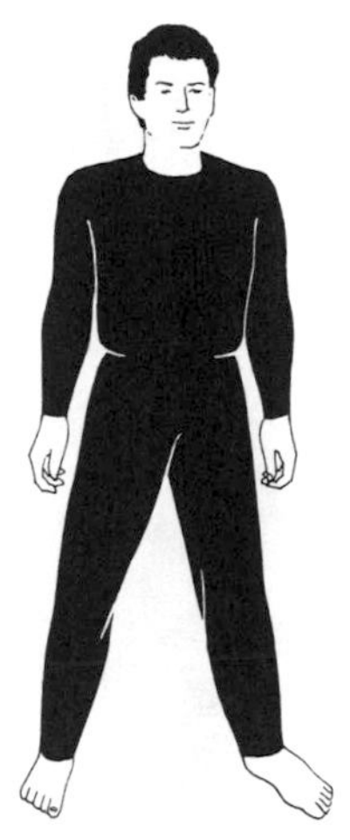

STARTING POSITION

PURPOSE: To develop flexibility of the spine, and prevent stiff neck.

STARTING POSITION: Stride standing (feet separated slightly more than shoulder width).

MOVEMENT: 1. Twist the trunk and head to the left until the heels of the feet are visible. At the same time swing the left arm to the left and place the right hand on the back of the head. Then return to the starting position. 2. Repeat this movement in reverse, twisting to the right, with the left hand on the back of the head. Then return again to the starting position.

Repeat this exercise 10–20 times.

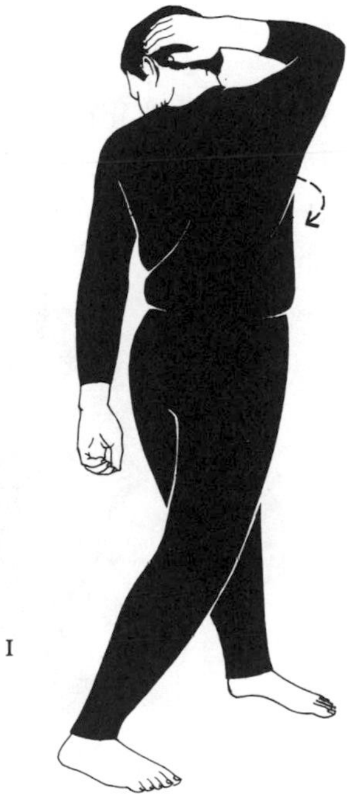

1

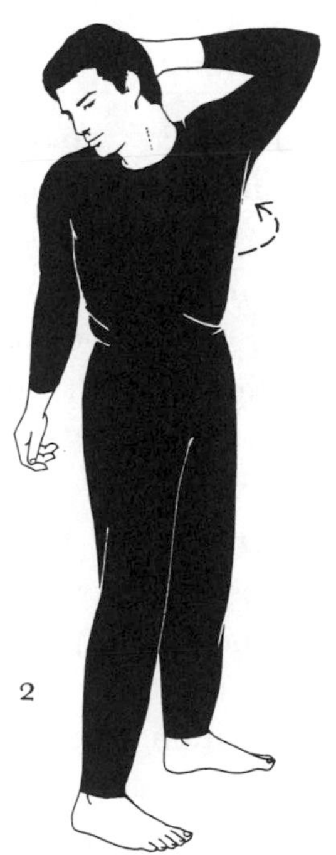

2

EXERCISE 3: *Pushing with the hands while riding a horse.*

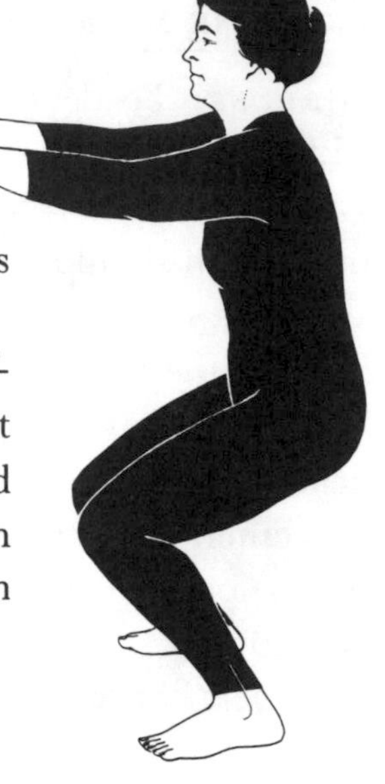

PURPOSE: To strengthen the arms and knees.

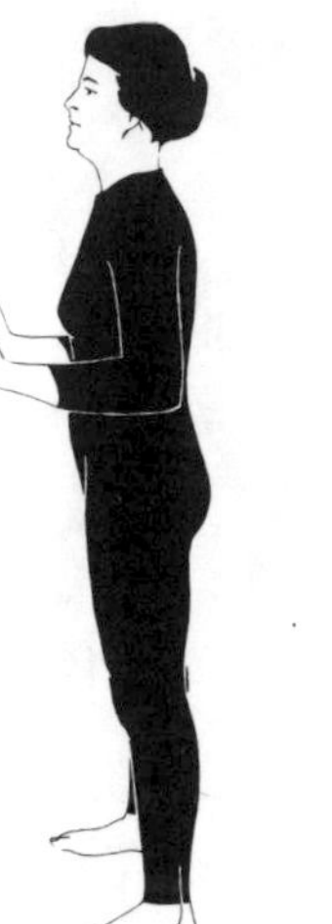

STARTING POSITION

STARTING POSITION: Stride standing (feet separated slightly more than shoulder width), arms at sides with elbows bent at a right angle, palms forward.

MOVEMENT: Bend the knees to a half-squatting position, as in riding a horse. At the same time stretch out the arms and push the hands forward slowly and with effort, as if pushing a heavy weight. Then return to the starting position.

Repeat this exercise 8–10 times.

EXERCISE 4: *Picking up beans.*

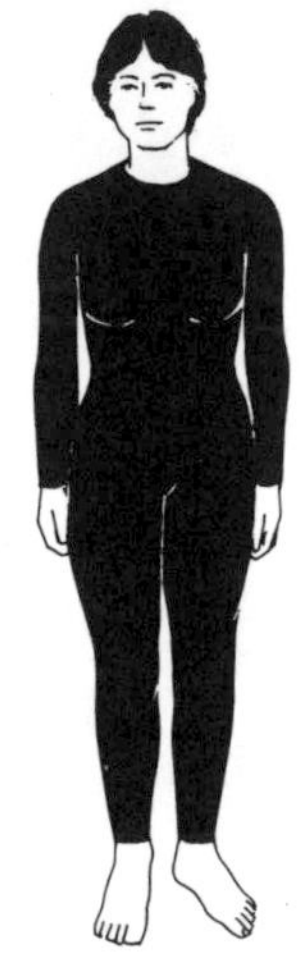

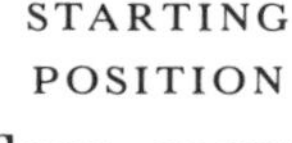

STARTING POSITION

PURPOSE: To develop general fitness, flexibility of the spine, and improve digestion.

Caution: This exercise should be avoided by those with lumbar intervertebral disk problems.

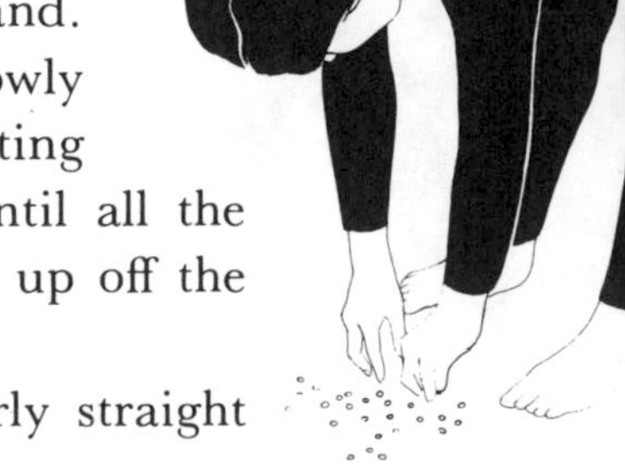

STARTING POSITION: Standing with feet slightly apart, 20–50 beans spread over the floor just in front of the feet.

MOVEMENT: Bend the trunk forward and pick up two beans, one with each hand. Then raise the trunk slowly and return to the starting position. Repeat this until all the beans have been picked up off the floor, or until you perspire or feel tired.

Note: Keep the knees straight or nearly straight when bending down.

EXERCISE 5: *Swaying from the waist and hips.*

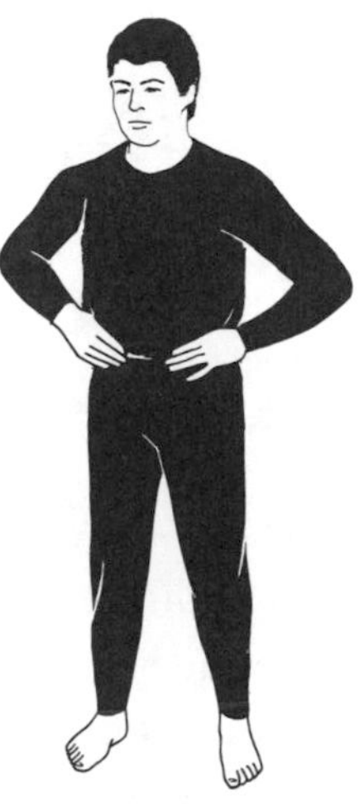
STARTING POSITION

PURPOSE: To develop flexibility of the lumbar spine and hip joints, and prevent lower back pain.
STARTING POSITION: Standing with feet apart about shoulder width, and hands on hips.
MOVEMENT: 1. Move the pelvis clockwise in a circular motion for 30 seconds. 2. Now, move the pelvis counterclockwise in a circular motion for 30 seconds.

Repeat this exercise 4–6 times.

Note: 1. This exercise should be performed in a relaxed manner. 2. The radius of swaying can be gradually increased.

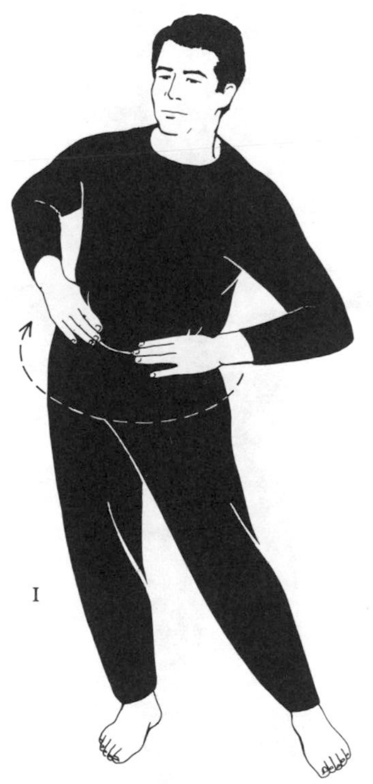
1

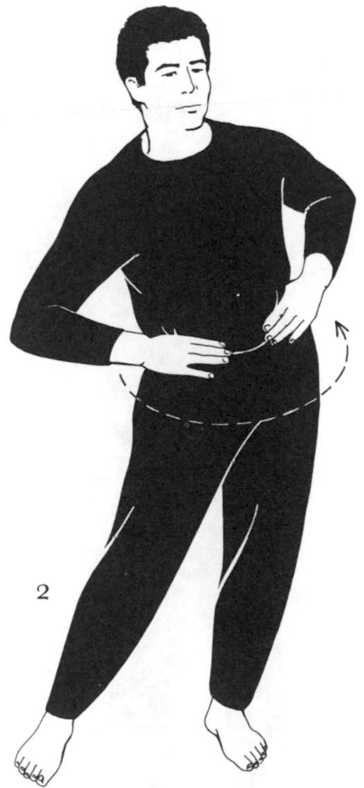
2

EXERCISE 6: *Walking like the wind.*

PURPOSE: To improve cardiorespiratory fitness.
STARTING POSITION: Standing.
MOVEMENT: Take a brisk walk. Move as swiftly as the wind, with arms swinging vigorously. Walk for 15–30 minutes.

EXERCISE 7: *Spreading the "wings."*

PURPOSE: To expand the chest and extend the trunk in order to counteract the effects of sedentary posture, and to develop deep breathing.
STARTING POSITION: Standing with feet apart about shoulder width, arms bent at elbows and crossed in front of the chest, palms downward.
MOVEMENT: 1. Extend the elbows and stretch the arms upward and outward. At the same time raise the heels as high as possible, and breathe in deeply. 2. Return to the starting position, and breathe out.

STARTING POSITION

Repeat this exercise 10–20 times.

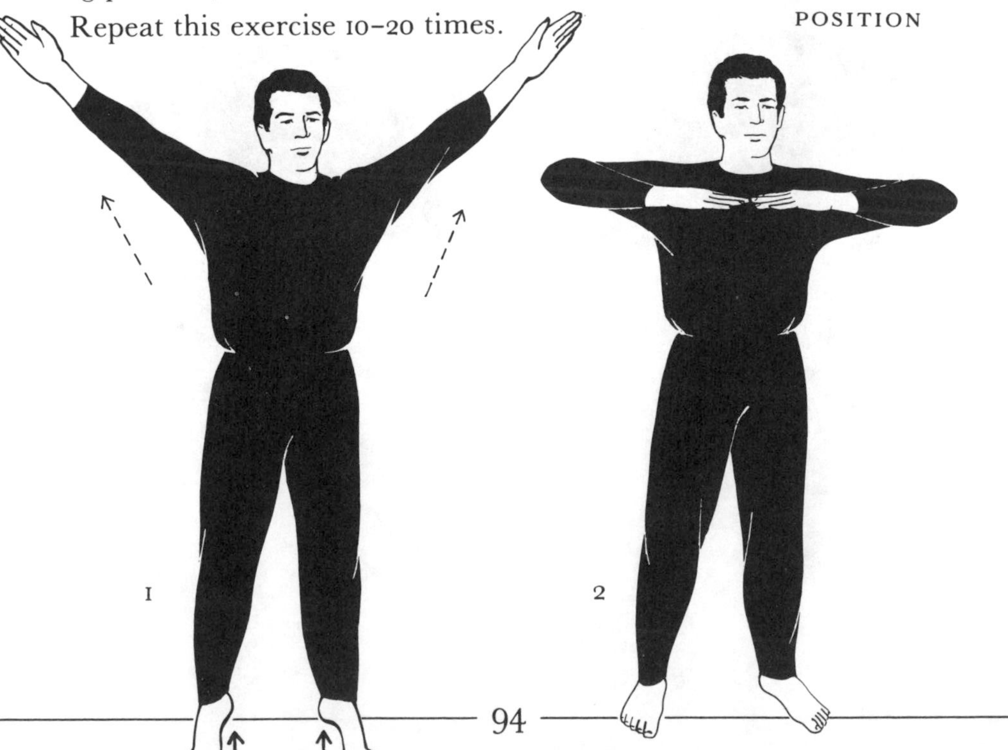

EXERCISE 8: *Kicking.*

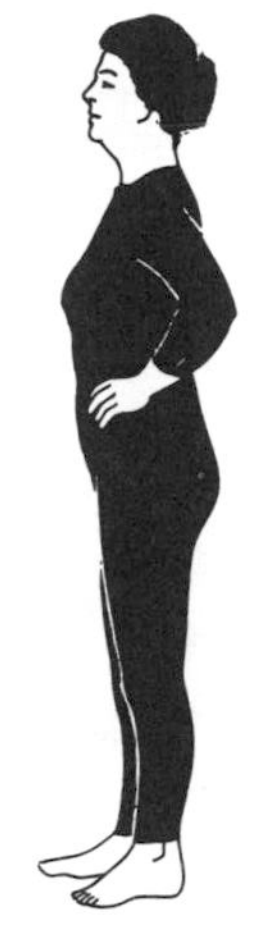

STARTING POSITION

PURPOSE: To stimulate blood circulation in the legs, and develop flexibility of the hip, knee, and ankle joints.
STARTING POSITION: Standing, hands on hips.
MOVEMENT: 1. Lift the right leg and kick forward. Then return to the starting position. 2. Lift the right leg and kick backward. Again, return to the starting position. Repeat this sequence with the left leg.

Repeat the entire exercise 8–10 times.

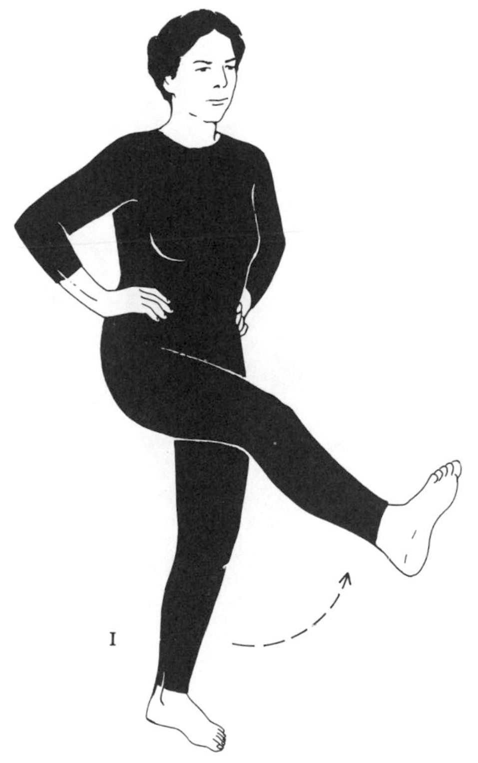

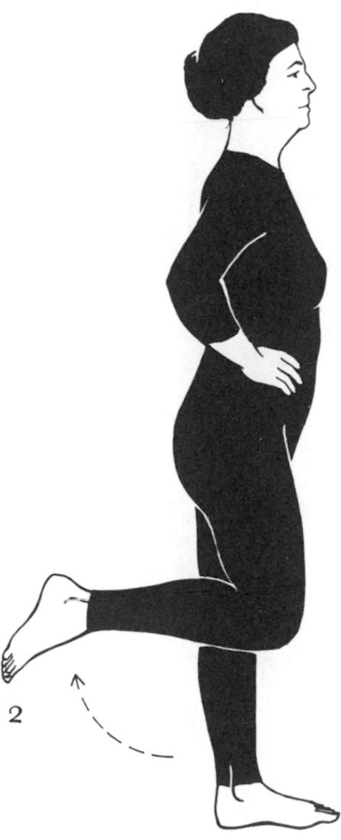

CHAPTER IX

Fitness Exercises for the Elderly

The following program is designed for the elderly with the purpose of improving physical fitness and preventing musculoskeletal problems such as weak feet, backache, and neck pain.

EXERCISE 1: *Swinging the arms.*

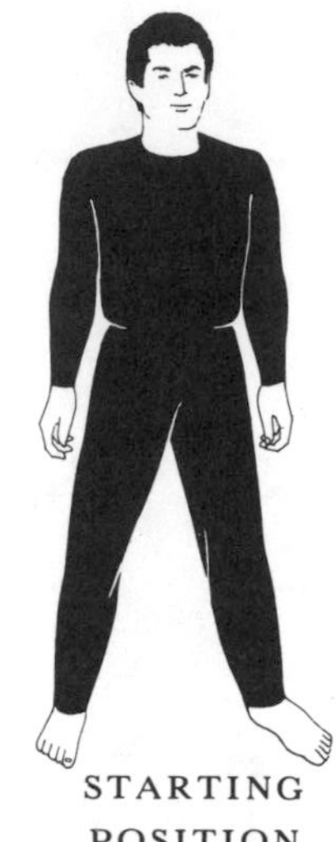
STARTING POSITION

PURPOSE: To improve digestion, blood circulation, and general well-being, and to keep the shoulder joints in good shape and prevent "frozen shoulders."

STARTING POSITION: Standing with the feet shoulder width apart. The trunk is straight, head erect but relaxed, mouth closed naturally, the tip of the tongue placed against the hard palate, eyes looking forward. Arms hang naturally at the sides. Fingers spread naturally.

MOVEMENT: Swing both arms forward and upward as high as the navel. Then swing them downward and backward naturally. With the continuing, rhythmic swinging of both arms, the lumbar region and the pelvis sway forward and backward with the same rhythm. Repeat this swinging motion 100–200 times (about 2–4 minutes), initially. Later, as the level of fitness improves, the number of swinging motions may be increased to 300–500.

Note: 1. Relax the entire body as much as possible during the exercise. 2. The swinging motion should be light, rhythmic, and effortless, performed at an easy and comfortable rate, about 50 swings per minute. 3. Continue to breathe naturally during the exercise.

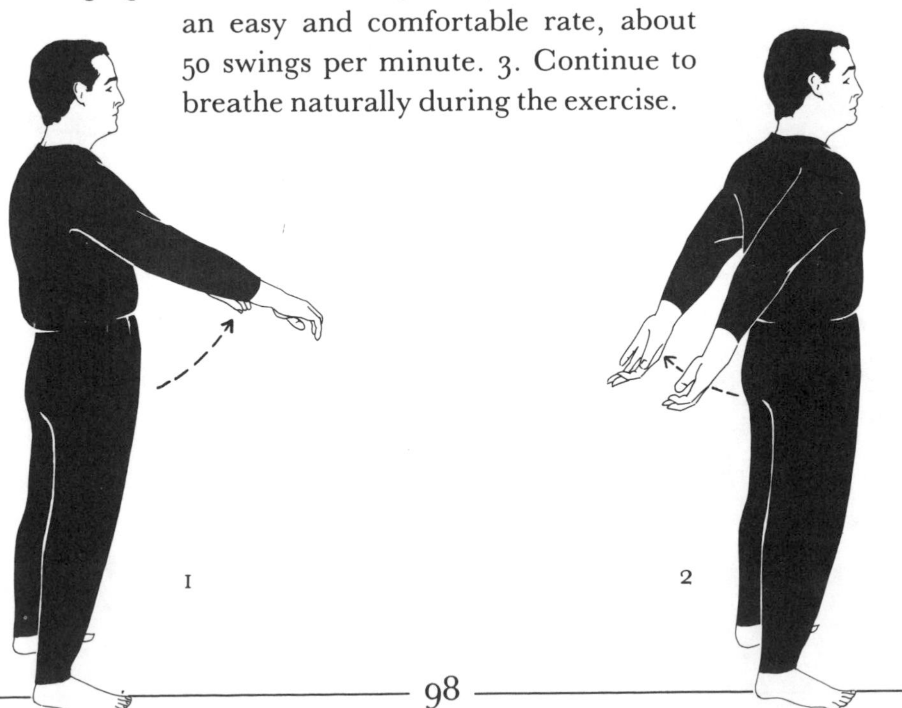

EXERCISE 2: *The cow looking at the moon.*

PURPOSE: To develop flexibility of the neck muscles and cervical spine in order to prevent a stiff neck.
STARTING POSITION: Standing or sitting.
MOVEMENT: 1. Bend the head to the right and twist it slightly up to the left, eyes looking toward the sky (or ceiling). Then return to the starting position. 2. Bend the head to the left and twist it up to the right, eyes looking toward the sky (or ceiling). And again, return to the starting position.

Repeat this exercise 8–10 times.

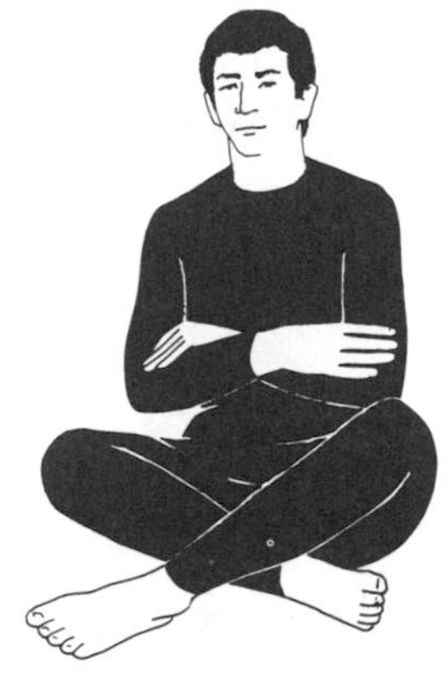

STARTING POSITION

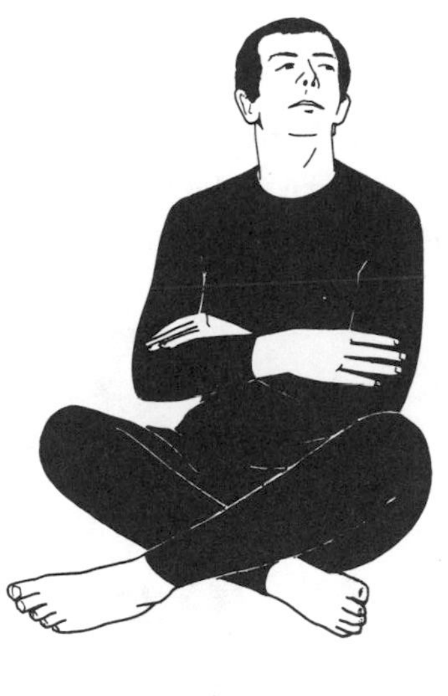

1

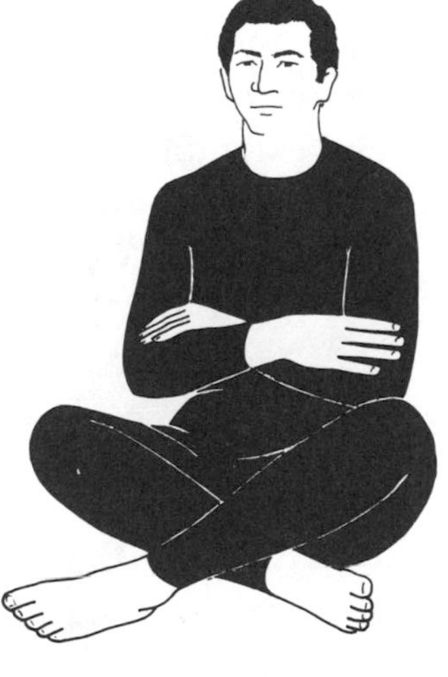

2

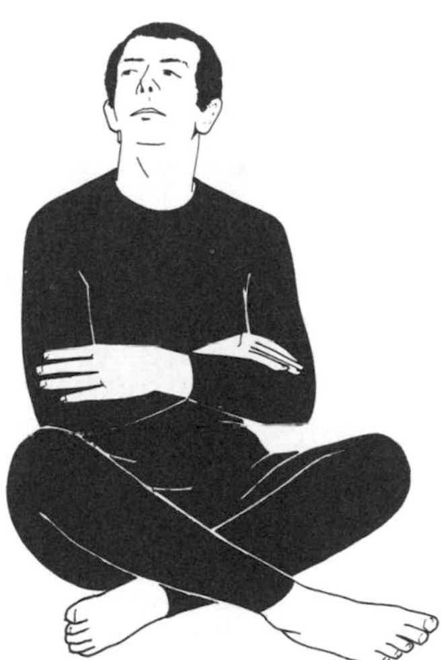

3

EXERCISE 3: *The dragon stamping on the earth.*

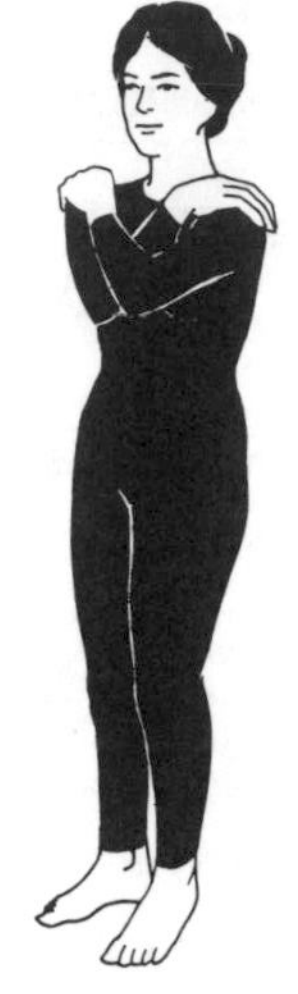

PURPOSE: To strengthen the feet and prevent loss of bone mass in the heel bone.

STARTING POSITION: Standing with feet slightly apart. Hands embrace both shoulders.

MOVEMENT: Grip the toes to the ground and stamp with the heels 24 times.

Note: The stamping motion should be moderate in effort.

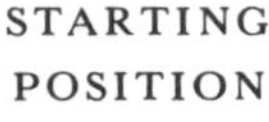

STARTING POSITION

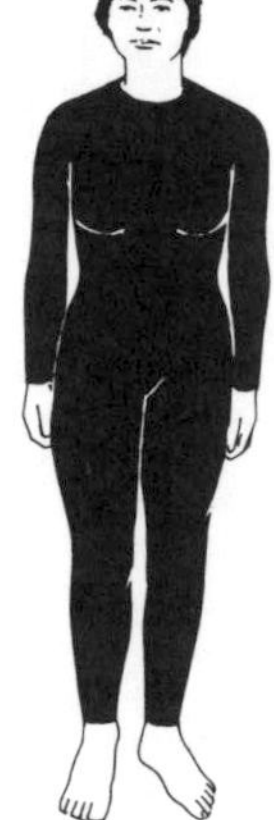

STARTING POSITION

EXERCISE 4: *Rowing.*

PURPOSE: To improve general fitness and develop the flexibility of the spine.

STARTING POSITION: Standing, feet slightly apart.

MOVEMENT: 1. Step forward with the left foot. Stretch both arms forward and upward, with the trunk falling slightly forward at the same time. 2. Then draw the hands downward and backward, with the trunk rising and extending slightly backward at the same time. Repeat this 8 times, then return to the to the starting position.

Stepping forward with the right foot this time, repeat the movements in steps 1 and 2, and again return to the starting position.

Repeat the entire exercise 8 times.

Note: The movement of the arms should be performed rhythmically as in rowing.

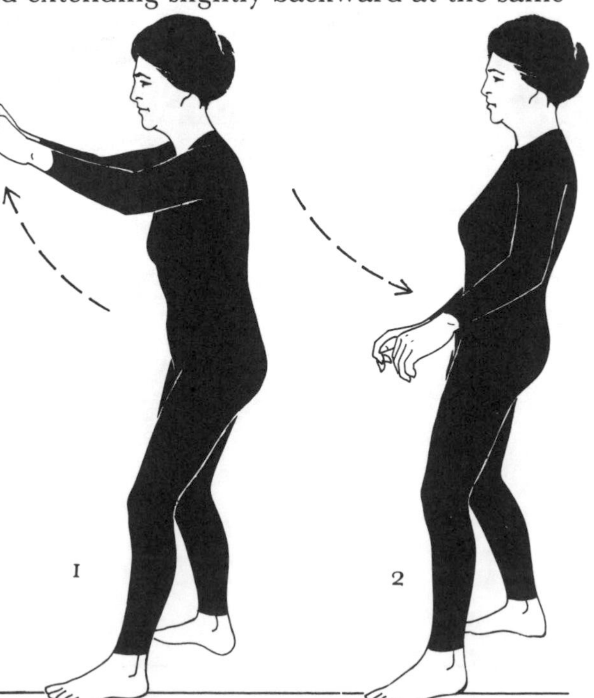

EXERCISE 5: *Handling two chestnuts with one hand.*

PURPOSE: To facilitate peripheral circulation in the upper arms, and develop flexibility of the finger joints.
STARTING POSITION: Sitting or standing.
MOVEMENT: Place two chestnuts (or small rubber balls, marbles, or smooth round stones) in the palm of the right hand. Move them around with the fingers of the right hand for 2 minutes. Then repeat this using the left hand.

Note: Handle the chestnuts with only one hand at a time, being careful not to let them slip off the palm.

EXERCISE 6: *Half-squatting.*

PURPOSE: To develop flexibility of the hip and knee joints, and strengthen the legs.
STARTING POSITION: Standing, arms at sides.
MOVEMENT: Take a step to the left with the left foot, while bending the knees and hips to lower the body to a half-squatting position. At the same time, bend the elbows and press the hands downward. Then return to the starting position. Repeat the movement, this time stepping to the right. Then return again to the starting position.

Repeat the entire exercise 8–10 times.

Note: Do the half-squatting in a relaxed manner.

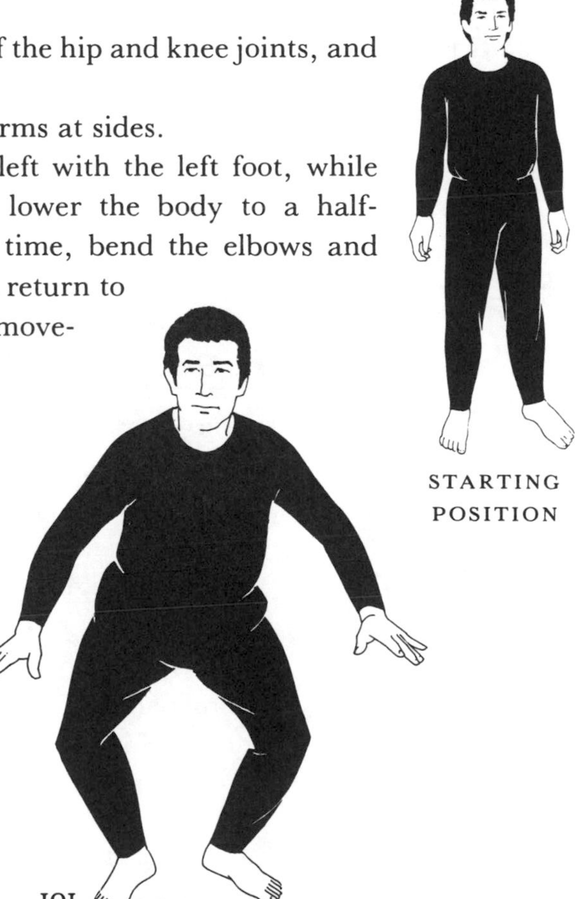

STARTING POSITION

EXERCISE 7: *Walking and massaging the abdomen.*

PURPOSE: To stimulate digestion and blood circulation, especially after having a big meal.

STARTING POSITION: Standing.

MOVEMENT: Walk 100–500 steps at a comfortable pace. Meanwhile, massage the abdomen with both hands in a circular stroking manner.

STARTING POSITION

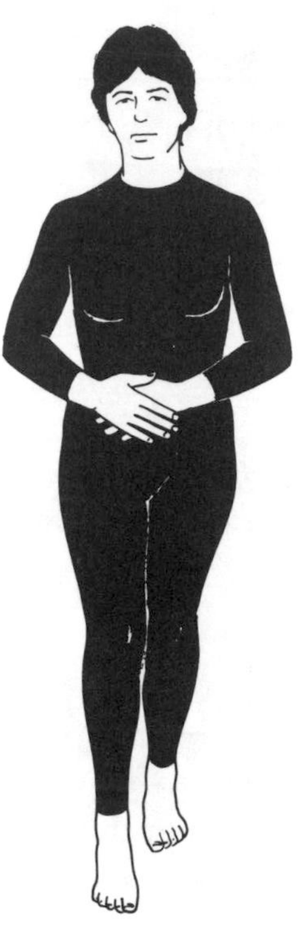

Self-administered preventive massage

I

1. *Hitting the arms and legs.*

PURPOSE: To stimulate peripheral blood circulation.

STARTING POSITION: Sitting.

MASSAGE: 1. Hit the left arm with the right open hand, then reverse. 2. Then slap the thighs and lower legs with both palms. Repeat this sequence for one minute.

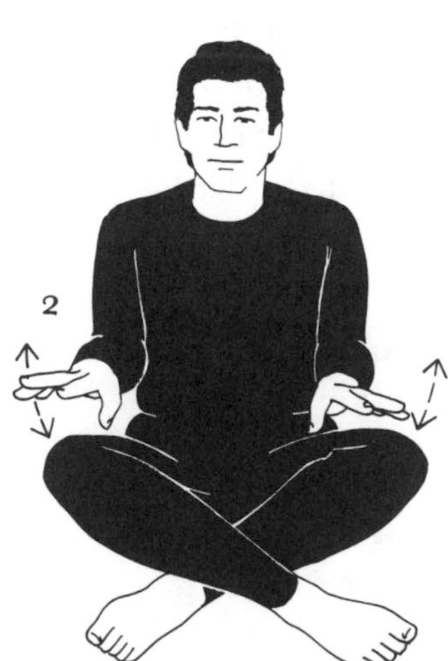

2. *Acupressure on* chu san li *(the point of longevity).*

PURPOSE: To improve general health and strengthen the legs.

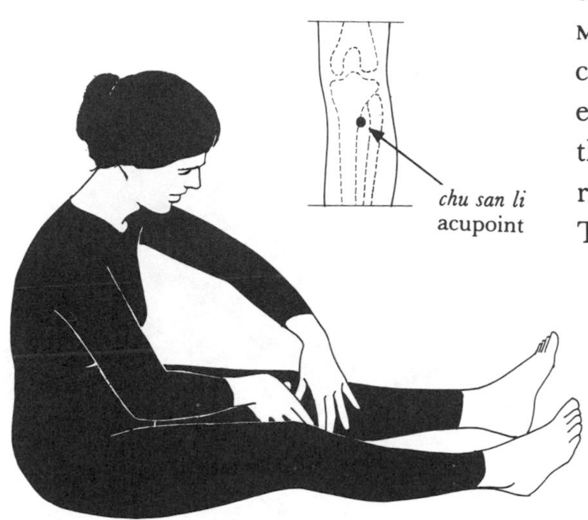

STARTING POSITION: Sitting.

MASSAGE: 1. *Chu san li* is located 2½ inches below the outer edge of the knee cap. Press the point with the thumb and rub it gently for one minute. Then repeat on the other leg.

3. *Stroking the point* shen shu.

PURPOSE: To prevent backache and increase vitality.

STARTING POSITION: Sitting.

MASSAGE: *Shen shu* is located in the lumbar region. Rub or stroke this area for 3–5 minutes.

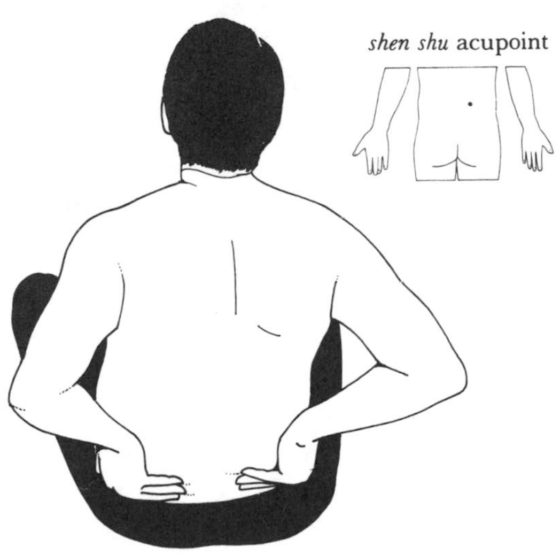

4. *Rubbing the knees.*

PURPOSE: To strengthen the knees.
STARTING POSITION: Sitting.
MASSAGE: Rub the surface of the left knee with both hands for two minutes. Then knead the back of the left knee for one minute. Repeat on the other leg in the same manner.

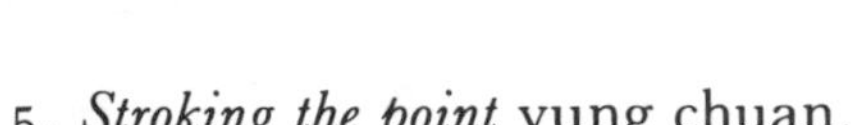

5. *Stroking the point* yung chuan.

PURPOSE: To strengthen the feet, induce sound sleep, and lower high blood pressure.
STARTING POSITION: Sitting.
MASSAGE: The *yung chuan* point is located in the middle of the sole. Rub this point on the left sole with the right thumb until there is a feeling of warmth in the area. Then repeat this on the other foot.

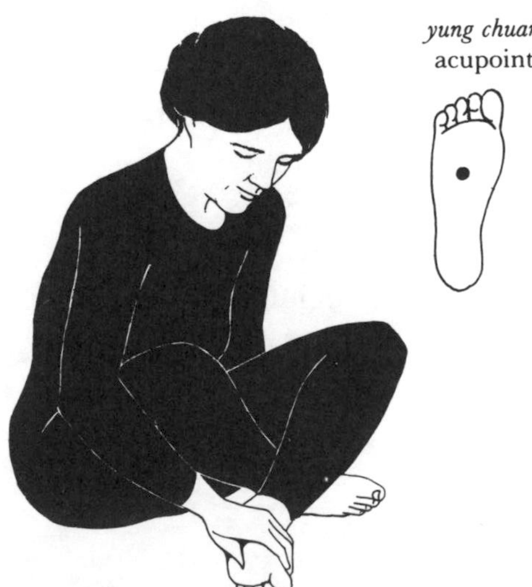

CHAPTER X

Fitness Exercises for Pregnant Women

Fitness exercises for pregnant women aim to promote relaxation, relieve pelvic pressure, and reduce swelling or edema in the legs. The following program is suitable for the expectant mother from the fourth through eighth month of pregnancy.

EXERCISE 1: *Abdominal breathing.*

PURPOSE: To promote relaxation and lift the abdominal wall off the uterus.
STARTING POSITION: Lying on the back, hands on the abdomen, knees bent at about 60°, and feet on the floor.
MOVEMENT: Breathe in slowly protruding the abdomen. Then breathe out slowly, allowing the abdomen to relax.

Repeat this exercise 8–10 times.

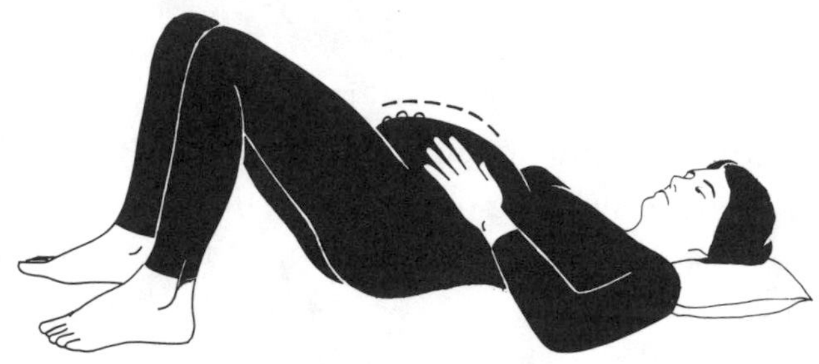

EXERCISE 2: *Pelvic rocking.*

PURPOSE: To prevent or relieve lower back pain.
STARTING POSITION: Lying on the back with knees bent at about 60°, arms at sides resting on the floor, palms down.
MOVEMENT: Raise the buttocks and hips off the floor. Then lower them returning to the starting position.

Repeat this exercise 8–10 times.

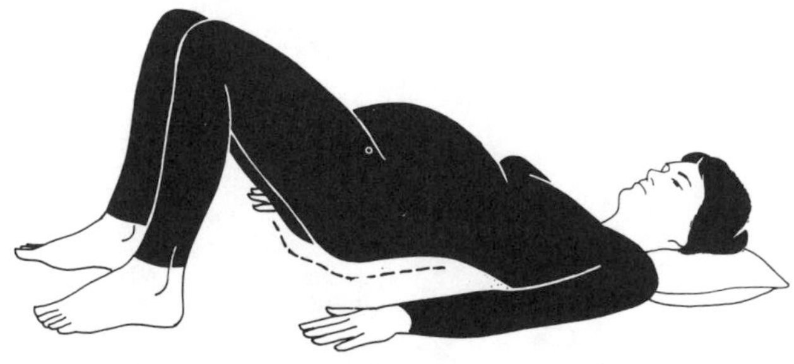

EXERCISE 3: *Knee bending and relaxing.*

STARTING POSITION

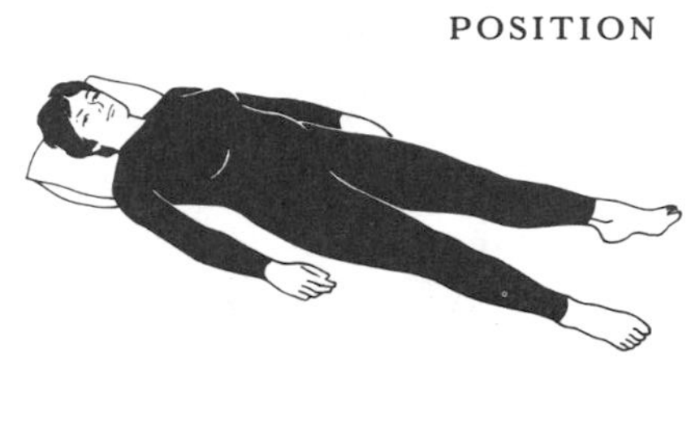

PURPOSE: To help relax the muscles of the pelvic floor.

STARTING POSITION: Lying on the back with legs extended, arms at sides resting on the floor.

MOVEMENT: 1. Bend the knees with the feet moving on the floor back toward the buttocks. 2. Then spread the knees apart, with the soles of the feet touching each other. Relax in this position for a short while. 3. Extend the legs and return to the starting position.

Repeat this exercise 8–10 times.

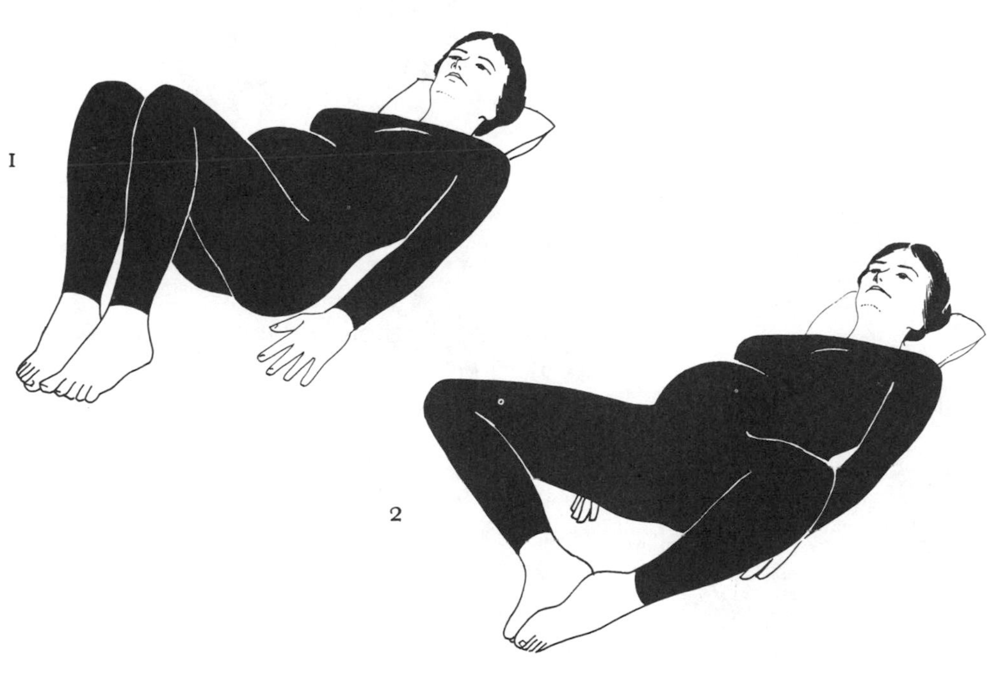

EXERCISE 4: *Half-sitting and relaxing.*

PURPOSE: To help relax the muscles of the pelvic floor.
STARTING POSITION: Half-sitting, leaning back against a pile of pillows, knees separated, feet touching the floor.
MOVEMENT: Open the knees wide with the help of the hands, and relax. Then return to the starting position.

Repeat this exercise 8–10 times.

STARTING POSITION

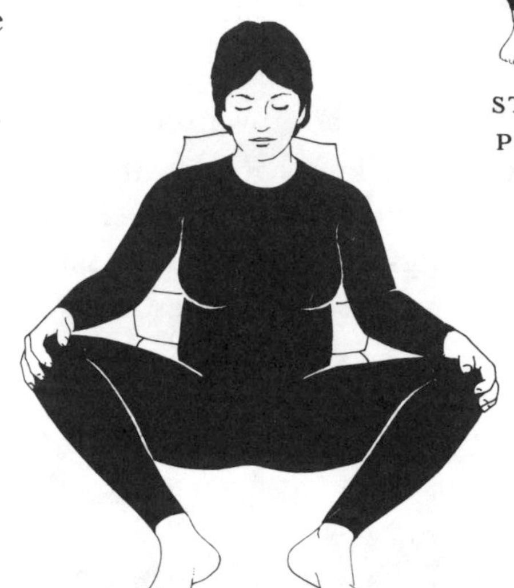

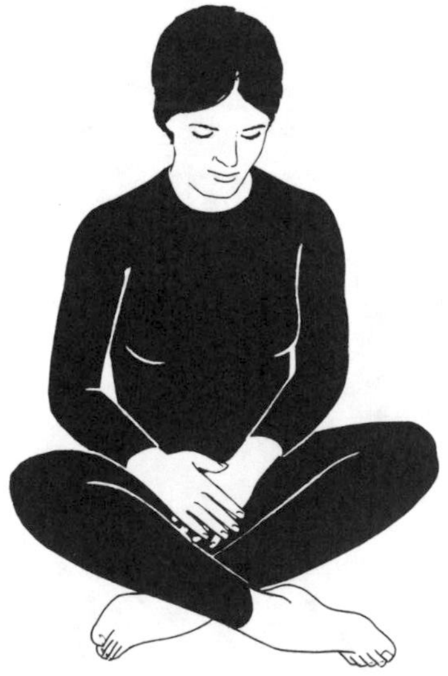

EXERCISE 5: *Tailor sitting (sitting cross-legged) and rhythmic breathing.*

PURPOSE: To help relax the muscles of the pelvic floor.
STARTING POSITION: Sitting cross-legged, with a cushion supporting the buttocks, hands clasped and placed on the lower abdomen in a relaxed manner.
MOVEMENT: Breathe in slowly and naturally. Then breathe out in the same manner, slightly moving the lower back to help relax the hips and buttocks.

Repeat this exercise 8–10 times.

EXERCISE 6: *Squatting and relaxing.*

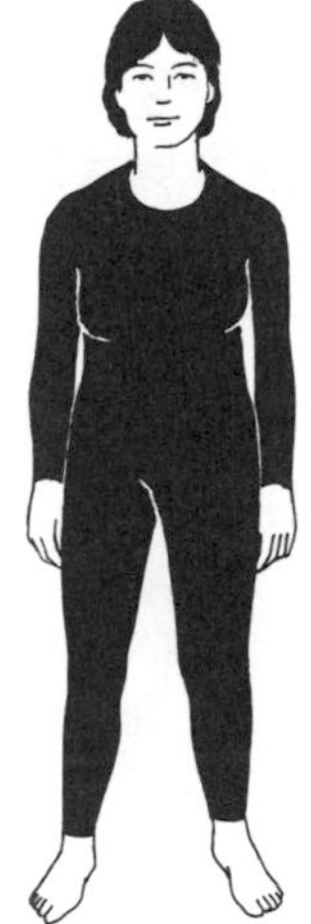

STARTING POSITION

PURPOSE: To help relax the pelvic floor.
STARTING POSITION: Standing with feet shoulder width apart.
MOVEMENT: 1. Bend the knees and take a squatting position with hands resting on the knees. 2. Raise the trunk and return to the starting position with the help of the hands.

Repeat this exercise 6–8 times.

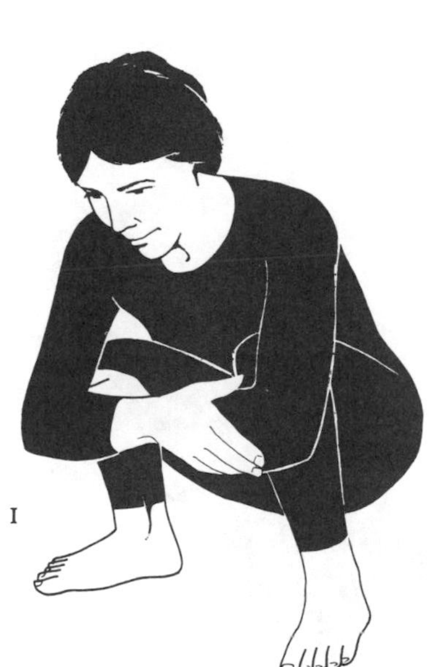

1

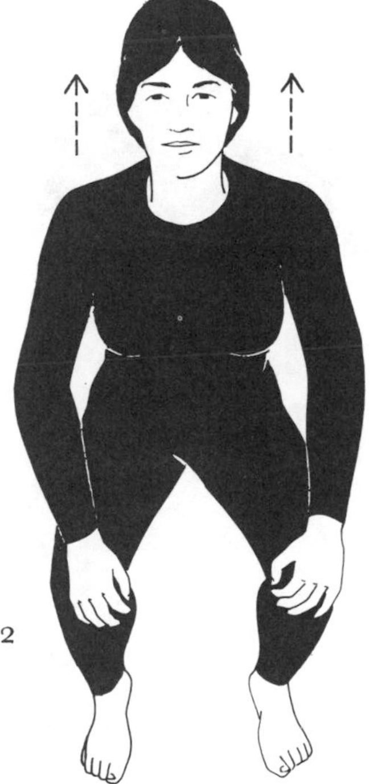

2

EXERCISE 7: *Walking.*

PURPOSE: To improve blood circulation and digestion.
MOVEMENT: Walk indoors, or, weather permitting, outdoors at a slow and comfortable pace for 5–10 minutes.

EXERCISE 8: *Stretching and relaxing.*

PURPOSE: To rest the legs and reduce swelling or edema.
STARTING POSITION: Lying on the back, arms at sides, legs bent, feet pointing at a wall.
MOVEMENT: Raise the legs and place the heels on the wall. Hold this position for one or two minutes. Then return to the starting position.

Repeat this exercise 3–5 times.

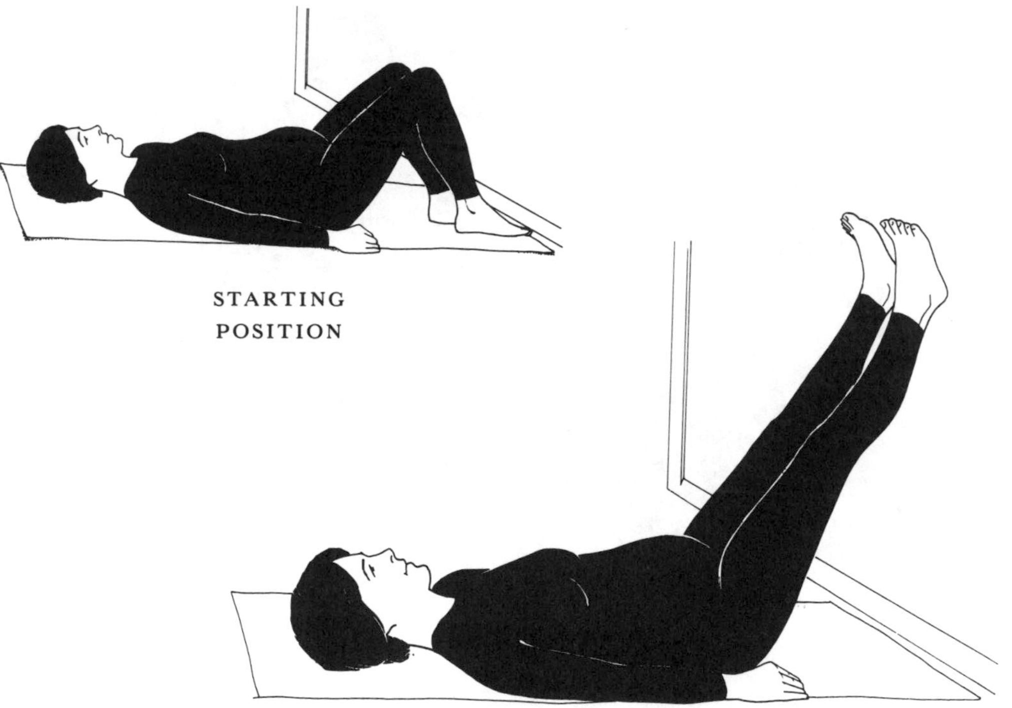

CHAPTER XI

Fitness Exercises for Athletes

The following program is planned for athletes to practice regularly in order to develop the back and knees, and to increase flexibility. It is designed to help in the prevention of sports injuries. When this program is followed after training workouts, the exercises and self-administered massage will facilitate the body's recovery.

EXERCISE I: *Riding a horse.*

PURPOSE: To develop the quadriceps and knees for the prevention of painful knees.

STARTING POSITION: Stride standing (feet pointing forward and separated more than shoulder width), trunk erect, elbows bent at the sides, fists clenched, and toes firmly touching the floor.

MOVEMENT: 1. Bend the knees, as if riding a horse, with thighs parallel to the ground. Hold this position for 2–3 minutes. Meanwhile, take deep breaths. 2. Return to the starting position. 3. Again, bend the knees as in riding a horse. Hold this position for 3 minutes. Meanwhile, stretch out and draw in the arms 6–8 times. When stretching out the arms, do it as if hitting a target with the fists. Then return again to the starting position. This exercise is to be done once or twice only.

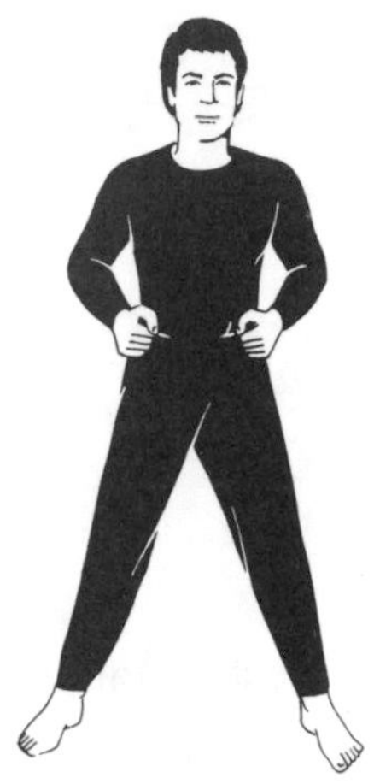

STARTING POSITION

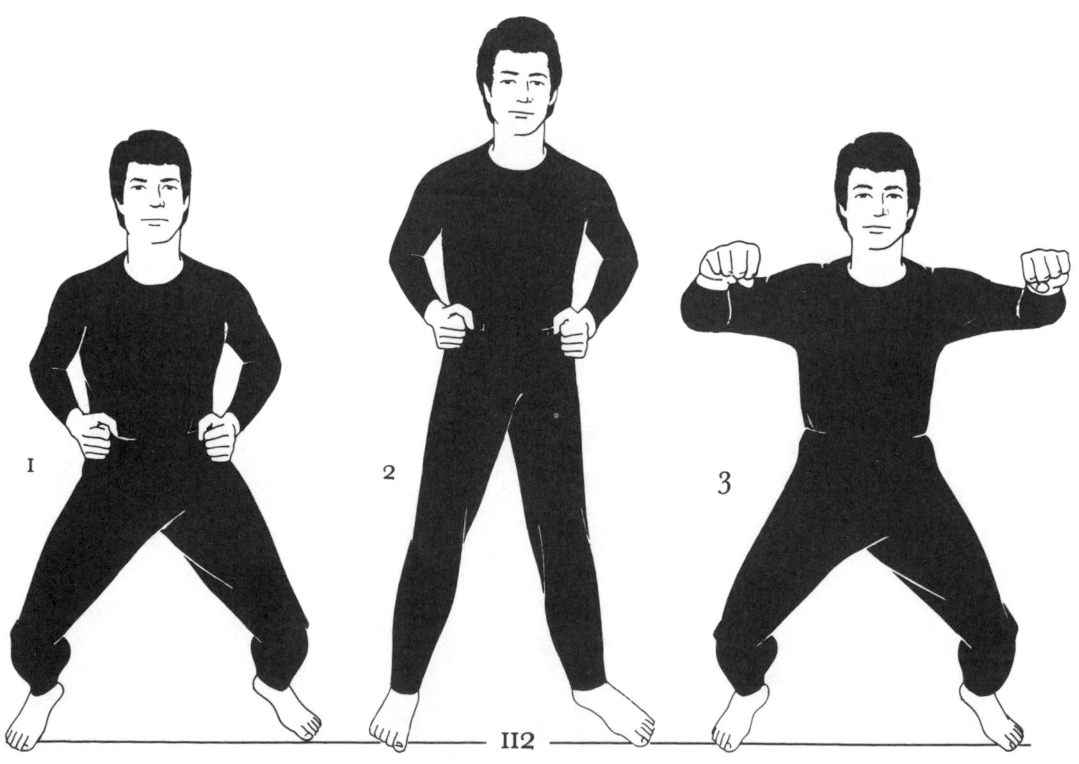

EXERCISE 2: *Tiger walking.*

PURPOSE: To develop the flexibility of the lower spine and hip joints.

Caution: This exercise is not suitable for those with back injuries.

STARTING POSITION: Standing with feet separated shoulder width.

MOVEMENT: 1. Bend the trunk forward, bending the knees so the back is almost parallel to the floor. Grasp the left ankle with the left hand, and the right ankle with the right hand. 2. Take a step forward with the right foot, while turning the head to the right. 3. Then take a step forward with the left foot, while turning the head to the left. Walk 8 steps in this manner. Then raise the trunk and return to the starting position. Breathe naturally in a rhythmic manner 8–10 times.

Repeat this exercise 2–4 times.

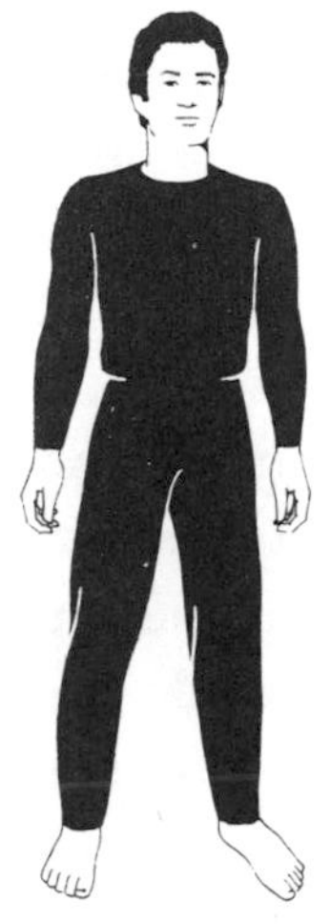

STARTING POSITION

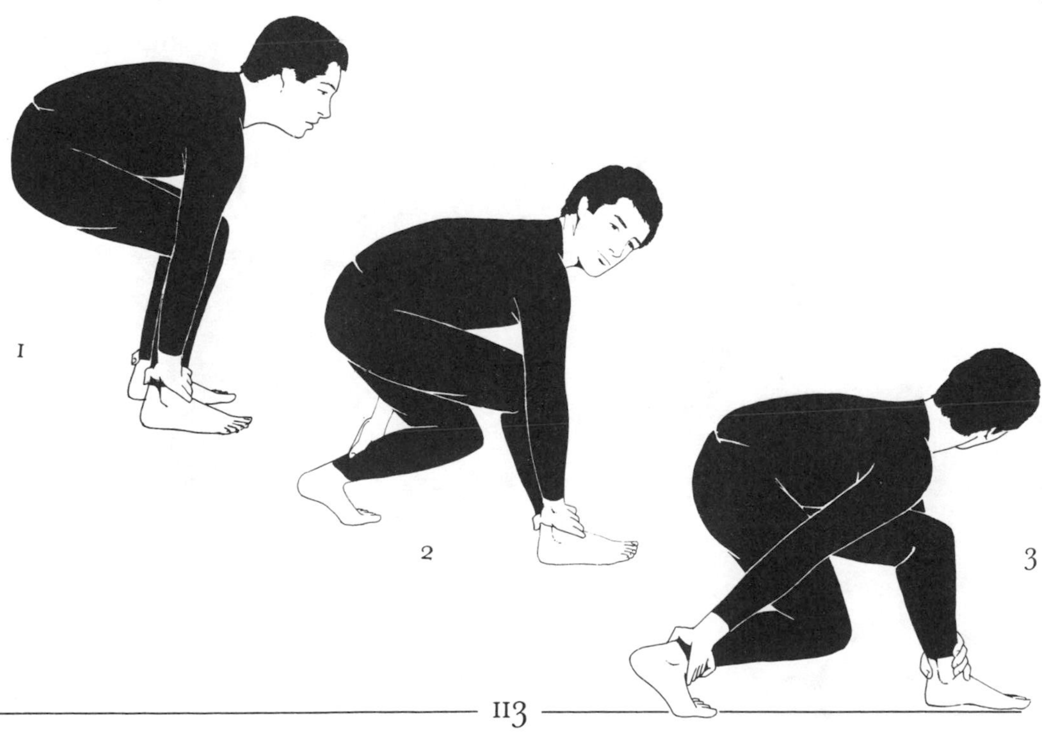

EXERCISE 3: *Forward thrust.*

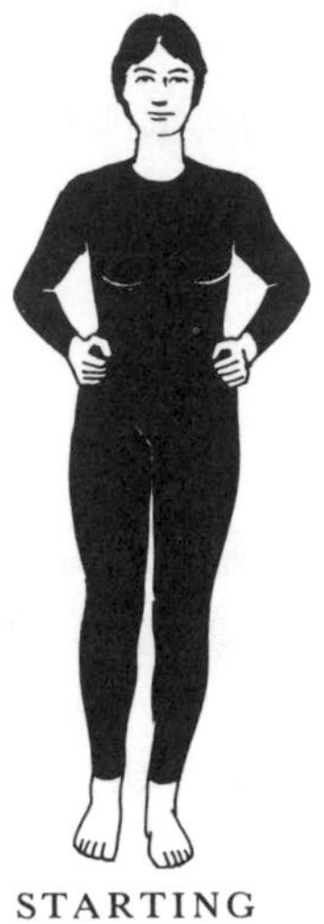

STARTING POSITION

PURPOSE: To develop the thighs and hips, the shoulders and arms, and prevent lower back pain.

STARTING POSITION: Standing with feet together, arms bent at sides, fists clenched firmly at the waist.

MOVEMENT: 1. Take a big step forward with the left foot, bending the left knee, while keeping the right foot in place, with the right knee straight. Meanwhile, stretch out the right arm and thrust the open hand forward with effort, palm facing inward, fingers together and pointing forward, while keeping the left fist in place. 2. Take a big step forward with the right foot, bending the right knee, while keeping the left foot in place, with the left knee straight. Meanwhile, stretch out the left arm and thrust the open hand straight forward with effort, palm facing inward, fingers together and pointing forward, while drawing in the right hand, fist clenched, to the side of the waist. Continue stepping forward in the manner described above for three minutes (about 100 steps).

Note: 1. Keep the back and head straight during the entire course of the exercise. 2. The knee of the leg which is behind must be kept straight. 3. The forward thrust of the hand should be forceful.

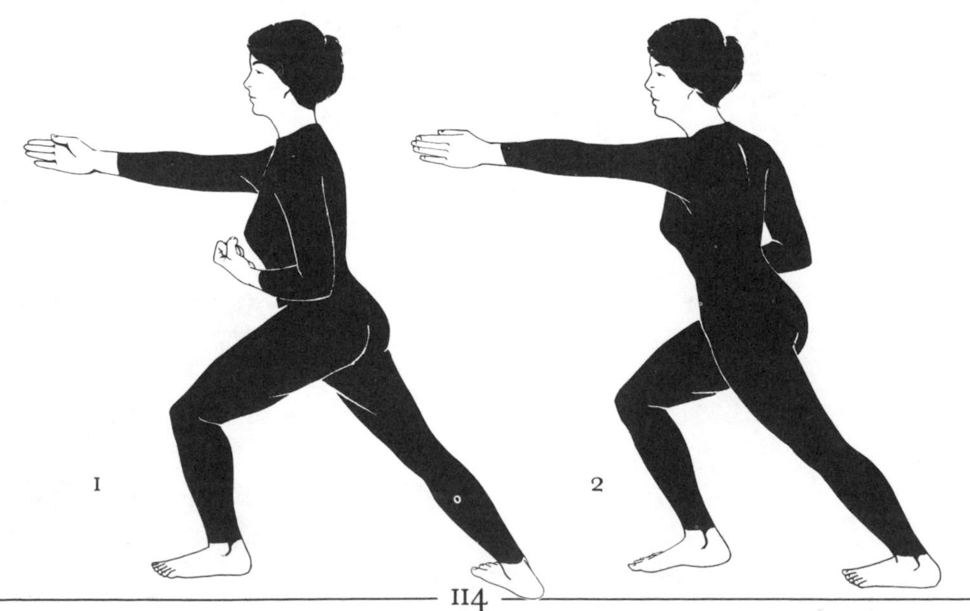

EXERCISE 4: *Swallow flying.*

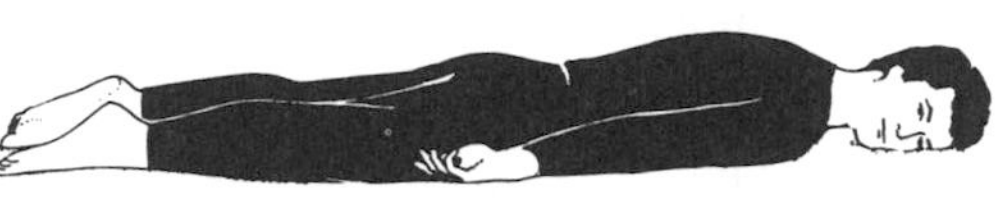
STARTING POSITION

PURPOSE: To develop the back muscles for the prevention of backache. This exercise is particularly appropriate before a workout.

STARTING POSITION: Lying on the stomach, arms at sides.

MOVEMENT: Raise the head, chest, and legs off the floor simultaneously, with arms swinging backward to assist the trunk movement. Then return to the starting position by dropping the head, chest, and legs to the floor.

Repeat this 8–10 times.

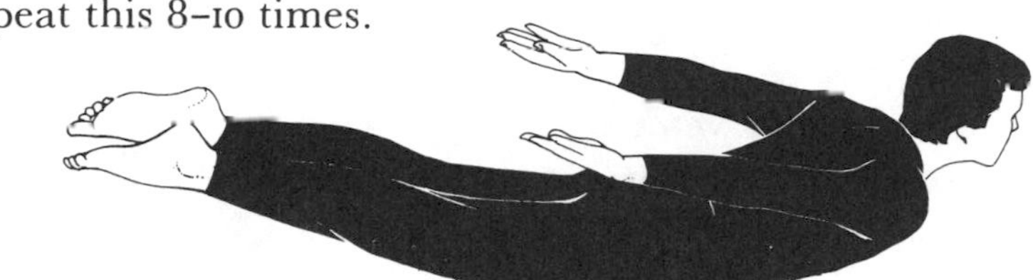

EXERCISE 5: *Wall pushing.*

PURPOSE: To develop the abdomen and the legs, and strengthen the knees.

STARTING POSITION: Standing with the back against a wall.

MOVEMENT: Bend the knees and move the feet out to lower the body to a half-squatting position with thighs parallel to the floor. In this position, push the back against the wall by pushing with the legs as hard as possible, and hold for five seconds. Then rest five seconds in the half-squatting position. Finally, return to the starting position.

Repeat this exercise 2–4 times.

Note: Hands should not press on the thighs at all.

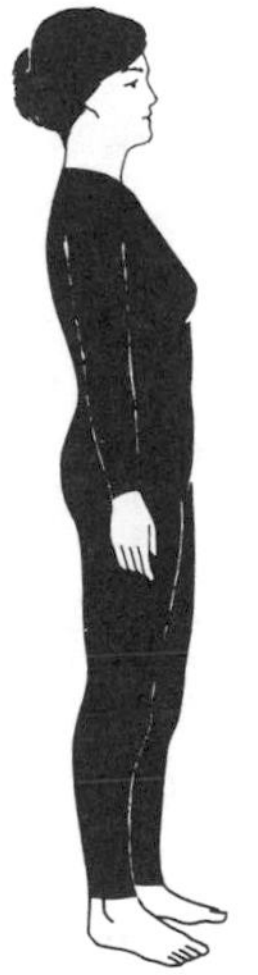
STARTING POSITION

EXERCISE 6: *Hanging and swinging.*

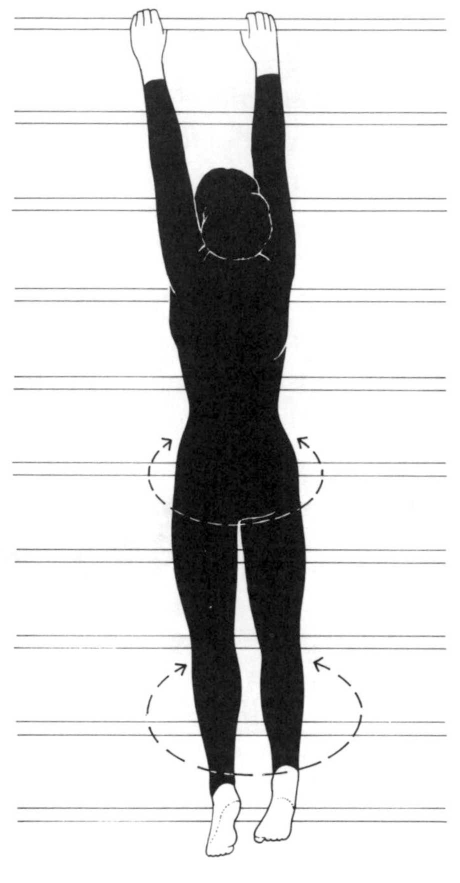

PURPOSE: To relieve strained back muscles and spine in order to prevent back pain. It is particularly suitable for athletes after a workout.

STARTING POSITION: Standing on toes with feet together. Hands reaching upward as far as possible, grasp an overhead bar in order to stretch the trunk. Elbows and legs are kept straight.

MOVEMENT: 1. Swing the waist ten times in a clockwise circular movement. 2. Then swing it ten times in a counterclockwise circular movement.

Repeat this sequence 8–10 times.

EXERCISE 7: *Relaxing the waist and tapping the body.*

PURPOSE: To aid in relaxing the body.

STARTING POSITION: Standing with feet apart, arms at sides, fists clenched slightly, body relaxed.

MOVEMENT: 1. Twist the trunk to the left, while at the same time swinging the arms easily to the left. Let the swinging right fist hit the left abdomen, and the left fist hit the lower

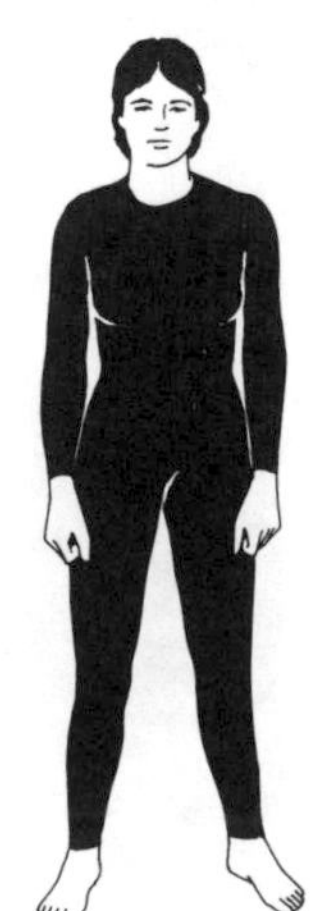

STARTING POSITION

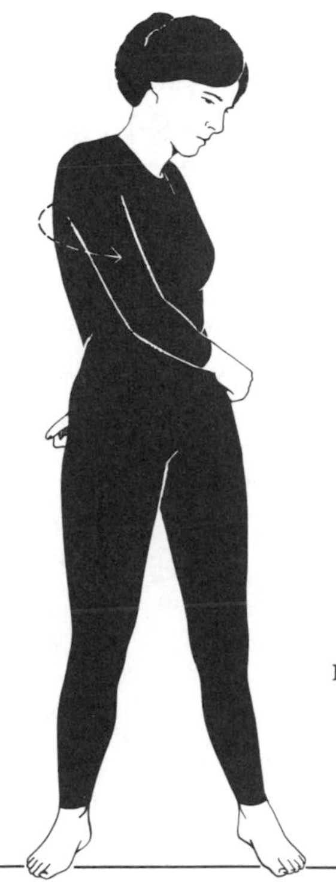

back on the right side. 2. Twist the trunk to the right, while swinging the arms easily to the right. Let the swinging left fist hit the right abdomen, and the right fist hit the lower back on the left side.

Note: The hitting should be moderate in effort.

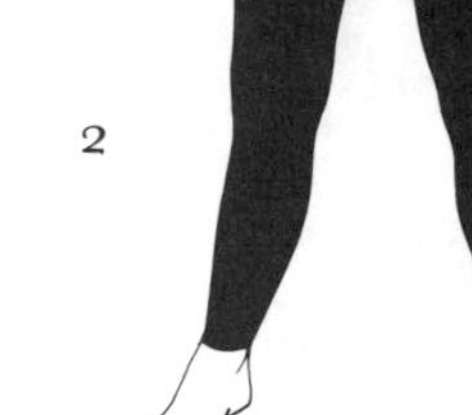

1

2

Self-administered massage

PURPOSE: To help prevent sports injuries, and facilitate the recovery of the body after a workout.

STARTING POSITION: Sitting on a chair.

MASSAGE SEQUENCE: 1. *Hitting the arms.* Hit along the length of the right arm with the left fist ten times. Hit along the length of the left arm with the right fist ten times.

2. *Hitting the thighs.* Hit the thighs with both fists 20 times.

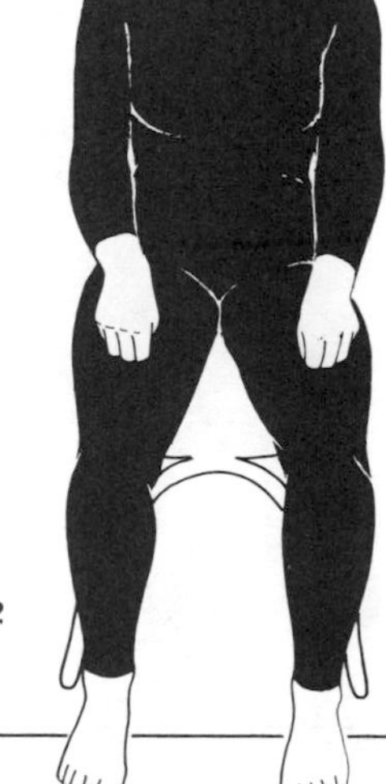

1

2

3. *Massaging the shoulders.* Stroke and knead the muscles around the left shoulder joint with the right hand for one or two minutes. Repeat on the other side. 4. *Massaging the knees.* Rub the surface of the left knee with both hands for two minutes, then knead the back of the left knee for one minute. Repeat on the other knee. 5. *Massaging the ankles.* Rub the left ankle joint with both hands for two minutes. Repeat on the other ankle.

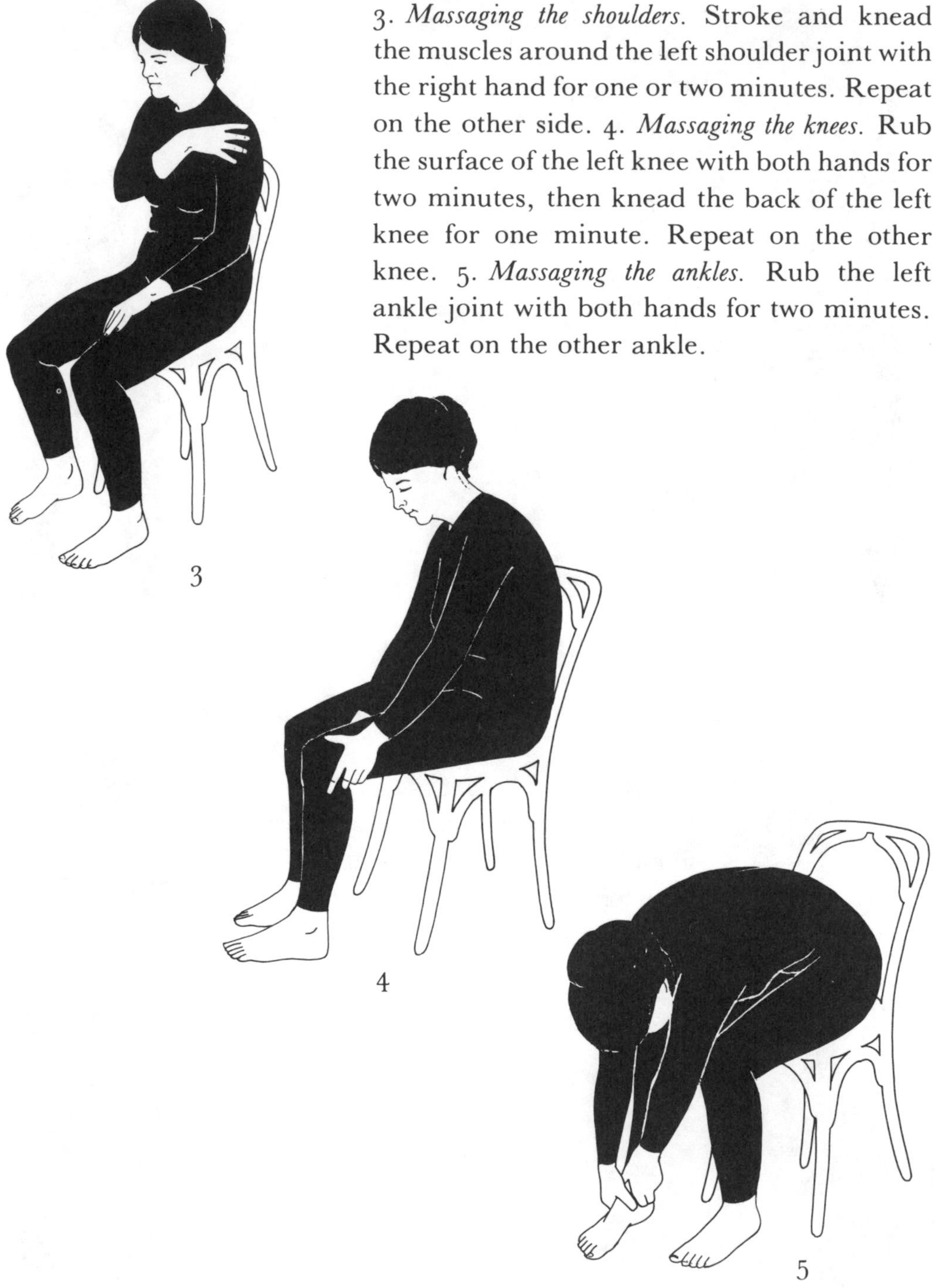

PART III

Chinese Therapeutic Exercises

CHAPTER XII

Exercises for Hypertension

Over the past three decades, Chinese exercise therapy has been used in the treatment of hypertension with favorable results. A comprehensive program for hypertension includes such exercises as *Chi Kung, Tai Chi Chuan,* walking, massage, therapeutic exercise, and remedial games. Any one of these can be used alone or along with one or two other forms of exercise therapy. The best combination would be *Chi Kung, Tai Chi Chuan,* massage, walking, and swimming.

It usually takes about three months to obtain significant therapeutic results. These may include lasting reduction in blood pressure, relief of symptoms (such as dizziness, headache, insomnia, palpitation), an increase in efficiency of heart and lungs leading to generally improved physical functioning, as well as the improvement of one's emotional and psychological state.

All the exercises should be performed at a comfortable pace and in a relaxed manner. Hypertensive patients respond to strenuous exercise in a drastic manner, with a sharp rise in blood pressure and heart rate, which may be accompanied by increasing headache and dizziness. In some hypertensive patients, angina—acute chest pain—may be triggered by vigorous exercise. Furthermore, when exposed to contact games, hypertensive patients, who are usually poor in balance and co-ordination, have to face the risk of falls and collisions resulting in internal bleeding. It is therefore important to avoid strenuous exercises and contact games in an exercise program for hypertensive patients.

Chi Kung

The effects of *Chi Kung* in the treatment of hypertension consist of lowering the blood pressure, decreasing the sensitivity of the body to mental stress, and reinforcing the therapeutic effect of hypertensive drugs. To achieve these results, hypertensive patients using *Chi Kung* therapy should try their best to attain relaxation, serenity, and "letting go" (letting the tension go and the blood pressure go down). The most commonly used techniques for this purpose are *Chi Kung for Relaxation* and *Standing Chi Kung.*

Chi Kung for Relaxation: Sitting on a comfortable chair or on a stool, the patient is to breathe naturally and use the cue words "relaxed" and "quiet" to induce a relaxation response. All areas of the body, including the heart and blood vessels, are to be relaxed in this way. (For detailed technique see *Chi Kung for Relaxation,* page 69.)

Standing Chi Kung: The standing posture has already been described in detail in the section, *Chi Kung for Fitness,* page 70. To induce quietness, and relax both mind and body, the patient is encouraged to utilize positive thoughts or imagery as auto-suggestion. For example, one may imagine that fresh rains are falling on the body from the head down to the feet giving a general feeling of freshness, coolness, and relaxation. Or, one may imagine oneself standing in a beautiful garden with fresh air, spring flowers, and other beautiful sights. These pleasant thoughts help the patient relax both mentally and physically, thereby lowering the blood pressure. *Standing Chi Kung* is indicated for those who are moderately fit. If a weak patient cannot stand too long, he may stand for a while and then sit for the remainder of the session. The length of each session starts at 3–5 minutes, then gradually increases to 15–20 minutes. If standing for this length of time cannot be sustained, he or she may rest for a few minutes before resuming the practice.

To achieve a therapeutic effect in hypertension, it appears that *Standing Chi Kung* is superior to *Chi Kung for Relaxation* or to *Chi Kung* in the sitting positions. The reasons for this are two-fold. First, in the standing position, in which the leg muscles are in a state of isometric contraction, the legs are strengthened, enabling the patient to walk at a steadier pace. Standing in that position, combined with steady breathing and auto-suggestion (focusing attention on the lower abdomen or on the soles of the feet), helps conduct blood congested in the region of the head downward. As a result, after a session of *Standing Chi Kung,* the patient will feel the head to be clear and lighter than before, the legs to be stronger, and the walking pace to have become firmer, with better balance. In addition, the standing position itself facilitates reduction in blood pressure. During the practice of *Chi Kung* it is important to observe the principle of descent. By descent is meant the flowing down of the blood and the *Chi* from the head towards the feet. It will be easier to achieve the above effects of descent if the patient practices *Chi Kung* in the standing position with the attention focused on the lower abdomen or on the soles of the feet. It has been shown by experimentation that during a session of *Chi Kung,* infusion of blood in the limbs increases as a result of expansion of the peripheral arteries. It has also been demonstrated that blood pressure drops when attention is focused on the lower abdomen, while it rises when attention is focused on the tip of the nose.

The influence of *Chi Kung* on blood pressure may be accounted for by its action on the autonomic (or "automatic") nervous system which unconsciously controls many of our vital functions. The autonomic nervous system exists in two parts, one speeding up certain physiological processes (such as the heart rate and respiratory rate) and the other slowing them down. It has been observed, in hypertensive patients, that *Chi Kung* therapy changes the balance of these functions, favoring those producing the slow down effects, thus lowering blood pressure by relaxing the muscle around the arteries. Responses to environmental stimuli such as light and sound, and also to internal stimuli such as limb and joint position and movement, are also lessened, thus producing a state of general relaxation that also contributes to reducing hypertension. Animal experiments suggest that a decrease in internal stimuli would result in a reduction in activity of the hypothalamus and visceral sympathetic nerves, and this, in turn, provides a basis for explaining the antihypertensive effect of *Chi Kung.*

Clinical observations have proved that the beneficial effects of *Chi Kung* on hypertension will be reinforced only when the patient keeps up the practice of this exercise. One cannot be satisfied with the transient blood pressure reduction observed at the end of a *Chi Kung* session, as this is simply the immediate result of relaxation and gentle breathing. Radical and lasting improvements in the condition can only be guaranteed by profound alteration in the functioning of the nervous system, which emerges through the long-term practice of *Chi Kung*.

Therapeutic exercise and sports

The best selection of exercises for a hypertensive patient is *Chi Kung, Tai Chi Chuan,* massage, walking, and swimming. Patients with only mild hypertension may take part in jogging as well.

Tai Chi Chuan: Tai Chi Chuan is an excellent exercise for hypertensive patients.

First, the gentle movement and the relaxed stance of *Tai Chi* can reflexively induce the dilatation of the small blood vessels and thus lower the blood pressure. We have observed that a decrease in systolic pressure by 10–15 mmHg was achieved in hypertensive patients immediately after practicing a set of *Tai Chi*.

Secondly, *Tai Chi Chuan* is a mental exercise which requires that the participant become concentrated and peaceful in mind—a good remedy for the distractedness and mental hypersensitivity seen in many hypertensive patients.

Thirdly, because many movements in *Tai Chi* are coordinative or balancing in nature, they are useful in improving the balance and coordination of hypertensive patients.

There are two programs of *Tai Chi Chuan*—Simplified *Tai Chi Chuan* and Old Form *Tai Chi Chuan*. It is advisable for the average hypertensive patient to take up Simplified *Tai Chi Chuan,* because it is much easier and less intense than the older form. For those whose physical condition is too poor to complete an entire sequence, individual movements may be selected. We have found some movements of *Tai Chi* to be particularly beneficial for the hypertensive patient. For example, a stretching exercise called "The white crane spreads its wings" and a coordination exercise called "Parting the wild horse's mane on both sides" are each relaxing and gentle enough to produce relaxation in hypertensive patients. They may repeat each movement 8–12 times and should benefit equally from these exercises. (See pages 23–24.)

Therapeutic exercise: The program of therapeutic exercise for hypertensive patients consists of a breathing exercise, relaxation exercise, head movement, stretching exercises of the limbs and trunk, and simple and complex walking. It should be practiced 2–3 times daily, 20–30 minutes for each session, either in class or individually.

Breathing exercise.

STARTING POSITION: Sitting on a chair, hands on thighs.
MOVEMENT: 1. Breathe in slowly and naturally. 2. Breathe out slowly and naturally.

Repeat this 6–8 times.

Relaxation exercise.

STARTING POSITION: Standing with feet apart shoulder width.
MOVEMENT: Swing the arms forward and backward, one moving forward while the other goes back. With the continuing, rhythmic swinging of the arms, swaying the lower back and pelvis forward and backward with the same rhythm.

Repeat the swinging motion 100 times (for about 2–3 minutes).

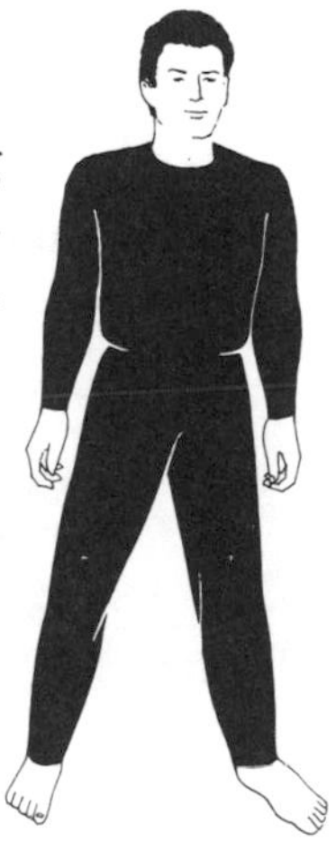

STARTING POSITION

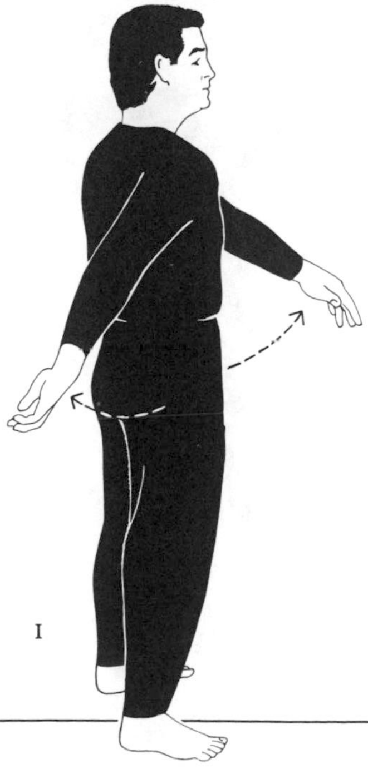

1

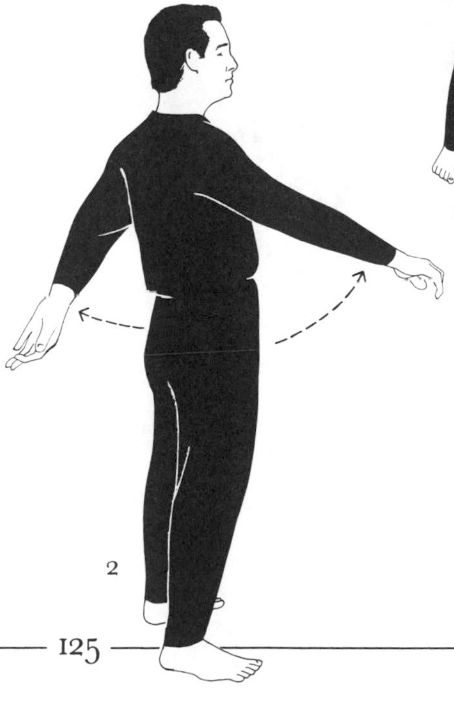

2

Head exercise.

STARTING POSITION: Sitting on a chair.
MOVEMENT: 1. Bend the head forward, then extend the head backward. 2. Tilt the head to the left, then to the right. 3. Turn the head to the left, then to the right.

Repeat each of the above movements 8–10 times, and then go on to the next.

Stretching exercise 1: *Sideward stretch.*

STARTING POSITION: Standing, feet apart shoulder width, hands on hips.
MOVEMENT: 1. Twist the trunk to the left and stretch the left arm horizontally backward, elbow straight, palm upward. Then return to the starting position. 2. Twist the trunk to the right and stretch the right arm horizontally backward, elbow straight, palm upward. And again, return to the starting position.

Repeat this 8–10 times.

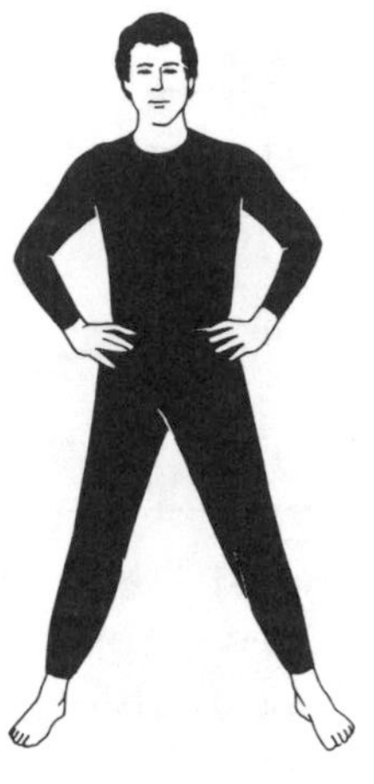

STARTING POSITION

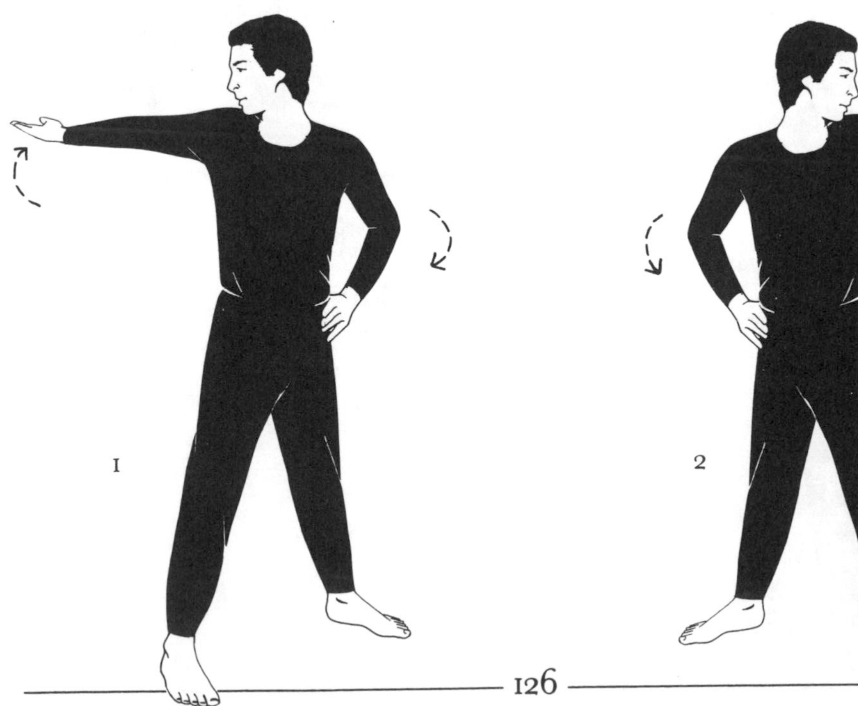

Stretching exercise 2: Upward stretch.

STARTING POSITION: Standing, feet together, arms at sides.

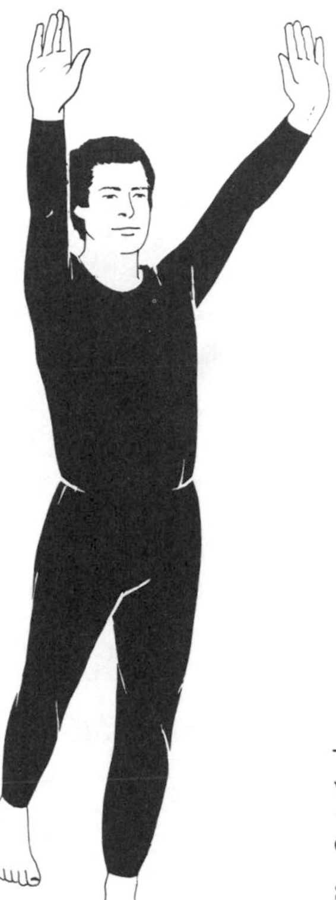

MOVEMENT: 1. Take a step forward with the left foot and stretch both arms forward and upward. And return to the starting position. 2. Take a step forward with the right foot and stretch both arms forward and upward. Again, return to the starting position.

Repeat this 8–10 times.

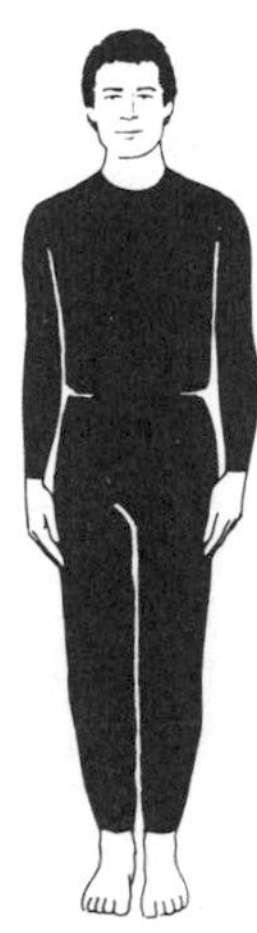

STARTING POSITION

Walking.

Walk at various speeds in the therapeutic gymnasium or or in a big room at home. Start with normal speed (80–90 steps per minute) for 3 minutes. This is followed by a brisk walk at a rate of about 110 steps per minute for 2 minutes. Then take a relaxed and slow walk to complete the exercise session.

Walking: It has been reported that walking on level ground for a prolonged period of time will cause a significant decrease in diastolic pressure. In general, walking is practiced in the early morning, in the evening or before going to sleep—once or twice daily, 15 minutes to an hour per session, at moderate speed. On the weekend, the patient may go on a longer journey on foot for sightseeing, or, if not too rigorous, he or she may go hiking in the hills.

Swimming: Patients who have already mastered this skill may swim outdoors on warm and sunny days or indoors in a warm pool. Therapeutic swimming must be practiced in a slow and relaxed manner, and for short distances only.

Games: Hypertensive patients may benefit from games that are simple, relaxed, non-competitive, and of low intensity.

Jogging: Jogging, properly prescribed and executed, may be helpful to improve the tone of the autonomous nerves. Since jogging may cause some drastic responses in the cardiovascular system of hypertensive patients, physicians should be cautious when prescribing jogging. It would be better to advise the patient to first participate in a brisk walking program, for example, walking ½ to 1 mile (1–2 km) at the rate of 3 miles per hour. If the patient responds well to the brisk walking, he may progress to jogging.

A chronic patient in poor physical condition should begin a jogging program at a very low intensity. One might start with short distance jogging, say, 50 yards, and then increase gradually to 100, 150, and then 200 yards at a speed of 100 yards in 30–40 seconds. Another form of easy jogging is jog/walk. The patient jogs for a short while, then walks for a short while, and then repeats jogging. For example, jogging for 30 seconds followed by walking for 60 seconds, the cycle can be repeated 20–30 times. Such a session would last 30–40 minutes. The speed is generally slow, and adapted to the participant's level of fitness. This form of interval jogging trains the heart at a lower intensity and guards against exhaustion.

Start the program by jogging short distance, and gradually increase both distance and speed. Patients should jog within the limits of their capacity, and stop jogging before they feel exhausted. Never over-stress the heart or exceed the target heart rate prescribed by the physician.

When jogging, breathing should be natural and rhythmic: an inhalation for two steps, then an exhalation for the next two steps, or three steps for each inhalation and exhalation.

It is best to practice jogging in the early morning. However, an afternoon session is acceptable for those who do not have time in the morning. A warm-up of 5 to 10 minutes and a similar cool-down should be included in each jogging session. Participants should be taught to constantly monitor changes in their pulse rate and to watch for other changes of subjective feeling. General health and physical fitness and the suitability of the jogging program should be reassessed regularly by a physician.

Hill climbing: Climbing up a 30–60 yard hill with a slope of 30–40 degrees is indicated for young hypertensives who are fairly fit and have no complications in the early stages of their illness. The climbing is usually done with periods of rest.

Massage

Chinese manipulation and massage: Following a session of *Chi Kung* or therapeutic exercise, a type of sedative massage will be given to the patient as an adjunctive measure to reduce the blood pressure, and to relieve headache and dizziness. For this purpose, the following techniques are commonly used:

Percussion of the head. Tap lightly and quickly on the top of the head or wherever there is discomfort. This is done with the tips of the five fingers.

Kneading the back of the knee (popliteal fossa). Knead the muscles and tendons in the back of each knee with the index, middle, and ring fingers. Knead one knee at a time.

Stroking the point yung chuan. Stroke gently on the point *yung chuan* in the middle of the sole. (See page 64.)

Sedative massage on the head: First, rub both palms to make them warm. Then 1. "Wash" the face with the palms (as in *Shier Duan Jin,* Exercise 3, page 60). 2. Next, stroke the forehead from the midline to both sides with palms and fingers, massaging the occipital region in the same way, and 3. finally, massage the back of the neck and the scapular region.

In a massage session, either or both of the above two techniques may be used. The length of such a massage session should be 5–10 minutes.

CHAPTER XIII

Exercises for Arteriosclerosis

Throughout adult life, the walls of arteries of all sizes become gradually less elastic and more rigid. These changes constitute arteriosclerosis. Chemical analysis has shown that there is also a gradual increase in calcium salts in the arterial walls. These changes alone have little effect on function. However, similar changes, but with some thickening of the arterial walls, are a feature of chronic hypertension. In people with diabetes, the calcific changes may be accelerated and severe. Peripheral circulation may be impaired. In addition, calcific arteriosclerosis is thought to predispose one to another type of arteriosclerosis, namely atherosclerosis, which is by far the most dangerous threat to human life in today's world. Therefore, from a preventive point of view, people with arteriosclerosis should seriously take up an exercise program for both prevention and therapy.

In recent years, a number of investigations have shown that patients with arteriosclerosis may benefit from exercise therapy in the following respects. First, regular exercise may help delay or limit the progression of this disease. It has repeatedly been observed that arteriosclerosis is much milder in laborers and physically active people than in the sedentary, and its severe forms much more common in those who are physically inactive.

Emotional tension and high circulatory lipid (fat) levels are also considered to contribute to the development of arteriosclerosis. Since exercise can relieve tension and can reduce the concentration of lipids in the blood, regular physical training is helpful in preventing the progression of the disease.

As well, exercise can improve blood circulation and relieve symptoms due to peripheral ischemia (deficient blood supply), such as numbness of the hands and feet, and muscular weakness.

Methods of exercise therapy for arteriosclerosis are much the same as for hypertension. In fact, a majority of arteriosclerotic cases are associated with hypertension. The intensity of exercise should be lower in those with severe arteriosclerosis. Typical exercises for arteriosclerotic patients include walking, *Tai Chi Chuan,* therapeutic exercise, and massage. The duration of exercise in one day should not exceed 30–45 minutes.

Walking: Slow walking for 300–1,000 yards on a fine day, preferably in the early morning or in the evening, can stimulate digestion and improve the quality of sleep. Hence walking is a good remedy for insomnia and dyspepsia, which are rather common in patients with arteriosclerosis.

Tai Chi Chuan: As a gentle and soft exercise, *Tai Chi* is particularly good for these patients. They may do the whole set of movements, half a set, or merely some individual movements, depending on their physical condition.

Therapeutic exercise: The goal of therapeutic exercise is to improve the blood circulation of the body in general, and of the limbs in particular. For this purpose, the following exercises and massages were chosen from a program of calisthenics developed in ancient China for the elderly. Preliminary observation of the effects of these modified exercises has indicated that they are of benefit to patients with arteriosclerosis.

EXERCISE 1: Sitting on a chair, clench the fists, and then open the fingers. Repeat this 20 times.

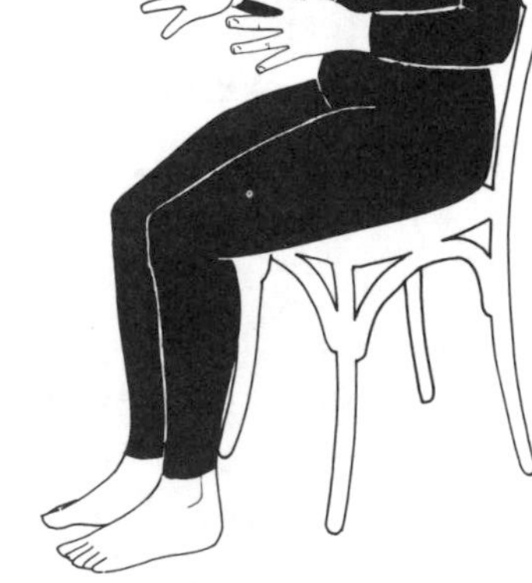

1

EXERCISE 2: Sitting on a chair, hold two small chestnuts (or small rubber balls, marbles, or smooth round stones) in one hand, and move them around with the fingers of the same hand. Be careful not to let them slip off the palm.

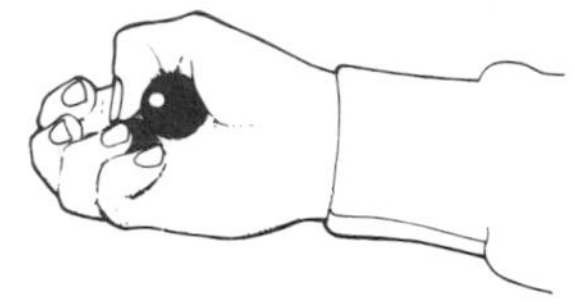

EXERCISE 3: Sitting on a chair, rotate the feet in circles. Repeat this 20 times.

EXERCISE 4: Sitting on a chair, with both hands placed on the back of the neck, 1. twist the trunk to the left, and 2. then to the right. Repeat 20 times. The twisting should be gentle and slow. The number of repetitions for patients with vertigo may be fewer.

2

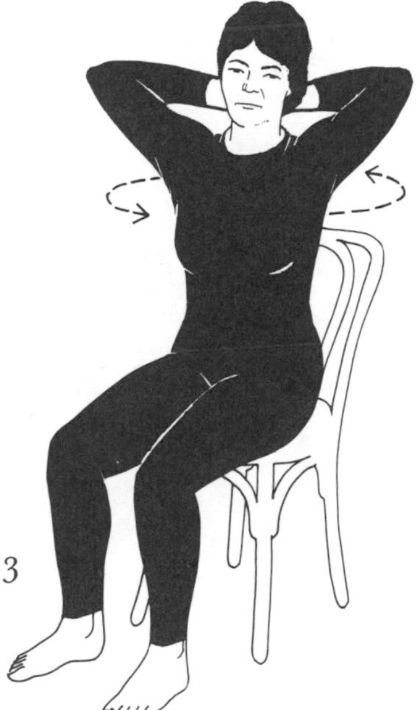

3

4

EXERCISE 5: Sitting, 1. bend the left knee, extending the leg, 2. then the right knee, extending the right leg. Repeat this 20 times.

The above exercises may be practiced several times daily.

Therapeutic massage: Sedative massage on the head, neck and shoulder, as for hypertension (see page 129). In addition, slapping the thighs with the palms and hitting the arms with the fists may be done. Such self-administered massage is preferably applied after getting up in the morning, before going to sleep at night, or after therapeutic exercise.

Hitting the arms: Hit the left arm and forearm with the palm of the right fist gently (as in diagram on page 117), then hit the right arm and forearm with the palm of the left fist.

Slapping the legs: Slap the thighs and lower legs with both palms while sitting with the trunk bent slightly forward.

CHAPTER XIV

Exercises for Coronary Heart Disease: Preventive and Therapeutic

Many western visitors to China have been much impressed by the fact that China has a much lower incidence of heart attacks than does the West. Some western physicians have ascribed this to the Chinese way of fitness, namely, doing *Tai Chi Chuan,* jogging, and living a life of moderation. In fact, it is quite true that Chinese exercise plays a part in the prevention and treatment of coronary heart disease.

In terms of the management of coronary heart disease, the strength of the Chinese exercise programs lies in their relaxation-producing effects. Since some types of heart attack and angina are stress-related, a combination of jogging or walking with *Tai Chi Chuan* or *Chi Kung* will result in more effective prevention of heart attack than the use of any of these alone.

Exercise programs presented in this section can be used both for preventive and therapeutic purposes. It is advisable for the patient to have a complete medical evaluation, and to obtain permission from a physician before taking up an exercise program. Once the program is started, general health and physical condition should be reassessed regularly. In addition, the participant in the program should watch carefully for any changes in his or her symptoms and heart rate.

Recent studies suggest that 65–85% of the maximum oxygen intake level is a safe and effective intensity for coronary heart disease patients. That means for a person 50 years of age, a target training heart rate of 110–145 per minute would be desirable. However, one should always remember not to push too hard to reach a target heart rate. It is the level suitable to one's capacity that is important and not a rigid target heart rate. Therefore, during exercise, take a look at the stopwatch from time to time, but do not become its slave.

The other important thing is to integrate exercise with daily life. One should try to use one's legs as much as possible. Again, a preventive life style is essential. Proper diet, adequate physical activity, and control of stress all contribute to the successful prevention and treatment of coronary heart disease.

Coronary heart disease (CHD), also known as coronary artery disease, is a common illness among the middle-aged and elderly. In CHD, the inside of the coronary artery becomes narrow and small, due to the deposit of fat in the inner arterial walls. In addition, the artery tends to be in spasm, reducing the blood supply to the heart muscle, and resulting in deficient blood supply (ischemia) to it. The patient with these pathological changes will suffer from an intense feeling of squeezing pain in the left chest region (angina pectoris). If the involved coronary artery is occluded rapidly, the heart muscle will suffer from acute, severe, and lasting ischemia, and a heart attack will occur.

It appears that lack of physical activity may have something to do with the development of CHD. Studies done in many regions of China have shown that the incidence of CHD in laborers over forty years of age is lower than in sedentary professionals of the same age group. It has been reported that physically active males have a lower incidence of heart attacks as well as a lower rate of mortality within 24 hours of such an attack than do males who are physically inactive. Such findings suggest that regular physical training is helpful in preventing the development of CHD.

Since the 1960's exercise therapy has been utilized with favorable results in treating CHD patients. According to studies done in China as well as in many other countries, exercise therapy may help patients with angina pectoris increase their tolerance for physical activities and improve their physical condition, thus relieving angina. For some patients an improvement in their electrocardiogram was observed. For patients recovering from an acute heart attack, exercise therapy may improve their subjective symptoms, shorten the duration of hospitalization, and increase their physical fitness, thereby promoting vocational rehabilitation.

The mechanisms accounting for the beneficial effects of exercise on CHD may be summarized as follows:

1. Increasing oxygen supply to the heart muscle: Physical activity may stimulate smaller arteries to supply blood to an area where a larger artery is narrowed or closed or it may increase the blood volume in these smaller blood vessels. As a result, blood circulation in the vascular network of the heart muscle may be improved and the oxygen supply to it increased.

2. Reducing oxygen consumption in the heart muscle: Since the adaptation of the blood circulation to exercise is improved by systematic physical exercise, the work of the heart becomes less intense, reducing, to a certain extent, the oxygen consumption in the heart muscle.

3. Improving metabolism of lipids: Experiments have shown that after long periods of physical training, the concentration of cholesterol in the blood is reduced. After eight months of systematic physical training, a steady decline in blood cholesterol levels was seen in a group of middle-aged and elderly people with high blood cholesterol. The improvement in lipid metabolism decreases the deposit of fatty material on the inner walls of the coronary artery.

4. Psychological regulation: Physical activity tends to modify the psychological state of the patient, by producing a more positive outlook and the motivation for maintaining a better lifestyle, as well as removing the preoccupation with CHD. Exercise will ease tension, bringing relaxation and peace of mind, thereby reducing attacks of angina.

5. Promoting fibrinolysis (anti-clotting effect) in the blood: It was reported that exercise of moderate and high intensity had the effect of enhancing fibrinolysis in the blood, thus impeding the progression of atherosclerosis.

There are a variety of exercises suitable for patients with CHD. Apart from the consideration of facilities available, they may choose those which are most suitable to their age, level of health and physical fitness, degree of skill and interest. No matter which exercises they decide upon, the appropriate intensity of the exercise is what counts most. Generally speaking, moderate exercise is preferred.

Walking: A brisk, vigorous walk is more valuable in training the heart than is slow walking. Brisk walking at the rate of 100 steps per minute will increase the heart rate up to more than 100 beats per minute. In brisk walking, it is important to maintain a steady stance and speed, and a smooth rhythm of breathing. If the walking speed is too fast for the body to tolerate, the walker will become breathless, very tired, and even get chest pain. If this occurs, the walking speed should be slowed down. For those for whom walking is their primary means of physical training, the duration of a walking session should be 45–60 minutes, once or twice daily. An alternate schedule is walking 800–2,000 yards a day at normal speed with intermittent sessions of brisk walking.

Jogging: It is recommended that a beginner start by jogging a distance of 50–100 yards, gradually increasing the distance by 100 yards each week. If he or she feels good following such a program, the distance can be increased to 1,000 or 2,000 yards, and, for those at a higher level of physical fitness, even to 3,000 yards.

Terrain cure: This is usually organized in a sanitorium or a large hospital. For those who are fairly weak, a walk of 800–1,000 yards on level ground at a rate of 50–70 yards per minute (i.e., 800–1,000 yards in 15–20 minutes) is recommended. Terrain cure of higher intensity, like the two routes below, may be prescribed for those in better condition.

1. Walking 3,000 yards (level): Walk the first 1,000 yards in 20 minutes, then sit down and rest for 5 minutes. The next 1,000 yards are walked in 16–18 minutes, with another rest, sitting down for 5 more minutes. The last 1,000 yards are to be completed in 20 minutes.

2. Walking 4,000 yards (level) and climbing up a small hill: First, walk 2,000 yards (level) in 40 minutes, then sit down and rest for 5–10 minutes. Follow this by climbing a small hill 30–50 yards high, with a slope of 30–45 degrees, in 30 minutes. After a rest of 5–10 minutes the return journey is resumed at the same rate.

Swimming: Those who have already mastered this skill and are fairly fit may be permitted to take part in swimming. It has been reported that swimming can enhance aerobic capacity in middle-aged people. The increase in oxygen intake after six months of swimming training is similar in effect to the same period of jogging.

Chi Kung: Chi Kung for Relaxation or *Chi Kung for Fitness,* performed in a sitting or lying position, is indicated for CHD patients, especially those undergoing emotional stress or those who are very sick. The following beneficial effects were observed in CHD patients receiving *Chi Kung* therapy: relief from dizziness, improved subjective feeling state, a lifting of depression and more positive general attitude, reduction in the frequency and severity of angina pectoris, and a warm sensation in the hands and feet.

Tai Chi Chuan: As a gentle and relaxed exercise, *Tai Chi Chuan* is suitable for CHD patients with coexisting hypertension or emotional difficulties. It may help lower the blood pressure and remove neurotic symptoms. To increase the degree of exertion, *Tai Chi* may be performed with a lowered stance and large-ranging movements, or else repeated several times in a session.

Comprehensive exercise program: This is generally carried out in a group setting, 2–3 sessions per week, for a half hour to an hour each, preferably scheduled in the afternoon. The content of a comprehensive exercise program includes warm-up, trunk and limb exercises, simple therapeutic sports (such as passing a ball, basketball shooting, bowling, badminton, etc.), walking/ jogging, and cool-down. Appendix I (page 141) contains a program used for CHD patients with controlled angina at Zhong Shan Medical College, Guangzhou, China.

Therapeutic exercise: For very sick patients, only simple trunk and limb exercises are prescribed. Avoid any starting position which may elicit angina. For example, if the patient has experienced angina during exercise in a standing position, then he or she is advised to begin a therapeutic exercise program in a lying position. Later, this may gradually be changed to a sitting or standing position, once the patient's condition is improving.

For patients who have recovered from an acute heart attack, simple therapeutic exercises may be prescribed in the initial stage, if the condition is stable. Appendix II contains a program of therapeutic exercise used in the early recovery period for such patients.

Appendix I

A program of therapeutic exercise for CHD patients
(*Moderate intensity*)

Each of the following exercises is to be repeated 8–12 times unless otherwise indicated.

EXERCISE 1.

Walking at normal speed 1–1½ minutes.

EXERCISE 2.

STARTING POSITION: Standing, arms at sides.
MOVEMENT: 1. Take a step to the left with the left foot and bend the elbows at the sides of the body, with fingers touching the tops of the shoulders. 2. Stretch the arms out to the sides at shoulder level, keeping the elbows straight. 3. Bend the elbows back to the sides, fingers touching the shoulders as in step 1. 4. Return to the starting position. Repeat, this time taking a step to the right.

STARTING POSITION

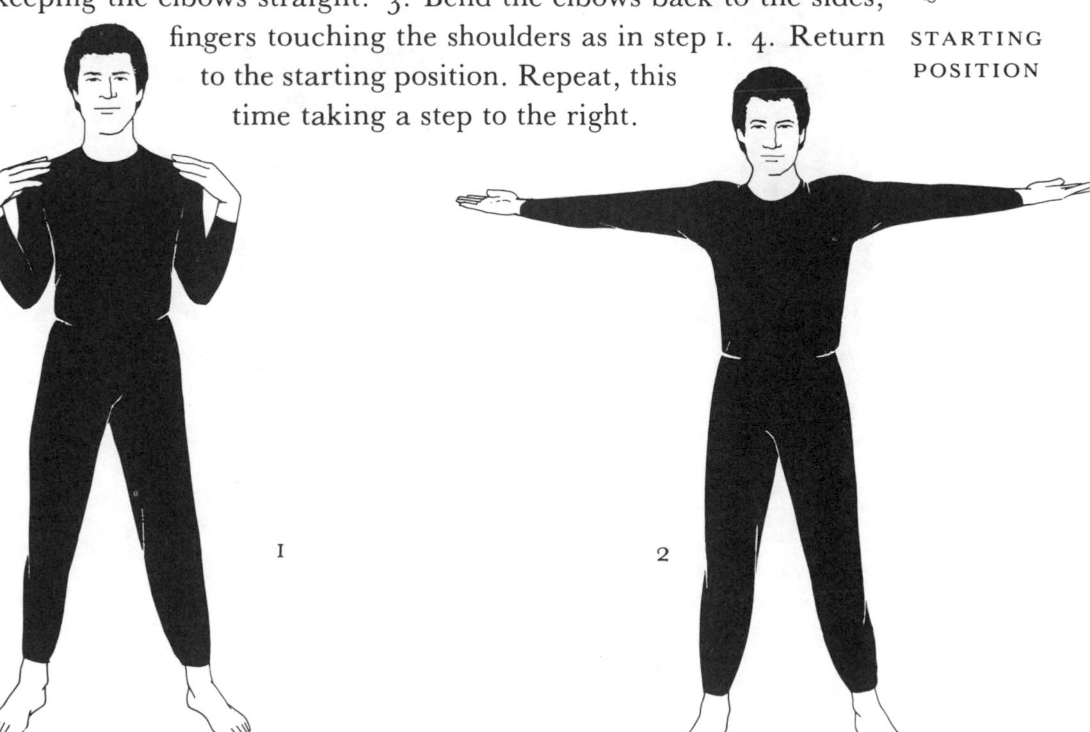

EXERCISE 3.

STARTING POSITION: Standing, arms at sides.
MOVEMENT: 1. Take a step forward with the left foot and bend the elbows at shoulder height so that the fingers meet in front of the chest, palms downward. 2. Stretch the arms out to the sides at shoulder level, elbows straight, palms upward. 3. Bring the arms back with elbows bent as in step 1. 4. Return to the starting position. Repeat, this time stepping forward with the right foot.

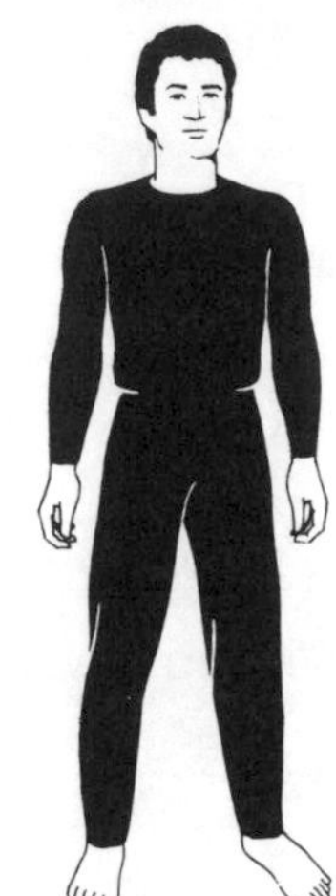

STARTING POSITION

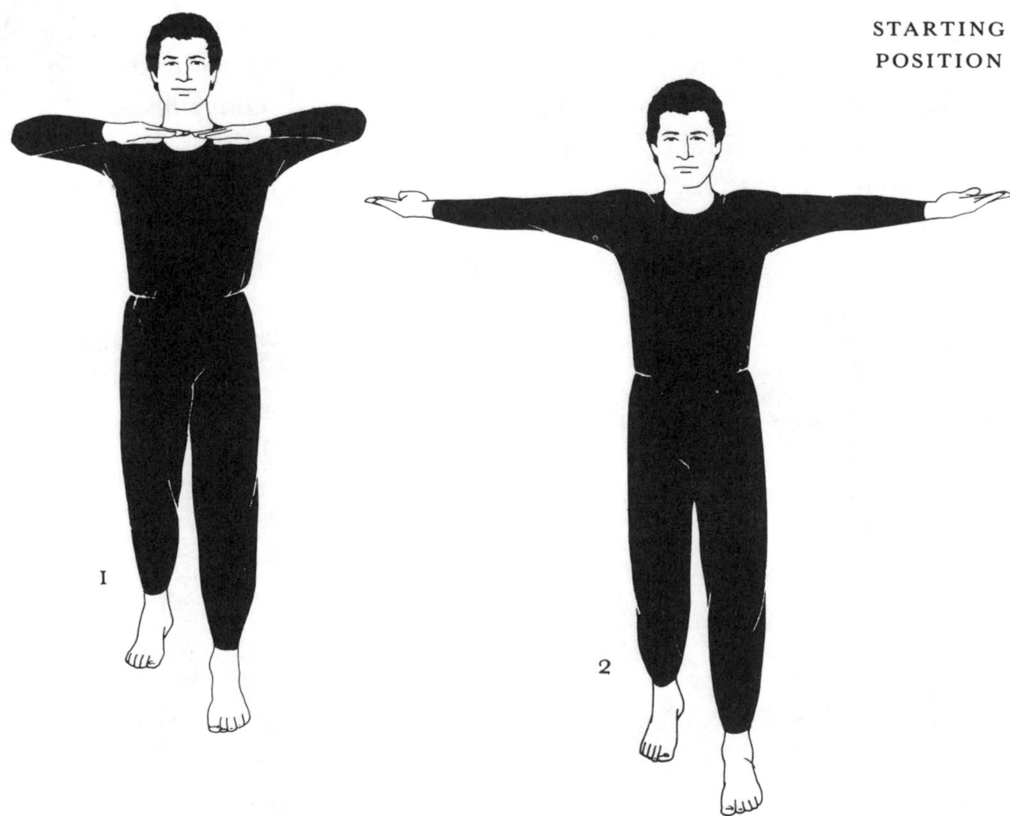

EXERCISE 4.

STARTING POSITION: Stride standing (feet apart more than shoulder width), hands on hips.

MOVEMENT: 1. Twist the trunk to the left and stretch the left arm back horizontally, elbow straight, palm upward, while the other arm remains on the hip. Then return to the starting position. 2. Twist the trunk to the right and stretch the right arm back horizontally, elbow straight, palm upward. And again, return to the starting position.

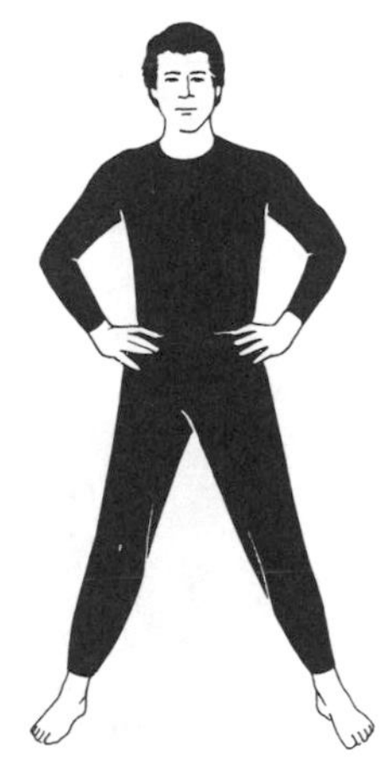

STARTING POSITION

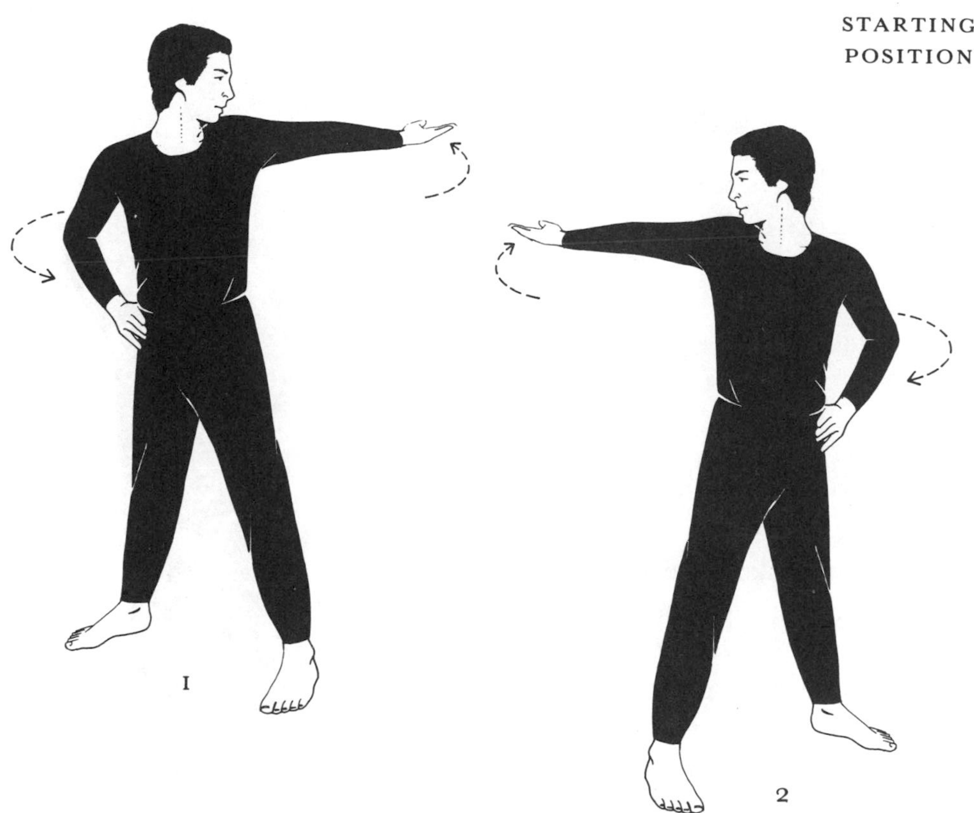

EXERCISE 5.

STARTING POSITION: Standing, feet together.

MOVEMENT: Take a step to the left with the left foot and bend both knees and hips to lower the body. At the same time bend the elbows at sides, fingers touching the top of the shoulders. Then return to the starting position, and repeat the movement, this time stepping to the right.

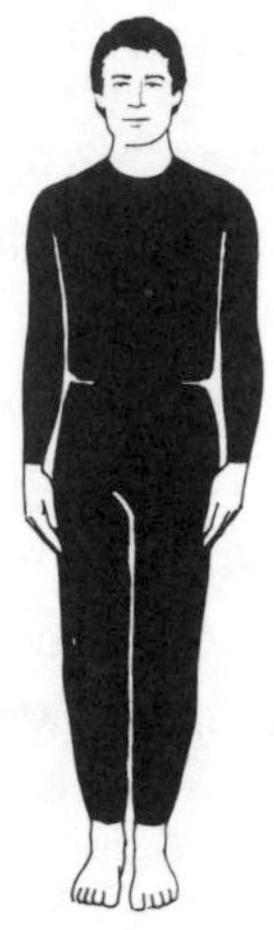

STARTING POSITION

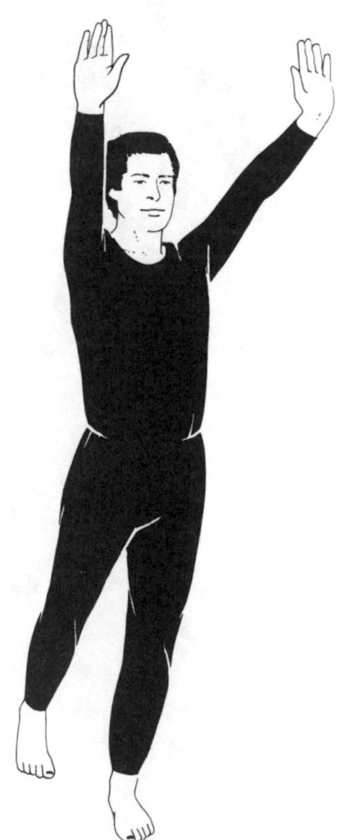

EXERCISE 6.

STARTING POSITION: Standing, feet together.

MOVEMENT: 1. Take a step forward with the left foot and stretch the arms forward and upward, palms facing forward. 2. Return to the starting position. 3. Take a step forward with the right foot and stretch the arms forward and upward. 4. Return to the starting position.

EXERCISE 7.

STARTING POSITION: Sitting, hands resting on thighs.
MOVEMENT: 1. Bend the head downward, then upward. 2. Turn the head to the left, then to the right.

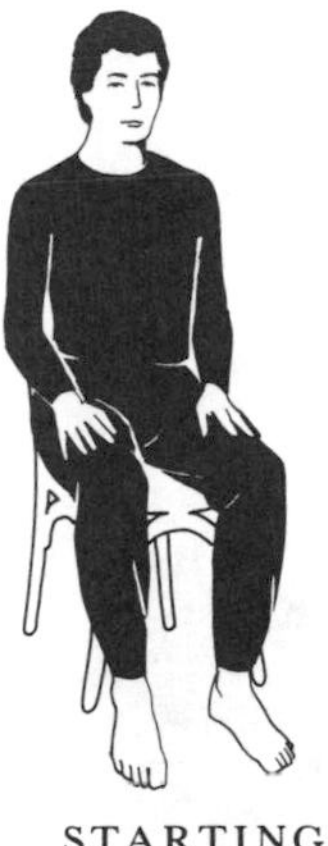

STARTING POSITION

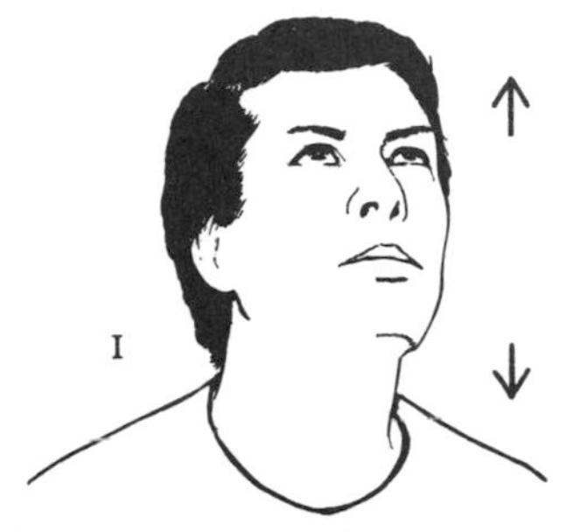

1

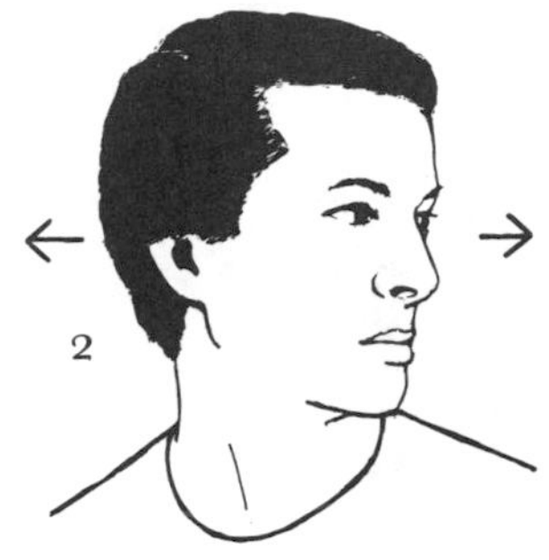

2

EXERCISE 8.

STARTING POSITION: Sitting, hands resting on thighs.
MOVEMENT: 1. Stretch the arms forward, and then to the sides at shoulder level, palms up, and simultaneously raise the bent left leg. Then return to the starting position. 2. Bring the arms forward and to the sides at shoulder level, palms up, and simultaneously raise the bent right leg. Again, return to the starting position.

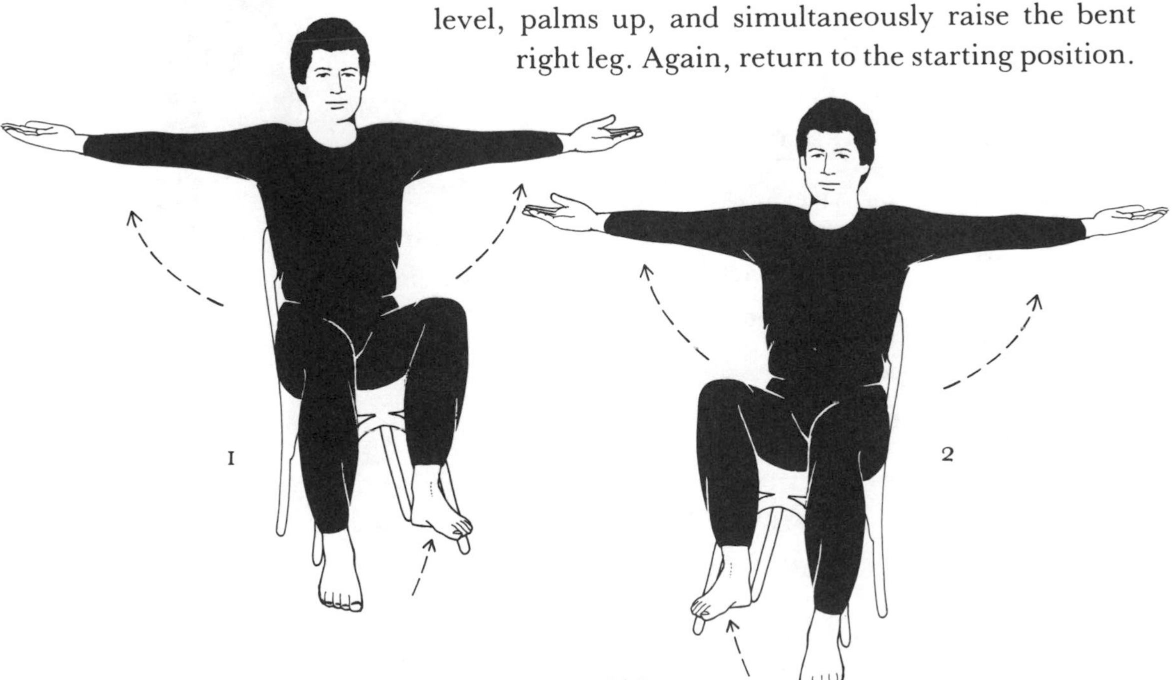

1 2

EXERCISE 9.

STARTING POSITION. Sitting, keeping hips firm.
MOVEMENT: 1. Bend the head and the trunk slightly backward. Then return to the starting position. 2. Bend the head and the trunk slightly forward. And again, return to the starting position.

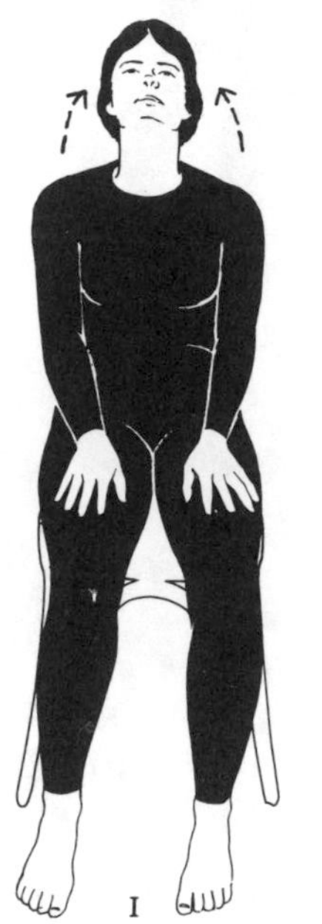

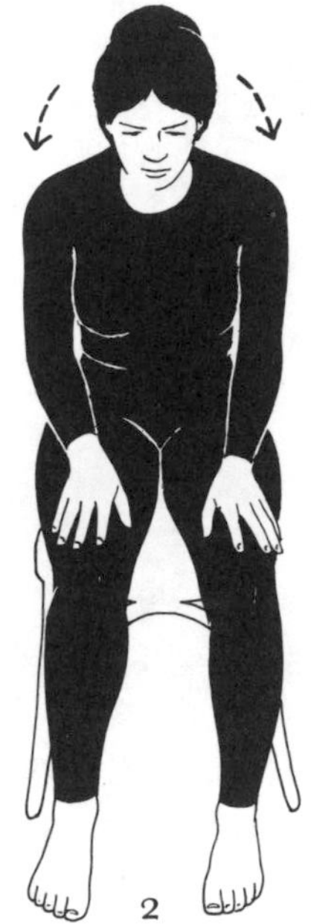

EXERCISE 10.

STARTING POSITION: Sitting.
MOVEMENT: Make a circle in front of the chest with both arms, elbows kept slightly flexed.

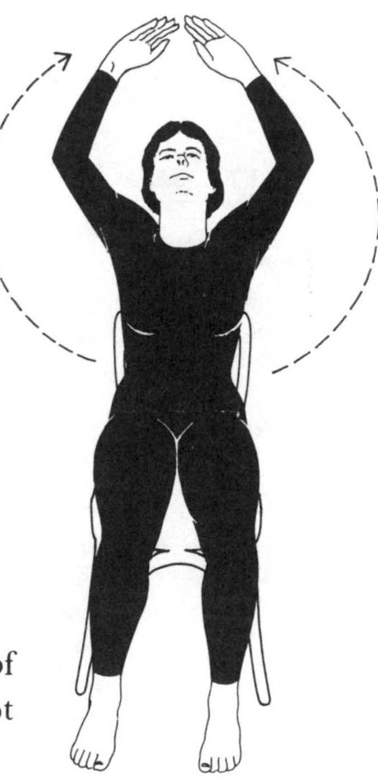

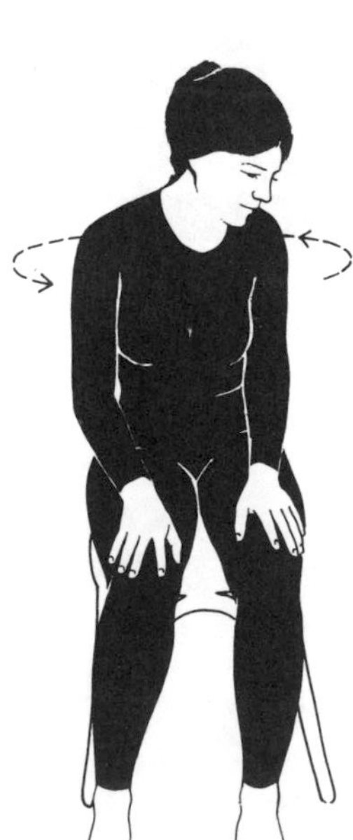

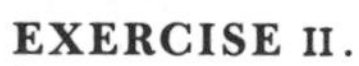

EXERCISE 11.

STARTING POSITION: Sitting, hands on knees.
MOVEMENT: Rotate the trunk in a small range.

EXERCISE 12.

STARTING POSITION: Sitting.
MOVEMENT: Stand up, raise the arms forward and stretch them up to the sides, with palms upward. Then return to the starting position.

EXERCISE 13.

STARTING POSITION: Standing.
MOVEMENT: Step in place for 30 seconds, at a rate of 80–90 steps per minute.

EXERCISE 14.

STARTING POSITION: Standing.
MOVEMENT: 1. Take a step to the left with the left foot and bend the elbows crossed in front of the chest, palms downward. 2. Twist the trunk to the left and stretch the arms out to the sides at shoulder level, elbows straight, palms upward. 3. Bend arms to position 1. 4. Return to the starting position. Repeat the sequence, this time stepping and twisting to the right side.

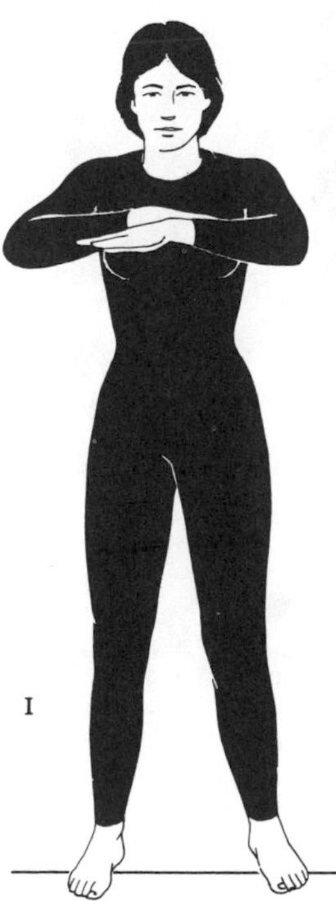

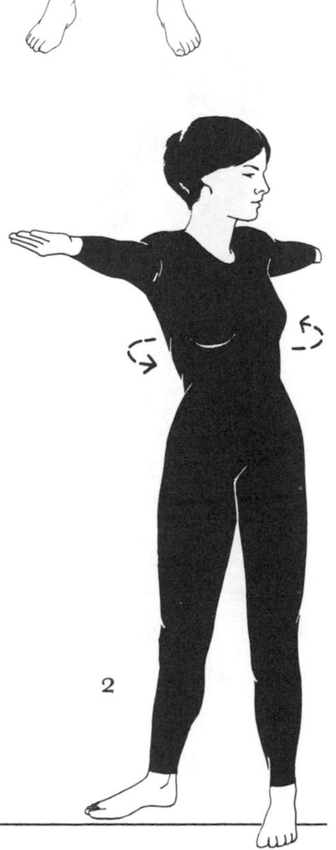

EXERCISE 15.

STARTING POSITION: Standing with feet separated shoulder width.

MOVEMENT: 1. Bend the trunk to the left and bend the right arm up gradually until the right hand, moving along the side, reaches the lower rib region. Then return to the starting position. 2. Bend the trunk to the right and bend the left arm up until the left hand, moving along the side, reaches the lower rib region. And again, return to the starting position.

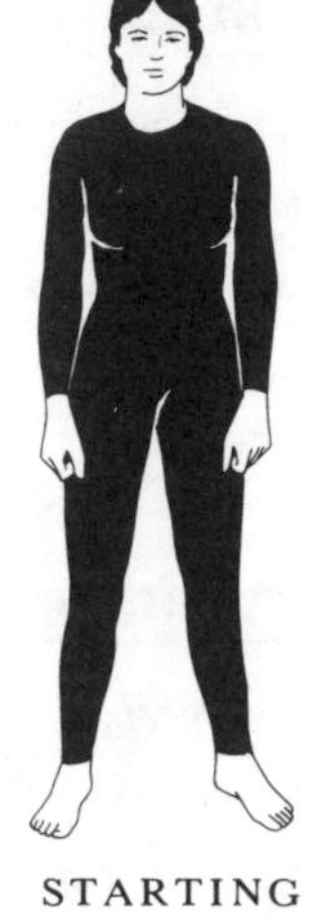
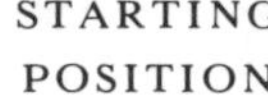
STARTING POSITION

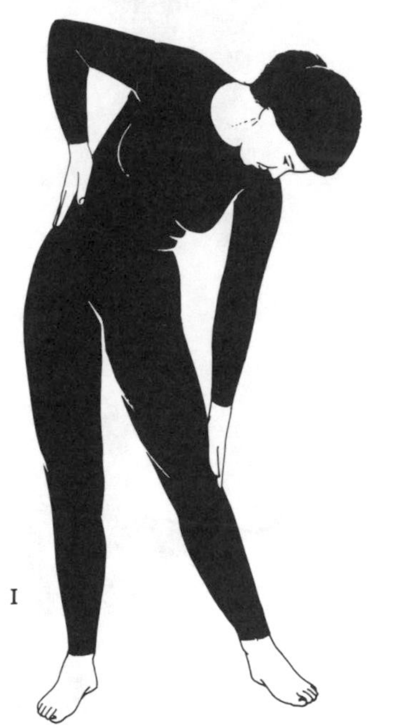
1

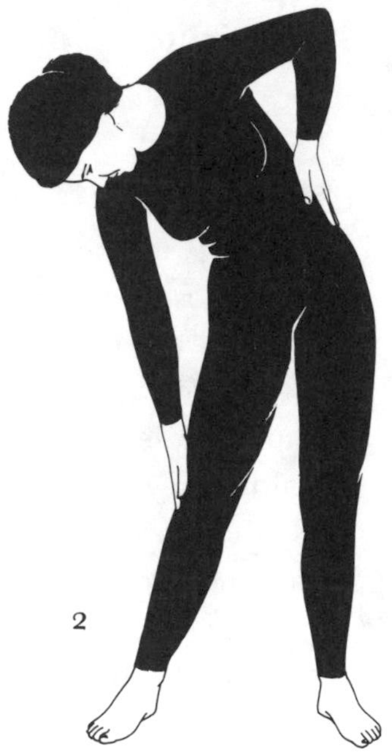
2

EXERCISE 16.

STARTING POSITION: Standing.

MOVEMENT: "Rowing." 1. Take a step forward with the left foot. Stretch the arms forward and upward, with the trunk falling forward at the same time. 2. Then draw the hands downward and backward, with the trunk rising and extending backward at the same time.

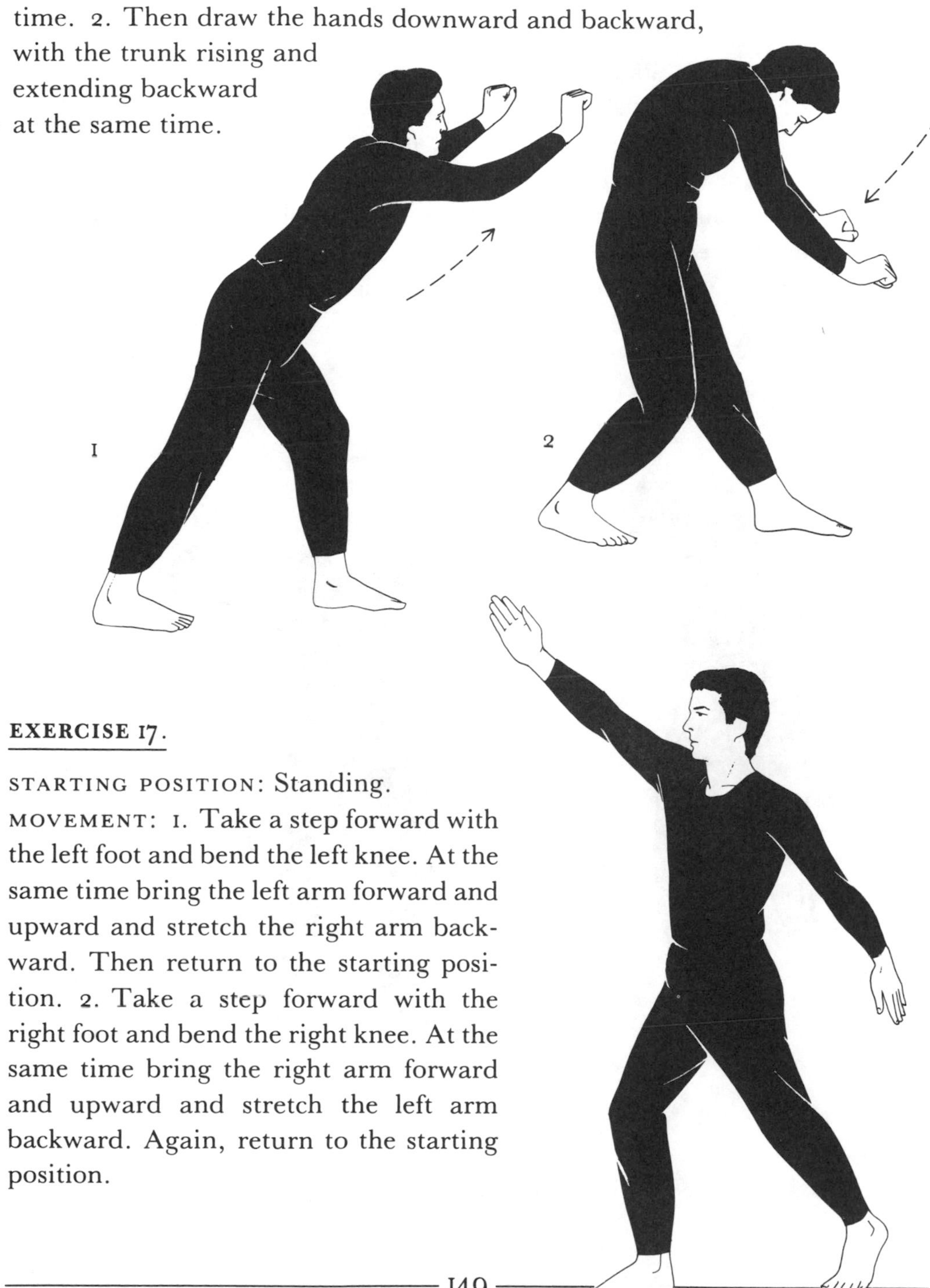

EXERCISE 17.

STARTING POSITION: Standing.
MOVEMENT: 1. Take a step forward with the left foot and bend the left knee. At the same time bring the left arm forward and upward and stretch the right arm backward. Then return to the starting position. 2. Take a step forward with the right foot and bend the right knee. At the same time bring the right arm forward and upward and stretch the left arm backward. Again, return to the starting position.

EXERCISE 18.

STARTING POSITION: Standing.

MOVEMENT: 1. Take a step to the left with the left foot. 2. Twist the trunk slightly to the left and bend the left knee. At the same time bend the elbows and raise the arms to the sides, touching the fingers to the tops of the shoulders. Return to the starting position and repeat the movements, this time stepping and twisting to the right side.

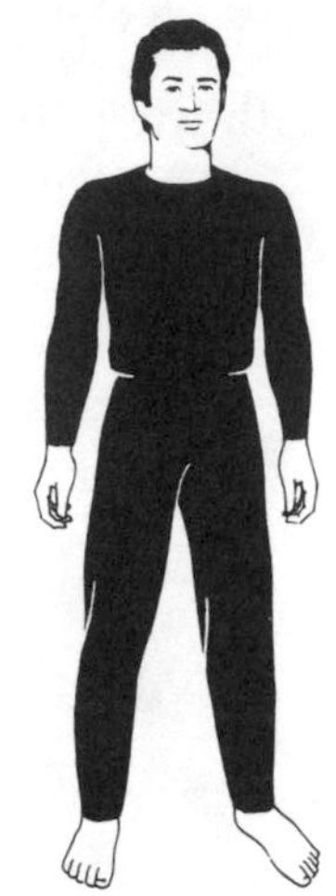

STARTING POSITION

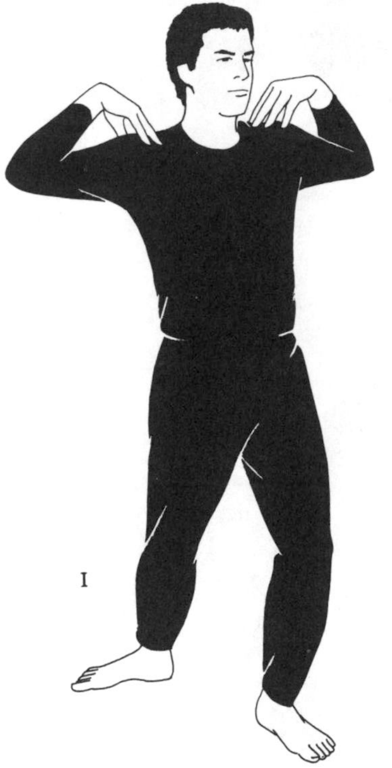

1

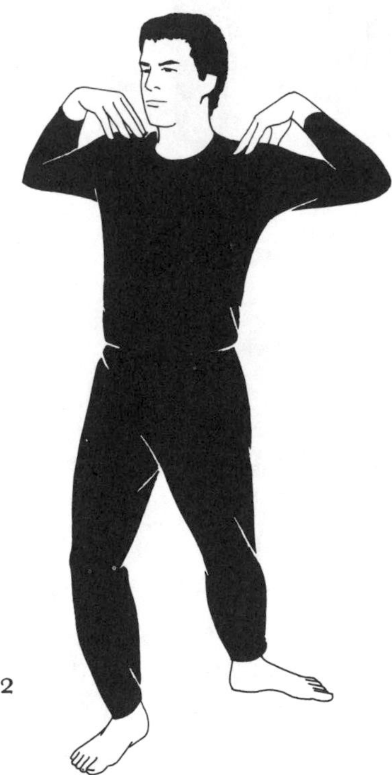

2

EXERCISE 19.

Try to shoot a basketball into a net, 10–20 shots.

EXERCISE 20.

Pedal a stationary bicycle without resistance 2–3 minutes.

EXERCISE 21.

STARTING POSITION: Standing.
MOVEMENT: 1. Take a step forward with the left foot and bring the arms upward, palms facing forward, with the trunk slightly extended and the head raised. Then, return to the starting position. 2. Repeat, this time with right foot stepping forward. And again, return to the starting position.

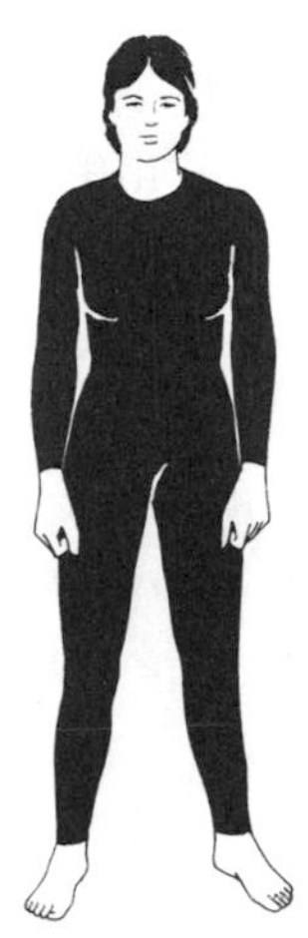

STARTING POSITION

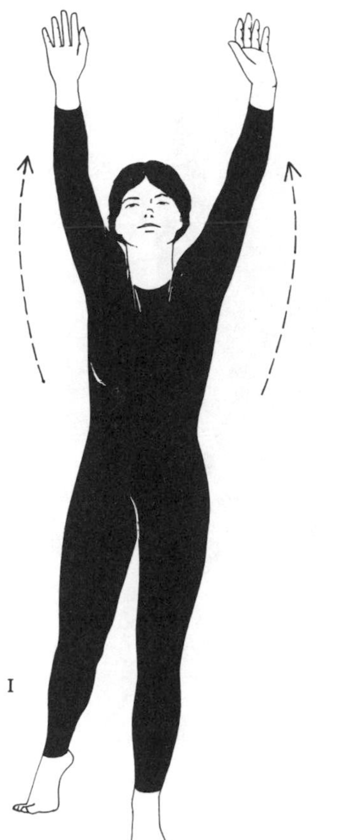

1

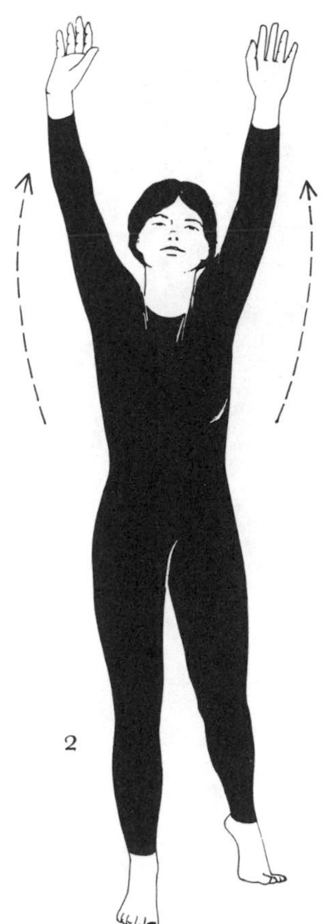

2

EXERCISE 22.

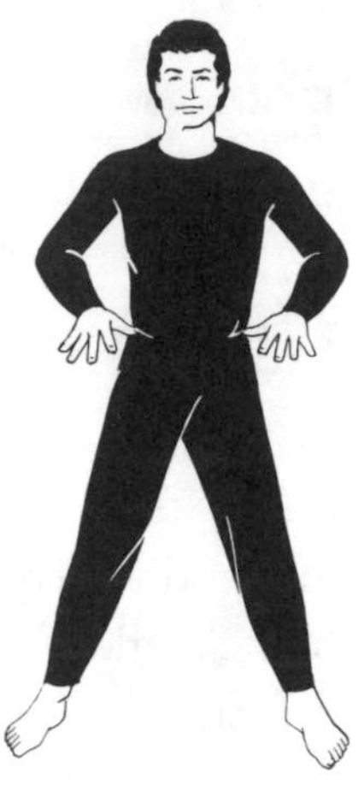

STARTING POSITION

STARTING POSITION: Stride standing (feet separated more than shoulder width), arms bent at the sides, palms down.
MOVEMENT: 1. Twist the trunk to the left, with the arms swinging to the left at the same time until the heels can be seen, then return to the starting position. 2. Now twist the trunk to the right with the arms swinging to the right until the heels can be seen. Again, return to the starting position. Repeat 10–20 times.

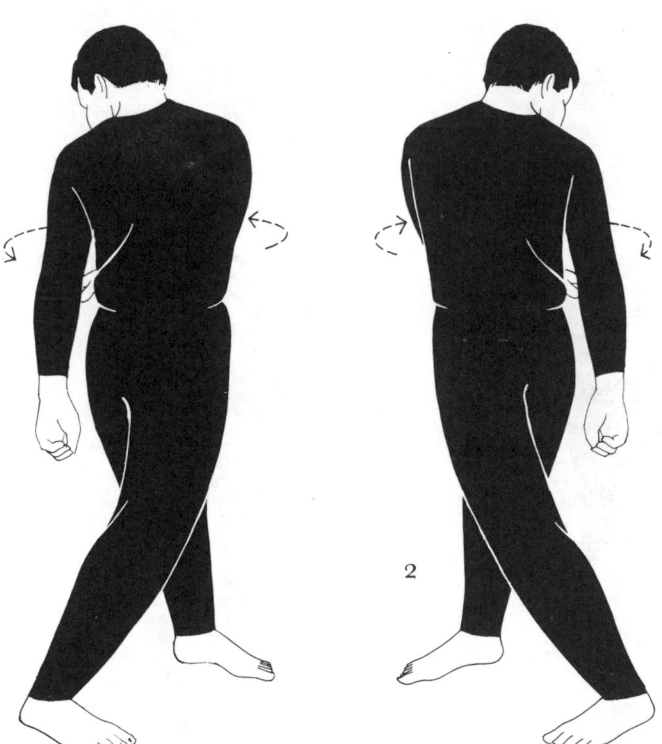

EXERCISE 23.

Walk at a normal rate for 1–1½ minutes.

EXERCISE 24.

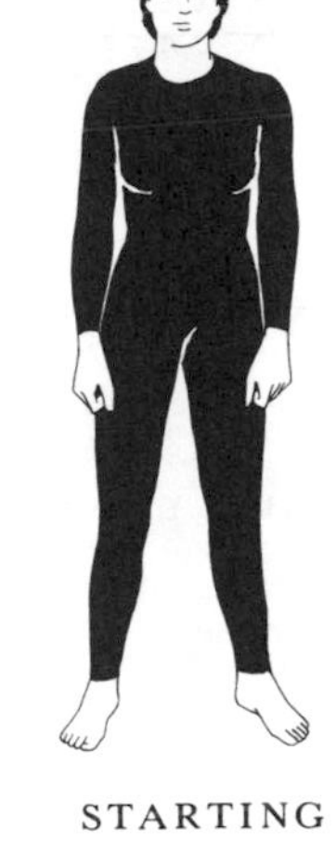

STARTING POSITION

STARTING POSITION: Standing, arms at sides.

MOVEMENT: 1. Raise the arms to the sides, at shoulder level, keeping the elbows straight. At the same time bend and lift the left leg. Then, return to the starting position. 2. Repeat the above, this time bending and lifting the right leg. And again, return to the starting position.

Note: The movements of the arms and legs should be done in a relaxed manner.

1

2

EXERCISE 25.

STARTING POSITION: Standing.

MOVEMENT: Shrug the shoulders and then relax.

EXERCISE 26.

STARTING POSITION: Standing, keeping hips firm.
MOVEMENT: Breathe slowly and rhythmically for one minute.

EXERCISE 27.

While sitting, massage the head, neck, face, and chest. Use soothing and gentle movements for 3–5 minutes.

Appendix II

A program of therapeutic exercise for patients recovering from acute heart attack

FIRST STAGE (duration: 1–2 weeks): Start with exercises 1 thru 3, then gradually add the other four exercises. In the initial stage, only one session of exercise is scheduled daily. Later, two sessions a day are scheduled. Each of the exercises is to be performed while lying on the back. Repeat each 5–10 times.

EXERCISE 1: Abdominal breathing (gently and easily).

EXERCISE 2: Bend the toes up, then curl them down.

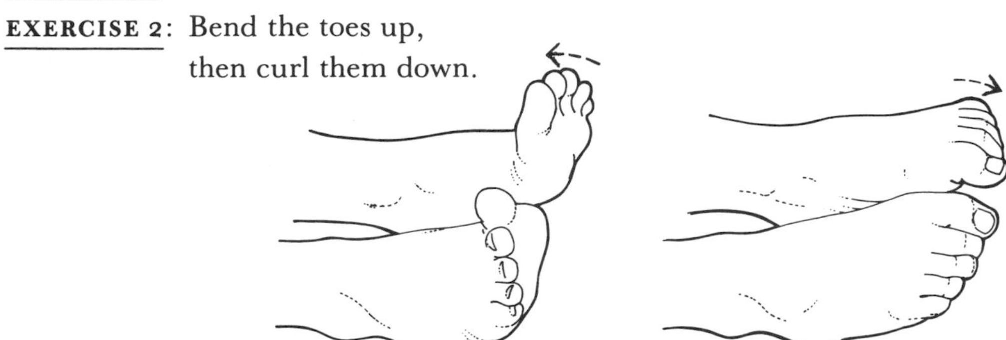

EXERCISE 3: Pull the feet up and then relax; push the feet down and then relax.

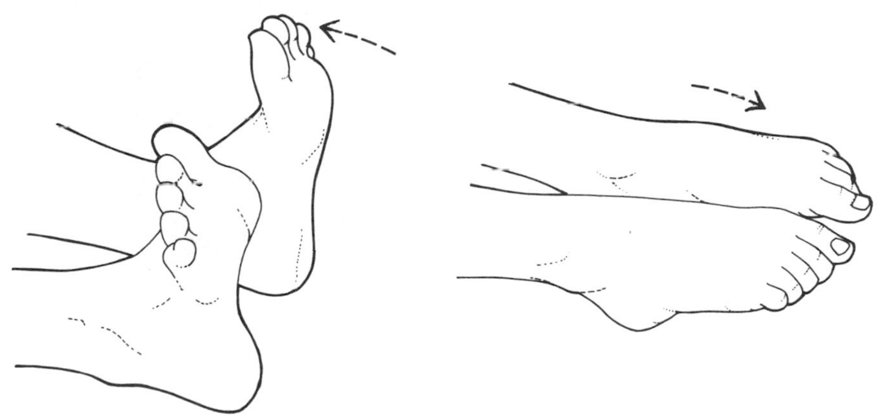

EXERCISE 4: Clench the fists, then relax.

EXERCISE 5: Contract the buttocks, then relax.

EXERCISE 6: Raise the arms above the head, then return them to the starting position.

EXERCISE 7: Bend the legs with the feet sliding on the floor.

SECOND STAGE (duration: 1–2 weeks): During this stage the prescribed exercise is essentially walking. First, walking by the bedside, 5 minutes each session, three times a day. Later, walking in the hospital corridor, 50 yards the first day, 100 yards the second day, 200 the third, and 300 yards the fourth day and thereafter.

In addition to walking, the following exercises done in sitting and standing positions should be practiced once or twice daily.

EXERCISE 1: Bend both elbows, then return to the starting position and relax.

EXERCISE 2: Bring the arms forward to shoulder level keeping the elbows straight. Then bring the arms down.

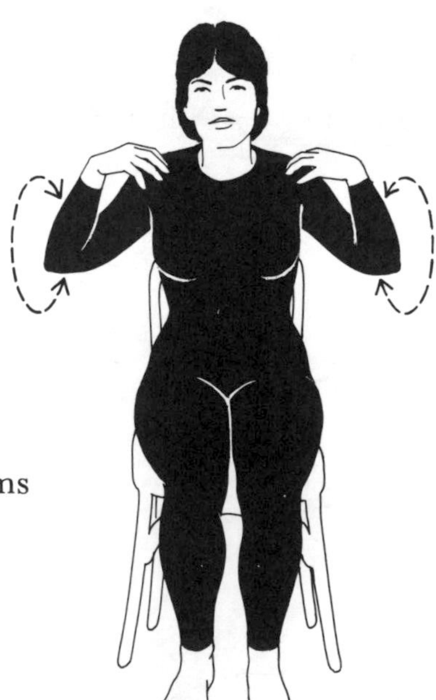

EXERCISE 3: Make a circle with extended arms and with the elbows bent.

EXERCISE 4: Bend the trunk forward slightly with the arms hanging loosely, then return to the starting position.

EXERCISE 5: Bend the trunk to the left and then to the right, in a small range, while breathing smoothly.

EXERCISE 6: Raise the heels and stand on tiptoe, then return to the starting position with heels resting on the floor.

EXERCISE 7: Raise the legs and step in place.

Finally, the patient may practice stepping up and down stairs, if the physical condition permits. At first, the patient is to step up and down four steps. Then the number of steps is increased in increments of four steps each day or two, up to a maximum of forty steps.

CHAPTER XV

Exercises for Gastrointestinal Problems

Improper life-style involving inactivity and overeating accounts for many gastrointestinal and metabolic diseases. Accordingly, the prevention and treatment of these diseases is largely a matter of improving the undesirable life style. In connection with this, exercise therapy is invaluable. For constipation, indigestion, obesity, and "potbelly"—all symptoms of gastrointestinal problems—a number of therapeutic exercise programs are given in this section.

As *Chi Kung* has been used successfully in China to treat peptic ulcer, it is also included in this section.

Since Chinese exercise therapy has traditionally been much concerned with the prevention of illnesses of the stomach and bowels, two kinds of preventive massage are presented.

However, in the treatment of the above-mentioned disorders, exercise therapy can be successful only when combined with rational dietary regulation.

Chronic constipation

Constipation arising from an irregular life-style, improper diet, and irregular habits of defecation is called chronic constipation. It is commonly seen in those facing a new environment requiring major changes in their life and work habits. However, lack of sufficient physical activity is the most common cause of this type of constipation.

Sedentary working conditions, an irregular life-style, lack of exercise, and ingesting refined, low-fiber foods, all contribute to constipation, because they do not provide adequate stimulus for the bowels to move normally. When these causes are removed, the constipation will be cured.

Exercise therapy is quite effective in treating chronic constipation. Dynamic exercises such as running and jumping can stimulate the movement of the bowels. Abdominal exercise strengthens the abdominal muscles which play an important role in the normal process of defecation. In addition, exercise can alter the neuropsychological state so that neurological regulation of intestinal activity can return to normal.

A variety of therapeutic exercises, therapeutic sports, *Chi Kung,* and massage are indicated for patients with chronic constipation.

Therapeutic exercises

The following exercises which are designed to strengthen the abdominal wall are very helpful:

EXERCISE 1: *Knee bending.*

STARTING POSITION

STARTING POSITION: Lying on the back, arms at sides, palms down. (Whenever lying on the back, a pillow under the head will relax the head and neck, and make breathing easier.)

MOVEMENT: Bend the knees and raise the legs back slowly as close to the chest as possible, then return to the starting position.

Repeat 16 times.

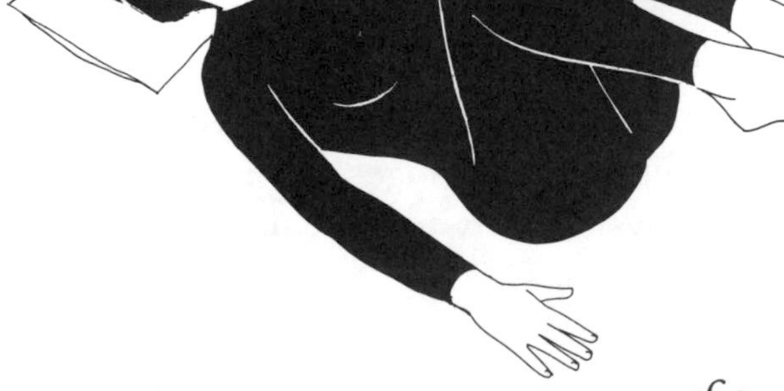

EXERCISE 2: *Leg raising.*

STARTING POSITION: Lying on the back, arms at sides with palms down, knees bent close to the chest.

MOVEMENT: Raise legs upward slowly from bent to a vertical position, to where the knees are straight, then return to the starting position. Repeat 16 times.

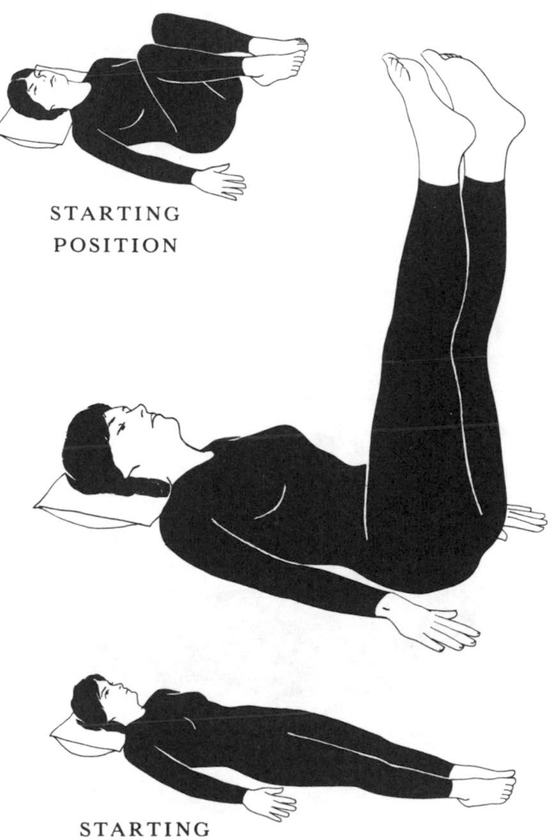

EXERCISE 3: *Cycling.*

STARTING POSITION: Lying on the back, arms at sides, palms down.

STARTING POSITION

MOVEMENT: Bend and stretch out the left and right leg alternately, as in cycling. The exercise should be performed quickly and in as large a range as possible. Keep this up for 20–30 seconds.

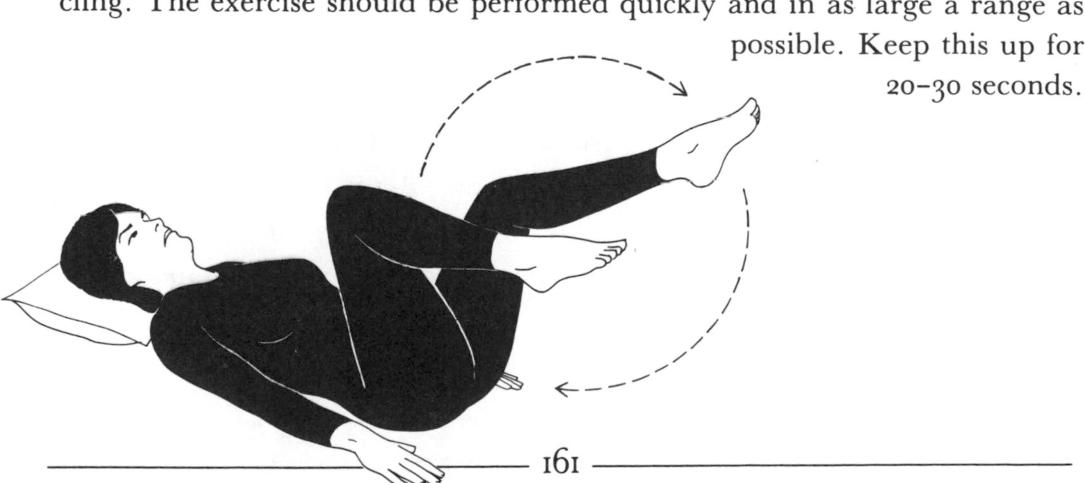

EXERCISE 4: *Sit-ups.*

Caution: This movement is contraindicated for those with back problems.

STARTING POSITION: Lying on the back, palms placed on the floor.

MOVEMENT: 1. Raise hands upward. 2. Then lift head and shoulders slowly and sit up, with the arms reaching forward as far as possible. Return to the starting position. Repeat 6–8 times.

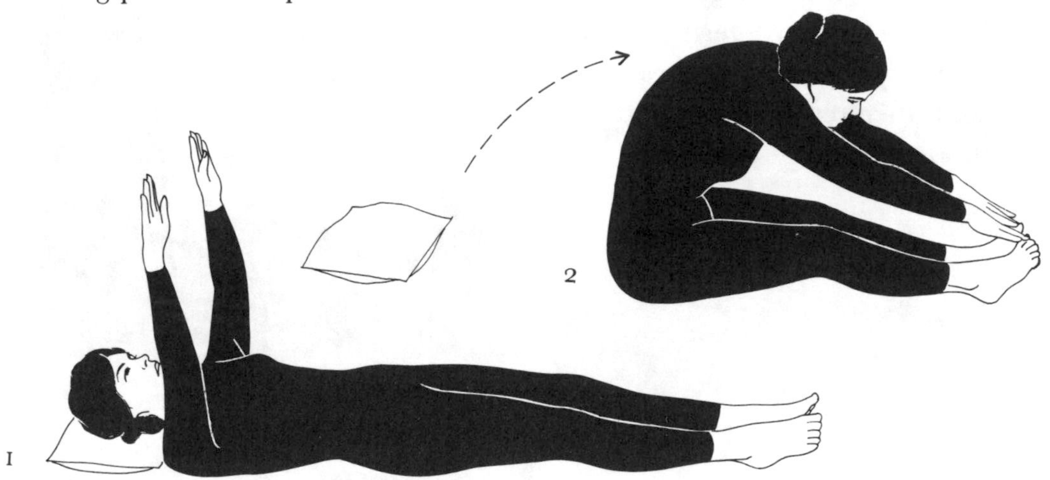

Therapeutic activities

Walking, running, and rowing are preferable.

Walking: Upon rising in the morning, walk briskly for 30 minutes. Then drink a glass of water and go to the toilet to move the bowels. In a sanitorium setting, long-distance walking (approximately 1 mile, or 2 kilometers) may be scheduled regularly for the patient.

Running: Running and jogging stimulate the bowels and promote peristalsis. If level of health permits, one may take part in these sports. Jumping and basketball can serve the same purpose.

Rowing: The movements of rhythmic rowing increase the intra-abdominal pressure, stimulating intestinal peristalsis.

Bathing: A cold water bath is preferable. It may be taken in the form of rubbing the body, a shower, or swimming, depending on the level of fitness and available facilities. If the patient cannot tolerate a cold bath, a hot bath may be taken. However, among these forms of bathing the cold shower is the most effective in stimulating the movement of the bowels. It is recommended that the bath be taken after exercise in the morning.

Chi Kung: For patients with constipation, *Chi Kung for the Internal Organs* is indicated. It should be performed while lying on the back with deep diaphragmatic breathing. This form of *Chi Kung* can "massage" the bowels through intermittent respiration. It has been reported that the range of vertical movement of the diaphragm during *Chi Kung* is 3–4 times greater than during ordinary breathing. This was supported by the finding that under the influence of *Chi Kung* the bowel sounds became louder. In addition, *Chi Kung* may improve the psychological condition, promoting recovery from excessive stress or anxiety, and modifying the bowels' neurological mechanism, return it to normal functioning.

Massage: Self-administered massage on the abdomen is beneficial in cases of chronic constipation. The best position is lying on the back with legs slightly bent, and the knees supported by a pillow. The massage is applied in a circular movement around the umbilicus with the hands on top of each other, starting from the lower right abdomen, moving upward to the upper right abdomen, then across to the lower left abdomen where deep and slow kneading is applied, and finally returning to the lower right abdomen. Repeat this clockwise massage for ten minutes. Upon finishing the massage, stand up, tap the lowest part of the back and the buttocks lightly with both hands. This massage may be applied twice a day after *Chi Kung.*

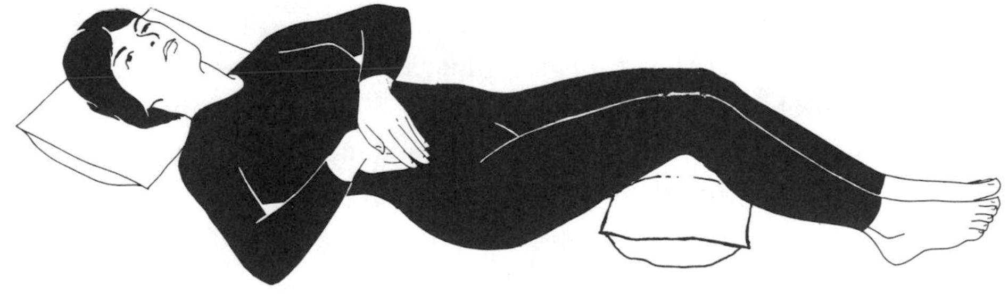

Note: Diet is another aspect in the management of constipation. One should eat foods rich in fiber such as whole grain cereals, fruit, vegetables, whole grain toast or rolls, preserves, and honey, and drink sufficient liquids. No other dietary regulation is necessary.

Gastroptosis

Gastroptosis, the downward displacement of the stomach, will go unnoticed as long as it is symptomless. However, symptoms will occur if the stomach moves down to the lower part of the abdominal cavity, or to the pelvic cavity. The patient usually complains of fullness of the abdomen, indigestion, headache, vertigo, fatigue, and constipation, all resulting from abnormal digestion and absorption, and the ensuing general weakness.

Bodily constitutional factors are said to have a bearing on the development of gastroptosis. It has been found that most patients with gastroptosis are thin and fragile. The ligaments of their abdominal organs are so weak and loose that they cannot keep the stomach in its normal position. Since their abdominal muscles are also very flaccid, the internal organs cannot be prevented from sagging. Other factors leading to gastroptosis are malnutrition, loss of fat tissue in the abdominal cavity, and changes in the shape and volume of the abdominal cavity, found in women after childbirth.

The basic treatment for gastroptosis consists of strengthening the body as well as the abdominal muscles, and improving nutrition. In this regard, *Chi Kung* and therapeutic exercise are very helpful. Therapeutic exercise for gastroptosis emphasizes building up the abdominal muscles (see pages 160–62).

Chi Kung is quite effective in modifying the constitution, increasing the appetite, improving digestion and assimilation of food, and improving the tone of the smooth muscles of the stomach. This, in turn, helps correct a flabby stomach. Clinical observation has shown that *Chi Kung* therapy can result in the ascent of the stomach and relief from such symptoms as indigestion, abdominal pain, fullness, flatulence, and heartburn.

Chi Kung for the Internal Organs is recommended in this regard. The patient is to lie on the back, buttocks supported by a pillow, with the knees bent at an angle between 45–90°. The breathing follows the pattern of diaphragmatic, intermittent respiration (see *Chi Kung for the Internal Organs,* page 74).

Flaccid abdominal wall

A person with a flaccid abdominal wall usually cannot control the bowels, and the abdomen tends to drop forward and downward (sagged abdomen). This sagging belly is often encountered in middle-aged people and in women who have given birth to two or more children.

A sagging belly itself is not a disease. However, it is an underlying factor in many diseases.

Chronic constipation may develop in those with a flaccid abdominal wall, because when evacuating, their abdominal pressure muscles (the external and internal oblique, and rectal muscles) fail to contract forcefully enough to compress the abdomen and stimulate bowel movement.

A great number of people with sagging bellies also complain of lower back pain. This type of functional backache arises from the faulty posture of the back—lordosis. Because of the condition of the belly, the center of their body weight shifts forward. Consequently, the forward curvature of the lumbar spine increases, straining the lower back muscles and causing lower back pain.

Indigestion also is not uncommon in those with a flaccid abdominal wall. It is the result of poor blood circulation in the abdomen as well as weakened peristalsis.

To correct a flaccid abdominal wall, exercise is indispensible. Abdominal exercises are recommended to strengthen the muscles in the abdominal wall. Simple exercises, as those described on pages 160–62, are useful. For those in better physical condition, more vigorous abdominal exercises such as sit-ups with dumbbells or sandbags held in the hands will be more helpful. Deep abdominal (diaphragmatic) breathing is also recommended, with particular emphasis on the strong contraction of the abdominal muscles when breathing out deeply.

CHAPTER XVI

Exercises for Anxiety and Depression

Chinese medicine presumes that physical exercise can have a significant effect on one's state of the mind. Since ancient times exercise has been used in China to foster a tranquil mind and to treat a number of mental disorders, such as depressive states, feelings of sadness, fears (phobias), and anxiety. Traditional Chinese exercise emphasizes training the mind through bodily movement, concentration, and relaxation. Therefore it is also known as "mental exercise" or "spiritual exercise." The traditional Chinese concept of the effect of exercise on the mind is consistent with recent findings by western scientists that exercise may reduce anxiety and depression.

The following section presents exercise programs for patients with anxiety or depression. In these programs, the time-honored Chinese "mental exercises" are incorporated with western remedial games and jogging. These latter activities have recently been reported to be useful in anxiety reduction.

It has been estimated that ten million Americans suffer from anxiety neurosis*, while mental depression is said to be as common as the common cold in the United States.** Various approaches have been tried in coping with these two problems. A century ago, rest therapy was enthusiastically advocated for mental disorders. However, research studies in China and North America over the past twenty years strongly suggest that people with anxiety or depres-

* Morgan, W.P., in Proceedings of the National College of Physical Education Association, p. 114, 1973.

** Lawrence, R.M., in Therapeutics Through Exercise (Ed. Lowenthal, D.T. et al), p. 213, 1979.

sion can benefit from exercise training. *Tai Chi Chuan, Chi Kung,* Chinese massage, and western style jogging and remedial games are all recommended for these common emotional disorders.

Tai Chi Chuan

This gentle exercise is particularly effective in training the mind of the exerciser to become quiet, relaxed, and concentrated. Because of this, individuals with anxiety or in low spirits may use it to develop composure and self-confidence. During the practice of *Tai Chi Chuan,* the patient is required to command every movement of the exercise while in deep thought. Irrelevant thoughts, and feelings of anxiety, sadness, and despair will give way to a definite awareness of the concrete benefits of body/mind training. In addition, the gentle and relaxing movements of the exercise can help relieve such physical symptoms as loss of appetite, fullness in the upper abdomen, flatulence, constipation, and vague pains or discomforts in various parts of the body.

Chi Kung

Chi Kung is of benefit to patients with anxiety. Deep and relaxed respiration throughout the practice, in conjunction with mental concentration, brings a sense of relaxation and ease. Furthermore, meditation plays a role akin to psychotherapy during the practice of *Chi Kung.* For example, in order to relieve mental stress and tension, it is recommended in a *Chi Kung* session to recite mentally some words or phrases with a positive connotation and self-suggestive meaning, such as "I am relaxed," "I am getting better day by day," "Worrying is harmful. I might as well take it easy," "I don't have to be so uptight. Everything is going well." On the whole, people with anxiety are recommended to practice *Chi Kung for Fitness* and incorporate the above-mentioned technique of meditation into the practice.

In the experience of Chinese physicians, those with mental depression tend to benefit much more from *Tai Chi* or remedial games than from *Chi Kung.* It seems that a more active and diversified program rather than *Chi Kung* is preferable for these people, as the former produces greater improvement in emotional state and motivation.

Massage

As a symptomatic treatment, massage can bring about a sedative effect. For headaches, massage the face in general and the temporal region in particular. For dizziness or vertigo, tap the occipital region (back of the head) as in "Beating the drum" (page 60). Massage can be self-administered or done by a therapist.

Walking

Clinical observations have shown that for patients with anxiety and depression, long distance walking (approximately 1½ miles, or 2–3 kilometers) can help modify the process of excitation and inhibition in the cerebral cortex. It will also relieve headache and pulsating pain over the temporal region caused by vasomotor dysfunction. Walking is also a refreshing exercise which can raise the spirits of a depressive patient. For older people with heightened tension, a brisk walk attaining a heart rate of about 100 beats per minute, has been shown more effective in reducing neuromuscular tension than was meprobamate, a common tranquilizer.

Jogging and running

Jogging and running are endurance exercises which, with long-term training (more than six weeks), have been shown effective in the treatment of depression and anxiety. In young men and women with moderate depression, running has been found to be just as effective as psychotherapy. A person with mental anxiety who is following a jogging program will become less preoccupied with symptoms and problems. A better subjective feeling, increased self-esteem, and better body image are achieved through participation in a regular jogging program.

The intensity of jogging and running should be adapted to the individual's physical condition. Generally speaking, jogging may be done three times a week, for 30 minutes, and at an acceptable rate—i.e., where the jogger feels relaxed and comfortable. In general, jogging at a rate of about a mile in 20 minutes would be acceptable for emotionally disturbed patients or people with neurotic symptoms.

Remedial games

Patients with depression or anxiety will benefit from stimulating games and sports such as table tennis, basketball, badminton, volley ball, and rowing. Light physical work such as gardening is also helpful.

Caution: 1. In the integrated treatment of anxiety or depression, exercise therapy must be combined with adequate rest, psychotherapy, and medication in order to effect a better cure. In the recovery stage of the illness, exercise alone can be used to keep the patient in a state of positive motivation.

2. Never exercise to the point of exhaustion. Start the exercise program with moderate intensity and increase the effort gradually.

CHAPTER XVII

Exercises for Insomnia

Insomnia has many causes. It is a condition commonly seen in patients with neurosis and transient emotional disturbance. This type of insomnia cannot be treated radically by prescribing a sleeping pill. However, symptomatic treatment of insomnia with exercise is quite simple and effective. What is needed is to calm the overexcited brain cells, leading the cerebral cortex into an inhibitive process, which, in turn, will cause the patient to fall asleep. In this connection, exercise therapy is useful. The following methods have been shown to have sedative effects. They may be regarded as natural "sleeping pills."

Walking

It is well known that walking is the best tranquilizer in the world. It has been reported that insofar as its sedative effect is concerned, 15 minutes of brisk walking is equal to a dosage of meprobamate. For those with insomnia, it is recommended that they walk for 10–15 minutes before going to bed.

Tai Chi Chuan

As a mental exercise, *Tai Chi* can help the patient relax. It is a natural sedative that brings serenity to the mind. Doing a set of *Tai Chi* 30 minutes before going to bed can help overcome insomnia.

Self-administered massage

Sedative self-administered massage is applied when lying in bed ready to go to sleep. The massage used for this condition involves rubbing and stroking the body with both hands by the patient herself or himself. It is also called "the dry bath." First, "wash" (rub) the face lightly with both hands. Next, stroke the left arm with the right hand and the right arm with the left hand. Then stroke the chest and abdomen slowly and lightly. Finally, massage the sole (stroking the point *yung chuan,* see page 64). With this massage, you will very soon become calm. Drowsiness usually occurs in response to a 10-minute session of massage. The next step is to stop the massage, relaxing further into sleep.

Chi Kung

It is recommended to practice *Chi Kung for Relaxation* or *Chi Kung for Fitness* before going to sleep. Lying on the right side is the preferred position. Relax the body, concentrate the mind using the method of "following the breath" (page 72). Practicing *Chi Kung* in this way for 10–15 minutes usually induces drowsiness. *Chi Kung* of this type is called *Chi Kung for Sleep.*

In addition, other adjunctive measures are beneficial, such as immersing the feet in warm water for 20–30 minutes before going to bed as well as stopping reading, writing, or other mental activity 30 minutes before going to bed.

If sleep is still intermittent by midnight, try the method mentioned above once more. It will assist in falling asleep again.

CHAPTER XVIII

Exercises Following Brain Concussion

Brain contusion may occur when the head is severely jarred. In societies with heavy automobile traffic, brain concussion from traffic accidents is not uncommon. Industrial and sports injuries also contribute to the incidence of brain concussion. Exercise therapy is helpful in hastening recovery from these conditions. Sometimes the patient can recover fully with proper rest and other treatment. Quite often, some sequela (after-effects) will remain, such as vertigo, dizziness, headache, absent-mindedness, depression, muscular weakness, or fatigue.

The above-mentioned symptoms may be relieved by exercise therapy in conjunction with medication. Methods of therapeutic exercise used for this condition are much the same as those for anxiety and depression, but with less intensity, because patients recovering from a brain concussion cannot tolerate vigorous exercise. Another valuable treatment is *Chi Kung for Relaxation,* helping to regulate the mental and psychological state of the patient. Walking and doing breathing exercises in the fresh air will make the patient alert and refreshed. Stimulating games such as table tennis and badminton are good for those patients in moderately good physical condition. Exercises accompanied by music can lift the spirits and relieve depression. As a symptomatic treatment, massage on the head performed either by the patient or by a therapist is helpful in relieving headache and vertigo.

CHAPTER XIX

Exercises for Paralysis

This section contains exercises for hemiplegia (paralysis of one side of the body) following stroke and paraplegia (paralysis of the lower half of the body) following spinal cord injury.

These programs are not only indicated for patients under medical care in a rehabilitation center, but also for those who have been discharged from a hospital or rehabilitation center and are now at home. A great number of exercises, such as the arm ad hand exercises for functional training, and a walking program in the later recovery stage, can also be performed by the patient alone.

It is the experience of Chinese physicians that it is best to combine exercise therapy with acupuncture in the initial stage of rehabilitative treatment (the first six months after the accident causing the paralysis). However, the exercise training should be continued as long as possible, over a period of months or even years.

Massage is a good adjunct to exercise training in the treatment of paralysis. For flaccid muscles, the method of deep kneading or stroking is recommended. For contracted or spastic muscles, soothing surface stroking is indicated.

Exercise therapy in hemiplegia

Cautions: 1. In cases of hemiplegia the intensity of exercise should be very low, so that an extra burden is not put on the cardiovascular system. 2. Pay attention to safety. When doing standing and walking exercises, the patient must be supervised by a therapist or an attendant for support and guidance.

FIRST STAGE: This stage generally begins in the early recovery period, about 3–4 weeks after onset of the attack. The goal during this stage is to restore the functions of sitting and standing. Apart from massage and passive movements applied to the paralytic limbs, the following exercises should be taught to the patient.

- Lying on the back, pull the foot and the toes up as far as possible, then relax.
- Lying on the back with legs extended, flex (bend) the hips and knees, then stretch them to return to the starting position.
- Sitting exercise: Sit up from a lying position, first with the help of a therapist, then gradually on one's own.
- Sitting on a chair, step in place, alternating with the right and left leg.
- Sitting on a chair, stand up from the chair, with hands firmly holding onto a stable object, then sit down.
- Standing exercise: Stand at bedside, with hands firmly holding onto a stable object for balance.
- Standing exercise: Stand alongside the bed, without holding onto any means of support.
- Standing exercise: Stand away from the bed, without relying on any object.

SECOND STAGE: The goal during this stage is to restore the function of walking and to improve the function of the upper extremities, especially the fingers. The ambulation program is as follows:

- Standing, with hands holding onto a stable object, move the trunk to the healthy side, then to the paralytic side. Rest weight alternately on the healthy, then the affected side.
- Standing, with hands holding onto a stable object, step in place.
- Standing, with hands holding onto a stable object, step sideward.
- Walk with the help of a walker.
- Walk with a cane.
- Walk independently.

At this stage, the hand program is as follows:

- Reduce the flexion contracture of the fingers by massage and passive movements.

- Separate the fingers as widely as possible. Try to keep the fingers straight and flat, and touch the surface of a table.
- Separate the fingers from each other, then close them together.
- Exercise the hands and fingers using various kinds of small apparatus.

THIRD STAGE: The goal of this stage is to restore the functions of everyday activity. Further ambulation training includes a variety of complex walking exercises such as walking over obstacles, walking up and down stairs, walking up a slope, and walking at various speeds. The hand program is much the same as that used in the second stage. Those who are recovering faster will do coordination exercises, agility exercises (e.g., grasping and releasing a ball, catching a ball), and other forms of occupational therapy.

Exercise therapy to help paraplegics stand

Paraplegia is the paralysis of the lower half of the body due to disease or injury of the spinal cord. Intensive treatment is important in order to give the paraplegic an opportunity to restore functioning as much as possible and enjoy a longer, more active life.

In the comprehensive treatment of paraplegia, exercise therapy plays a very important role in improving motor function, preventing complications, and maintaining general health.

The following program is applicable to paraplegics in the recovery period, in particular those who have suffered mild spinal injury. In cases of severe spinal injury, surgical intervention is usually indicated, followed by exercise therapy in the postoperative period.

Sitting exercise

The patient is helped to sit up from the supine position. At first, he or she can only assume a half-sitting position with the back leaning against a tilted headrest. This is followed by self-training, with supervision, for maintaining long sitting on the bed (i.e., legs extended flat on a bed or the floor). Finally, the patient is taught to sit on the side of the bed with both feet hanging over the edge. Sometimes the patient will experience a sense of syncope (faintness) when sitting up straight, particularly during several of the earlier sessions. This is due to ischemia (deficient blood supply) in the brain as a result of poor vasomotor response. It may be overcome by preparatory training, in the form of turning the body around and changing position frequently while lying in bed. When doing the sitting exercise, it is recommended that a belt be fastened to the abdomen to prevent a sudden influx of blood into the abdomen from the brain.

Preparation for getting off the bed

Before transferring from the bed to a chair or wheelchair, the patient is taught to do conditioning exercises to strengthen the muscles of the back, arms, and shoulder girdle. A kneeling exercise is also very important to train the knees to bear weight.

- Lying on the stomach, raise the body to an elbow-knee position, and crawl forward on the bed my moving the hip joint.
- Elbow-knee position ("four point" kneeling). Supported by two cut-down crutches (half the length of regular crutches), raise the body to assume a kneel-standing position. Then move the hip joints forward and backward to prepare for walking on the knees.

Standing exercise

The following procedures are training for standing.

- Prone standing, the trunk leaning on a bed, with the chest supported by pillows.
- Standing on a tilt table for 30 minutes at an angle of 45–70°.
- Standing with crutches, the back leaning against a wall and the knees supported by the hands of a therapist.
- As above, but without the support of a therapist.
- Standing between parallel bars with hands firmly holding the bars.

- Standing with the support of crutches.
- Standing with the support of a therapist.
- Standing independently.

Walking exercise

When the patient can stand with crutches or with the support of a therapist, he or she may be taught to walk according to the following program:

- Walking between parallel bars or with a walker, the hands holding firmly onto the bar.
- Walking with crutches, the knees supported by a therapist or by a brace.
- Walking with crutches.
- Walking with two canes.
- Walking with one cane.
- Walking independently.

For other exercises used in training patients to stand and walk, see *Exercise therapy in hemiplegia: third stage* (page 176).

The patient must be given help and supervision during both the standing sessions and walking exercises to prevent falling.

In spite of the fact that most paraplegics can benefit to varying degrees from exercise therapy, a great number still have to rely on the support of crutches or braces. Consequently, they must be taught to walk properly with crutches. There are two basic types of crutch gait for paraplegics:

1. The "four-pointed" gait. When walking with this type of gait, one crutch is advanced, then the opposite foot, then the other crutch, and then the other foot. This is a very stable gait, moving slowly, always leaving three points on the floor at one time. However, for patients with high spastic lesions, this type of gait is extremely difficult to perform.

2. The "shuffle-to and swing-to" gait: This consists of advancing both crutches forward at the same time and then dragging the feet toward the crutches. The feet are always behind the crutches.

The preceding principles and methods of exercise therapy are also applicable to paraplegics recovering from transverse myelitis.

Therapeutic sports

In recent years an increasing number of paraplegic patients in wheelchairs have taken part in various sports, not only at continuing care centers or at the spinal centers, but also at the international athletic meets especially organized for the handicapped.

Indeed, patients with paraplegia are capable of playing a variety of games and sports. Participation in some sports is actually a necessity to the paraplegic's life and health. Since they have lost the ability to run, jump, and walk, they have lost the opportunity to participate in many of the physical activities which healthy people enjoy daily. If they do not exercise their remaining healthy limbs, their general health as well as their arm and trunk muscles will be weakened. Therapeutic sports can develop muscle tone, increase the strength of the muscles in the arms, back, and abdomen, and improve general physical condition. Well developed arms and shoulder girdle are valuable assets to paraplegics, which will help them overcome many inconveniences encountered in their daily wheelchair life. Anyone who watches paraplegics in wheelchairs playing therapeutic sports in high spirits and with impressive vitality will realize that they can and should take part in physical training.

Many games involving the use of the arms and trunk are of value to persons with paraplegia. For example, dumbbell exercises, ball-throwing, table tennis, archery, and basketball-shooting are good for building up the muscles in the shoulder girdle and back. Among these, archery is particularly valuable, because of its effect of strengthening the muscles in the trunk and upper arms that are very important for daily activities. As well, archery can help correct scoliosis (when the thoracic curve is on the right side, the right hand should be used to draw the bow) and can improve sitting balance.

Therapeutic sports may be done individually, at home, or in a group setting at a rehabilitation center.

CHAPTER XX

Exercises for Sciatica and Lumbar Disk Problems

Sciatica is a condition characterized by pain, tingling, and other abnormal sensations in the hip, thigh, leg, and foot, caused by impairment of the sciatic nerve. A variety of conditions are responsible for this. Of these, inflammation of the sciatic nerve, intervertebral disk problems, and lumbosacral arthritis are among the most common.

Inflammation of the sciatic nerve (sciatic neuritis) is commonly caused by exposure to cold, toxicity and infection of the adjacent tissues, and sacroiliac arthritis. When the acute symptoms of sciatic neuritis have lessened, the patient may start massage and therapeutic exercise. The following program offers therapeutic exercises for sciatica of this type.

The treatment is also useful in recovery (post-operative of non-operative) from lower back and leg pain due to lumbar disk problems.

Massage

Tap the lower back, buttocks, and the posterior aspect of the thigh with one end of a stick which is fitted with rubber or cloth for 5–10 minutes, 3–5 times daily. This is generally self-administered by the patient, in a standing position. It may also be performed by a therapist.

Therapeutic exercise

During the initial recovery period, do the following four exercises.

EXERCISE 1:

While lying on the back, with legs bent at the knees, open and close the knees. Resistance may be applied on the lateral sides of the knees.

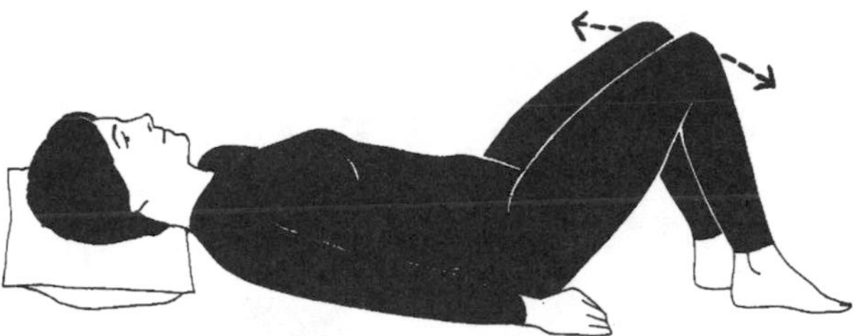

EXERCISE 2:

While lying on the back, with legs bent at knees, stretch the legs alternately (heels remain touching the floor).

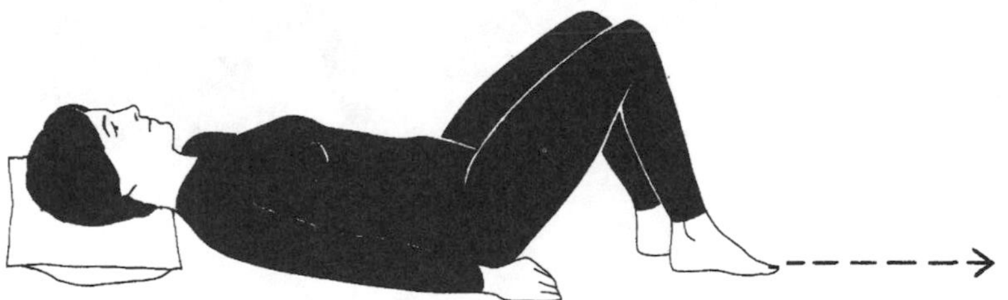

EXERCISE 3:

While lying on the healthy side, flex the knee and extend the affected leg. The hip is kept slightly flexed.

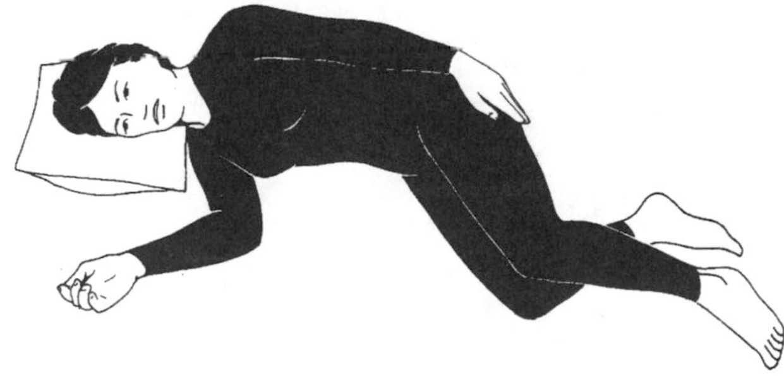

EXERCISE 4:

While half raised, supporting the body with the hands on the bed behind the body, 1. flex the left knee, extending the leg, 2. then do the same with the right knee and leg.

When the condition has improved, the following exercises may be added:

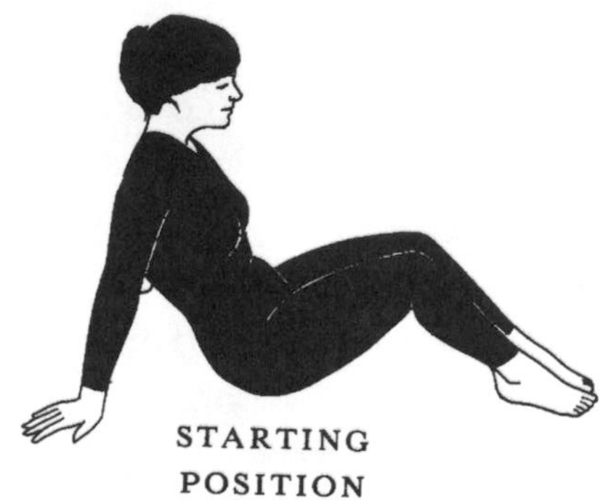

STARTING POSITION

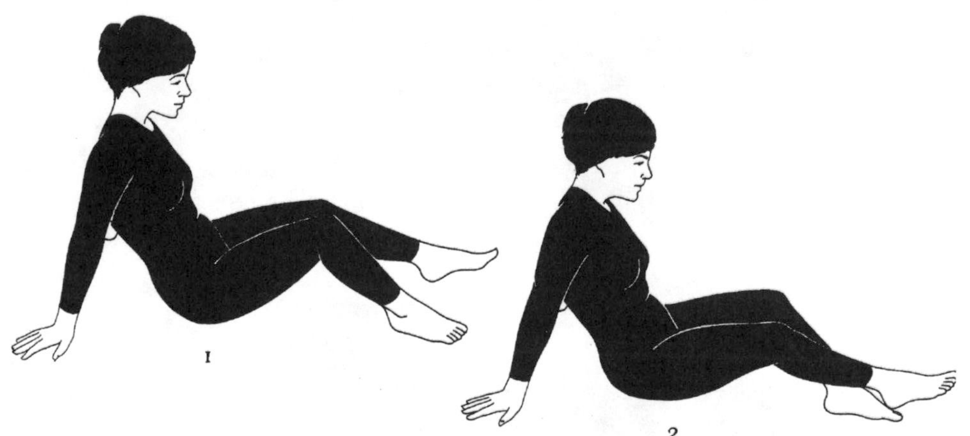

EXERCISE 5:

While sitting on a chair, with knees and hips bent at a right angle and hands on the thighs, bend the trunk forward and slide the hands down the front of the legs simultaneously.

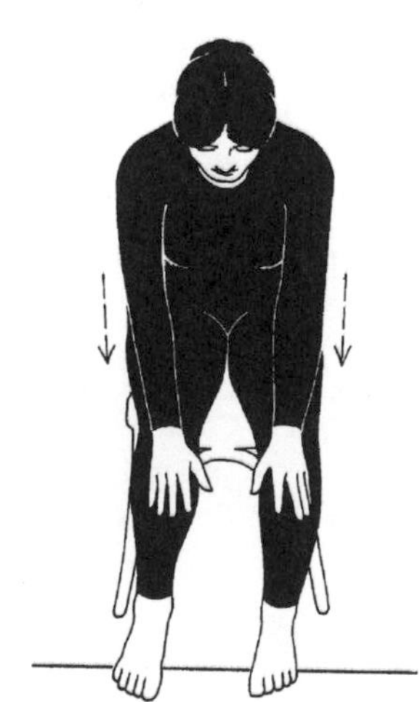

EXERCISE 6:

While sitting with legs extended, bend the trunk forward and push the hands toward the toes.

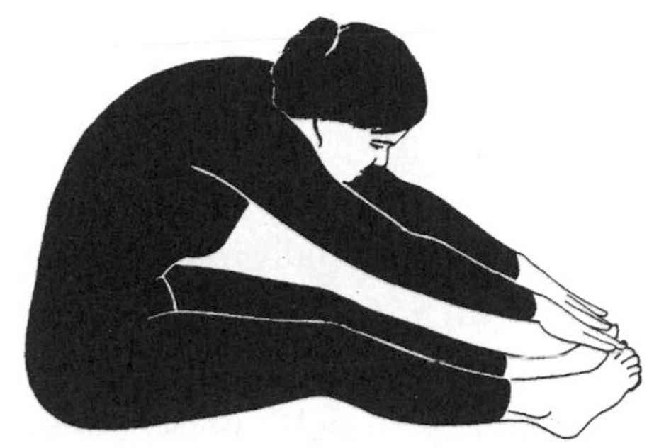

EXERCISE 7:

While standing with one hand holding onto a stable object, swing the affected leg forward and backward.

EXERCISE 8:

While standing, feet together, hands on hips, hips firm, 1. take a step to the left with the left foot. 2. Next, bend the left knee, keeping the right leg straight. Then return to the starting position. Repeat the above, this time stepping to the right.

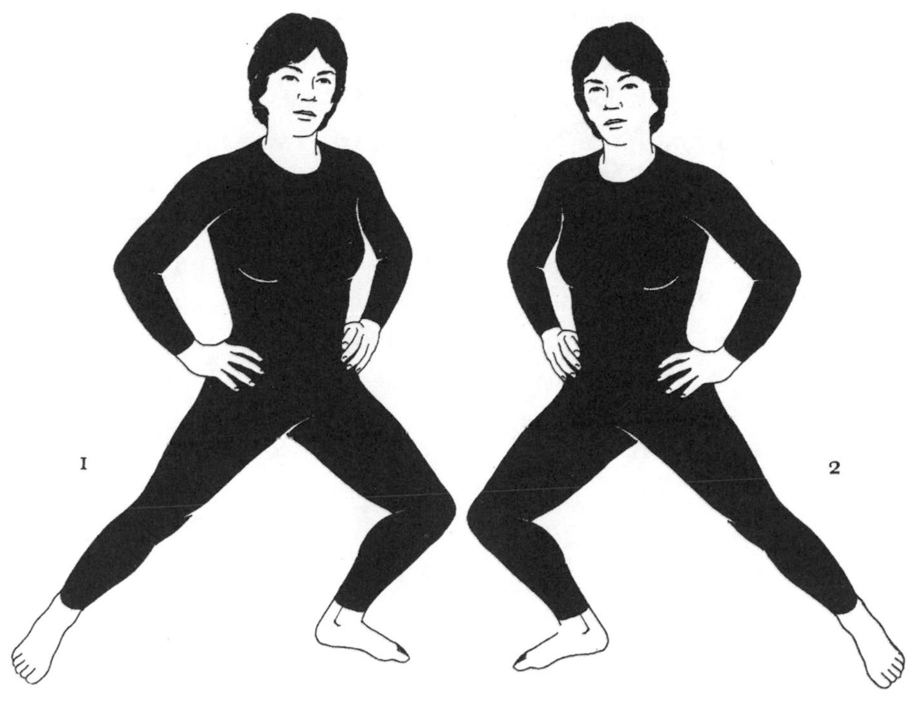

EXERCISE 9:

While standing, feet apart about shoulder width, hands on hips, hips firm, bend the trunk forward gradually with the knees kept straight.

Sciatica that is due to disk problems (disk degeneration or protrusion) can sometimes be relieved by proper rest followed by therapeutic exercise.

If the protrusion of the nucleus in the intervertebral disk is slight, bed rest for a few days (occasionally more than ten days) will help the protruded nucleus return to its normal position. The sciatica will then disappear. At such time, stretching exercise in a standing position is of help. The trunk is never to be bent forward with the legs straight. Physiotherapy, in the form of a hot pad or infrared radiation, will relieve tension in the back muscle sand its attendant pain.

If the protrusion of the nucleus is severe, manipulation and simple stretching exercises may be tried in addition to bed rest. Chiropractic manipulation should be performed by an experienced and skillful professional. One of the simple stretching exercises used in traditional Chinese medicine is "Hanging and swinging" which is done with a wall bar. Standing with feet together, the patient raises the hands upward as far as possible and grasps the bar overhead in order to straighten the trunk. Elbows and legs are also kept straight. The patient then twists the waist 10 times in a clockwise circular movement, then 10 times in a counterclockwise circular movement. This is to be repeated 2–3 times daily. This stretching exercise may help the nucleus return to its normal position. If the pain is not relieved after 10 days of bed rest, stretching exercise, and chiropractic manipulation, these treatments should be discontinued, and the patient advised to consult an orthopedic surgeon for surgical intervention, or other forms of therapy

PART IV

Principles & Techniques of Massage Therapy

Introduction

Massage therapy is simple and easy to use and its particular effectiveness in treating certain common ailments has gained it wide acceptance.

How does massage cure disease? It is generally considered that massage therapy has the ability to regulate nerve function, to strengthen the body's resistance to disease, to flush out the tissues and improve circulation of blood, and to make the joints more flexible.

1. *Regulating nerve function:* The nervous system links all parts of the body, influencing the function of every part and every organ. Imbalanced nerve function, or increases in nerve excitement or nerve inhibition can all cause the malfunctioning of certain organs, resulting in disease. The underlying pathogenic principle: "If *yin*[1] predominates over *yang*[2], then a *yang* disease appears; if *yang* predominates over *yin*, then a *yin* disease appears." The use of massage therapy techniques has a reflexive effect on nerve functions, causing the excitatory and inhibitory processes of the nervous system to reach a relative equilibrium (i.e., bringing the *yin* and the *yang* into relative equilibrium). And this, in turn, produces a medical effect. For example: when a headache or toothache is present, massage applied on a corresponding acupoint[3] (such as the *hegu*[4] point) kills the pain immediately. This occurs because the massage creates a new stimulation point, easing or dispelling the sensation of pain in the original location. This phenomenon is called the "pain-shift-

1. *Yin:* The negative principle associated with cold and quiescence.
2. *Yang:* The positive principle associated with heat and activity.
3. Acupoint: one of the large number of specific points on the body at which massage or acupuncture are applied to produce specific system effects.
4. *Hegu:* an acupoint located on the back of the hand between the bones of the thumb and index finger. See Diagram 59.

ing method." With hypertensive patients who exhibit such symptoms as dizziness and headache (said to be caused by too much *yang* in the liver), massage brings about a temporary drop in blood pressure. This is because the massage techniques cause the peripheral blood vessels to dilate through nervous reflex action. This type of regulative process is called "suppressing the liver's *yang*."

Also, for example, where there is a common cold or flu caught due to wind or cold, the pores of the skin are blocked, so that no perspiration can pass through them. Consequently, the body temperature rises and there is tiredness all over the body, as well as headache and discomfort. After massage is applied, the whole body reacts with perspiration, and the symptoms abruptly disappear. This phenomenon is called "relieving the surface of the body."

In the case of acute urine retention, applying massage on the lower abdomen and on a corresponding acupoint (such as the *qihai*[5] point) triggers bladder contraction, and the discharge of urine.

In recent years, there has been some experimental evidence to substantiate that massage therapy does produce such results as those mentioned above. For example, massage applied to the neck and upper back or lower back regions did increase the flow of blood to the internal organs associated with the corresponding section of ganglia. We have made some experimental investigation of the effects of massage on gastric activity. These showed that massage applied to the *weishu,*[6] *pishu*[7] and *chu san li* or *zusanli*[8] acupoints did indeed increase the strength of gastric activity. Where gastric activity has already been functioning in a fortified state, and the same method of massage is used, it leads conversely to the inhibition of gastric activity. This demonstrates the regulatory use of massage, which produces different effects when applied in different states. We have investigated these experimental observations in our clinical practice and obtained further verification. When the above method was applied in a post-operative patient suffering from

5. *Qihai:* an acupoint point just below the umblicus. See Diagram 58.
6. *Weishu:* an acupoint on the back, beside the lower end of the spinous process of the 11th vertebra. See Diagram 59.
7. *Pishu:* an acupoint on the back, beside the lower end of the spinous process of the 11th vertebra. See Diagram 59.
8. *Zusanli:* an acupoint on the outer edge of the tibia, just below the knee. See Diagram 60.

intestinal obstruction, the intestinal peristalsis returned to normal. Also, the use of this method has slowed intestinal peristalsis and dispelled the pain in a patient affected with enterospasm.

2. *Strengthening the body's resistance to disease:* Massage therapy can improve general physical condition, and strengthen the body's resistance, resulting in the prevention and curing of disease. The underlying principle of treatment is "support the good and expel the bad." For example, in the case of a patient with rheumatoid spondylitis, not only does massage therapy make the stiffened vertebral column more flexible and lessen pain, but after a period of massage treatment, the patient's complexion turns from gray to rosy, and better appetite and weight gain occur. Again, in certain cases of infantile pneumonia, though there was a long course of treatment with antibiotics, a murmur in the pulmonary area persisted, and the whole body was weak. After massage therapy, the murmur soon died out, and general condition also gradually improved. This illustrates how massage therapy mobilizes the body's internal defenses against disease.

Based on the fact that after massage treatment the skin in the area appears reddened, we made experimental observations of skin temperature before and after massage. The findings showed that skin temperature rose both in the local area, where the massage had been applied, and in areas distant from the massaged spot. This implies that massage can accelerate metabolism, and cause dilation of peripheral blood vessels, increased blood circulation, and strengthened resistance against invasion by noxious influences. In addition, observations were made of the effects of massage on red blood-cell count, white blood-cell count, the ability of the white blood-cells to destroy bacteria, and the serum complement values. The results demonstrated that, after massage was applied, each of these indices was raised above its previous level. This shows how massage can help the body to protect itself against disease.

3. *Flushing out the tissues and increasing circulation of the blood, making the joints more flexible:* The direct effects of massage therapy are most easily seen externally in the treatment of localized ailments. For example, for sprained limbs, bruises and local hematomatic pain, massage therapy can flush out the tissues and improve circula-

tion of the blood, replacing spilled blood cells with new ones, completely removing the localized collection of the leaked blood and causing the swelling pain to fade. In clinical observation, we found that to reduce a swelling means, in effect, to stop pain. This accords with the principle: "Where the blood does not flow, there is pain; where the blood flows, there is no pain."

In all types of paralysis resulting from muscular atrophy, massage therapy can speed up the restoration of normal muscle tone, and strengthen the muscles. This is known as: "Clearing the energy-system and strengthening the flesh and bones." Also, in cases of joint stiffness due to any variety of causes, massage can directly increase the degree of activity in the stiffened joints. In the case of articular rigidity caused by rheumatoid spondylitis, our clinical observations show that the joint is not irreversibly stiff as mistakenly believed in the past. In fact, the joint is as if "rusted," and therefore some of the passive methods of manipulation used in massage will gradually loosen the rusted joints.

We have also studied a comparatively large number of cases of protruding lumbar intervertebral disk ("slipped" disk). We found that the mechanical force applied during massage returned the protruding area to its proper place. Based on these findings we have improved the methods used in this massage, and have further advanced the effectiveness of the treatment.

The above represents an introduction to the basic principles of treatment by massage therapy. Just as matter evolves, so does human knowledge. Through actual practice our knowledge is continuously developed and increased, making massage therapy an even more effective method for the prevention and cure of disease.

Furthermore, it must be pointed out that the successful outcome of massage therapy will be greatly enhanced by a positive relationship between the practitioner and the patient. In massage therapy, it is necessary to have close coordination between them. This is especially true for certain ailments where the patient has to undertake a long-term program of self-massage and exercise to go along with professional treatment. These consolidate and improve the therapeutic effect of the treatment. Therefore, in the course of treatment, it is important to bring the subjective motivation of both practitioner and patient fully into play, and to establish confidence in the treatment and healing processes.

CHAPTER XXI

Fundamental Techniques for Effective Massage

by Joe Wong, Tui Na Therapist

The first principle for effective massage is that the patient must be relaxed. To accomplish this, the patient is placed in a comfortable position to induce initial relaxation, and the practitioner begins by massaging the limbs of the body. An indication of relaxation is that the patient is breathing abdominally rather than thoracically and the patient's face will appear more relaxed. When relaxation has been achieved, the patient's body becomes receptive to the practitioner and to the massage process, permitting positive physical changes to occur. It is equally important that the therapist be comfortable throughout the massage. If he is uncomfortable or tense, his touch will feel hard or painful to the patient, as well as tiring for the therapist.

Once the practitioner has learned *how* to touch the patient, he or she has learned the most important thing of all. The key to effective touch is that it be *slow*, that the pattern of movements remains always *circular*, and that a *rhythm* is established and adhered to. Here "circular" movement means that a roughly circular path is followed by the therapist's hands, or thumbs, or fingers. Also, the therapist's hands must be constantly touching the patient without interruption. Lastly, neither the therapist's nor the patient's limbs are ever held rigidly straight (producing tension and resistance) but are always loosely curved.

Practitioners may vary in their approach and methods. While some will be firm, others will be more gentle. To prevent the practitioner's becoming fatigued, a rhythm should be followed during the massage. The rhythm should be one that is comfortable and easy to maintain. It is most important that the practitioner maintains his or her own strength, endurance, and general high level of energy.

Daily practice of *Tai Chi*, for example, has been found very helpful in this regard. At the end of a massage session, the patient usually feels relaxed and energized—sometimes even euphoric.

After a session a patient will know if a massage was effective through a special feeling of well-being.

When a patient's condition has improved following a series of massage sessions, self-massage can be very helpful to maintain these benefits. Of course, the individual's life style—diet, exercise, rest—will also contribute to ongoing well-being, and new habits may have to be learned. With this type of treatment the patient must assume responsibility for his or her own health, together with the massage practitioner, and must be prepared to meet the practitioner halfway.

In all, the basic techniques described above are surprisingly simple, yet they are very powerful in their effects on the body. Using them, the practitioner can improve the patient's sense of well-being. Without these basic skills, he or she will be unable to give an effective massage, despite extensive knowledge of the acupoints and the various massage methods.

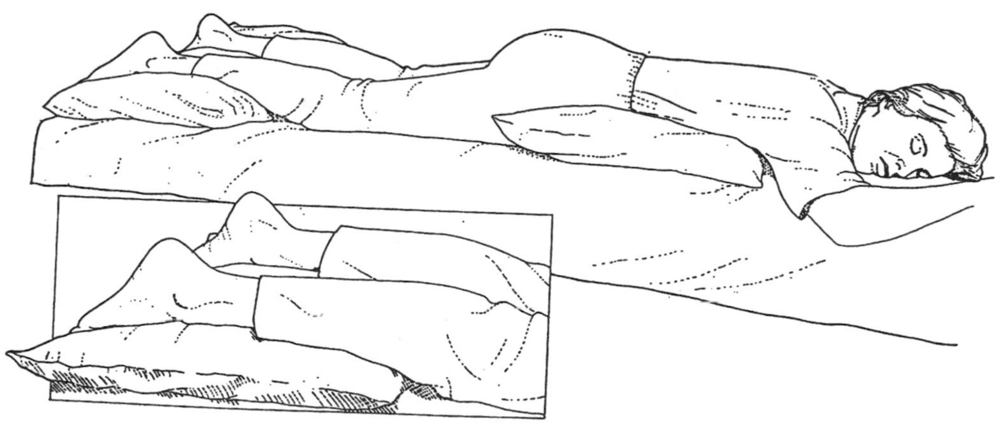

CORRECT PILLOW POSITIONS

Section 1: Commonly Used Techniques

In Chinese medical literature there is abundant information about massage techniques. Massage therapists from all parts of China have combined their clinical experience, and in the primary or secondary aspects of these techniques, each one has his own particular way of doing things. Below is an introduction to our commonly used techniques.

1. Press Method

The press method is a form of massage which uses the palm or the fingers to press on a certain part of the body. There are various ways to apply the press, such as with one hand, both hands, elbow, etc. When the press method is used one must gradually go from light to heavy, so that the patient feels a definite pressure, but no pain. At the close of the press method it is not desirable to release the pressure too suddenly. Instead, the pressure should be gently reduced. The press method may be applied continuously for a comparatively long space of time, or intermittently, at a fixed rate. After the press method has been applied, some other techniques must be added in combination with it. The effects of the press method can be felt as shallowly as just on the surface of the skin, or as deeply as in the bones and internal organs. The amount of pressure used can be adjusted as necessary.

The press method is divided into three different forms: palm press, thumb press, and elbow press:

Palm Press Method: The palm press method involves using the palm to apply pressure to an affected area of the body. Included are the single-palm press, two-palm press, and two-palm opposed press. The palm press is generally applied where there is an extensive area of pain, as in lumbago, or abdominal pain. (See Diagram 1.) If the entire head is in pain, then the two-palm opposed press (see Diagram 2) is used. In pressing on the abdomen, the pressing hand must follow the rise and fall of the patient's respiration. Doing so will prevent the patient from feeling discomfort. Sometimes the practitioner first rubs his palms until they become very hot, and then presses on the painful area. This has been found effective.

DIAGRAM 1

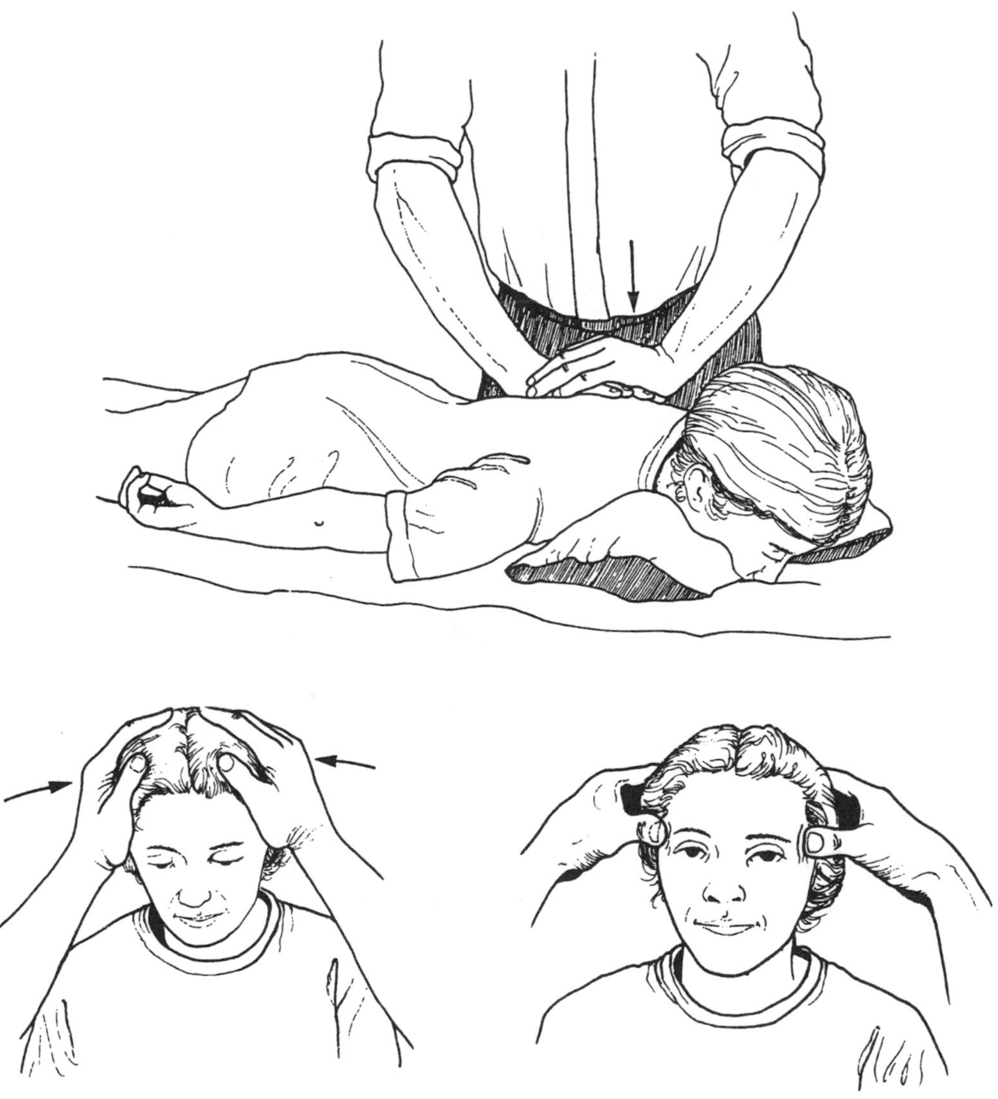

DIAGRAM 2

DIAGRAM 3

Thumb Press Method: When applying the thumb press method, press the flat of the thumb on a meridional acupoint (an acupoint situated on a meridian of the body's energy system) or on the site of the pain. While pressing, a suitable force must be applied, trying to avoid as much pain as possible. In the thumb press method, the single-thumb press and the two-thumb opposed press may be used. For an ache in the forehead, for example, the two-thumb opposed press is applied to the *taiyang*[1] acupoints in the temples. (See Diagram 3.)

Elbow Press Method: The elbow press is applied either at an acupoint or at a site of pain. It is properly applied to the lower back, buttocks, or to certain acupoints such as the *huantiao*[2] point. (See Diagram 4.)

DIAGRAM 4

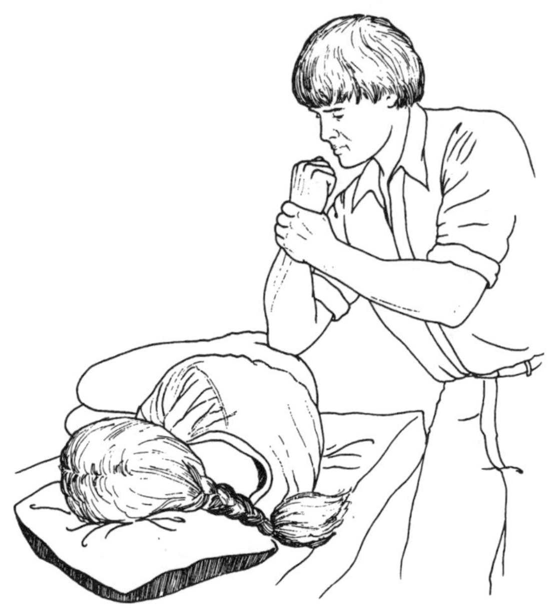

1. *Taiyang:* an acupoint in the depression about a finger's width outside a point between the outer canthus of the eye and the tip of the eyebrow. See Diagram 57, p. 246.
2. *Huantiao:* an acupoint on the buttock, between the highest point of the trochanter and the sacral hiatus. See Diagram 59, p. 250.

2. Rub Method

The rub method uses the fingers or the palm. There are single-handed and also two-handed rub methods. They involve rubbing the surface of the skin with a circular motion. Only enough force is applied to affect the skin and the subcutaneous tissues. The force of the rub should go from light to heavy, and the rate of the rub movement depends on what the condition of a disease requires; it should be somewhere between 30–40 and 200 times a minute.

The rub method is often used at the beginning of a massage, or performed just after the press method. Rub techniques generally include thumb, palm, and palm-heel rub methods.

Thumb Rub Method: This refers to rubbing with the flat of the thumb on a certain area of the body, or on an acupoint. It can be done with one thumb or with both thumbs at the same time. When using both thumbs, attention must be paid to coordinating their action, and their pressure must be identical. Be sure that the thumbs meet the skin squarely. Have the other four fingers slightly spread apart, with knuckles slightly bent so that during the rubbing the fingers do not touch the skin. Rub with a circular motion, moving mainly from the wrist. Generally, this method is used for headache, or poor eyesight, rubbing on the head and face, the back of the neck, and on the *fengchi*[3] acupoints at either side of the base of the skull. (See Diagram 5.) On the back and the abdomen, the two-thumb circular rub can also be used. (See Diagram 6.)

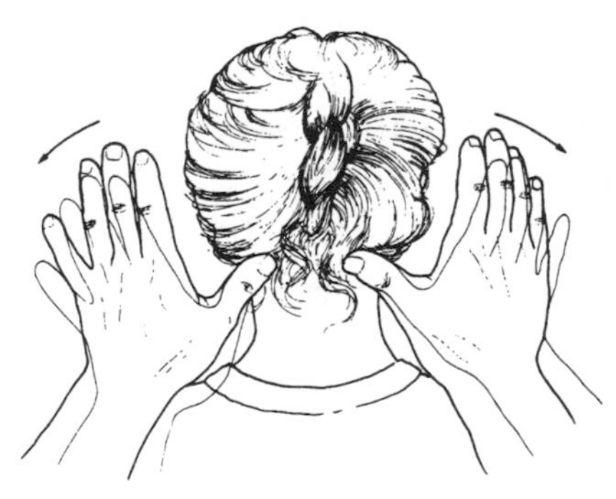

DIAGRAM 5

3. *Fengchi* acupoints: the depressions located at the base of the skull between the mastoid bone and the trapezius on each side. See Diagram 59, p. 250.

DIAGRAM 6

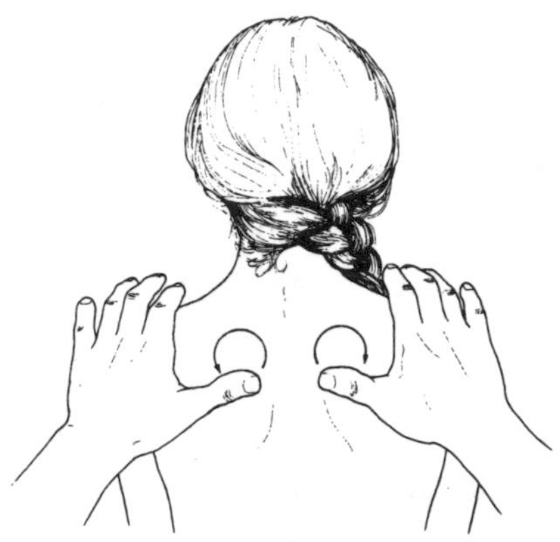

Palm Rub Method: The palm rub method is carried out with the palm of the hand lying flat on the body. Generally only one hand is used. Rub slowly in a clockwise direction, maintaining even pressure. (Diagram 7.) The palm rub is generally suited for larger areas of the body, and is used mostly on the chest, and abdomen, and the back. When indigestion occurs in children and the chest and ribs are bulging, the second rib section is rubbed. When a child has pain from overeating, the abdominal area can be rubbed. For lumbar strain, the lower back region can be rubbed.

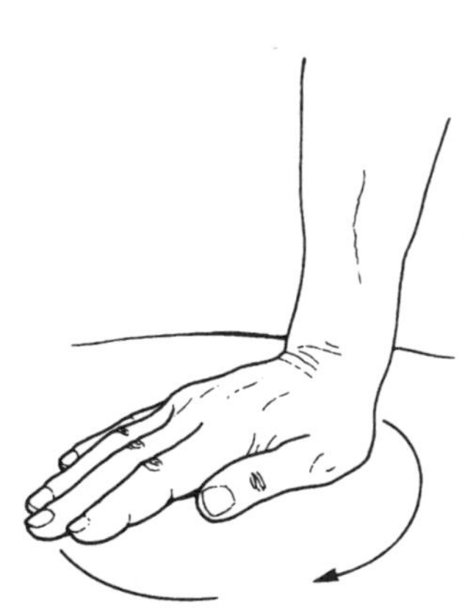

DIAGRAM 7

Palm-Heel Rub Method: Rub with some force, using the muscular pads on either side of the base of the palm. Keep the fingers and the thumb raised upward off the skin surface, with all the finger joints slightly bent. Swing left and right from

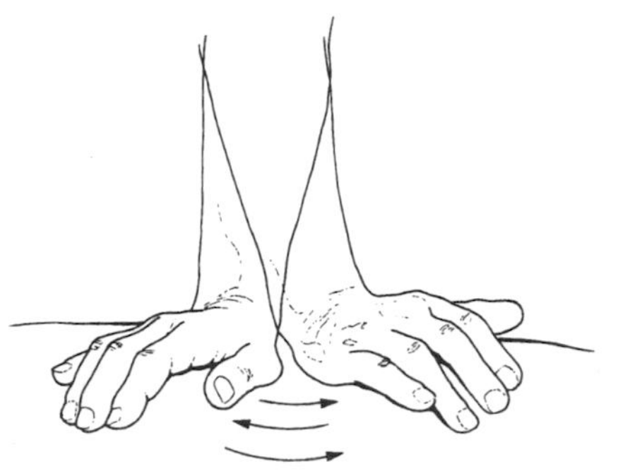

DIAGRAM 8

the wrist. (Diagram 8.) Both hands can be used alternately. Push forward at the same time as you swing from left to right at a rate as fast as 100 to 200 times a minute. The palm-heel rub is good for the lower back region, as in cases of backache or flu. When these are present, the lower back region is massaged up and down. This technique produces a sensation of warmth, making the patient feel comfortable and relaxed.

3. Push Method

In the push method either the fingers and thumb or the palm is used to push back and forth or left and right on the skin. The depth that the massage reaches will depend on the degree of force used. It can be as shallow as the subcutaneous tissues and the muscles, or as deep as the bones and internal organs. During massage, the force applied should be gradually increased from light to heavy. The amount of force used is determined by the nature of the ailment and the individual characteristics of the patient. Especially with those who are receiving their first massage treatment, frequent inquiries about how the person feels should be made, as well as observations of his or her reactions, in order to allow the proper adjustments. Frequency is generally 50–150 times a minute, beginning slowly, and gradually increasing speed.

Flat-Thumb Push Method: The flat-thumb push method is also called the "spiral push method." The pad of the thumb is used to stroke the skin surface, moving forward in a single direction. While pushing forward, the thumb has to exert pressure. But when moving back, the knuckles of the thumb must be slightly flexed and the back of the thumb carried back along the skin to the starting place. On the forward push, the knuckles of the other fingers should be slightly bent. On the return, extend them straight. Do not apply any force with the fingers, but use them only to help maintain position. (See Diagram 9.) Repeat over and over again, increasing speed.

DIAGRAM 9

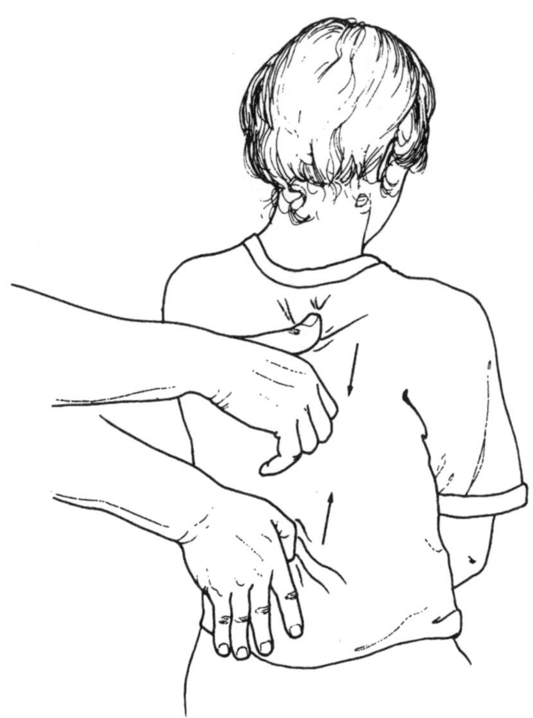

Skill in this technique must be developed with long practice, so that the fingers and the thumb become strong enough, and the joints of the fingers, the thumb, and the wrist become very flexible. Then the force of massage can be varied exactly as desired. The flat-thumb push can be done with one hand or with both hands alternately or simultaneously. When both thumbs are used simultaneously, they go to the left and to the right from a meridional acupoint. This technique is also called the "divergent push method."

The flat-thumb push method has wide application. It can be applied to the head, the back, or the limbs. In general, it is most often used in the head and back areas, as shown in Diagrams 9 and 10. Where pain is present in the forehead, the divergent push method can be applied at the *yintang*[4] and *zuanzhu*[5] acupoints of the brow ridge. The divergent push method is also applied on the shoulder and at the *dazhui*[6] acupoint. There is another type of divergent-push method called the "muscle-dividing" method. This utilizes a force deep enough to reach the muscular layer. In this case the divergent push follows the direction of the musculature. This pushing technique has been found most effective in sprains of the back and the loin.

DIAGRAM 10

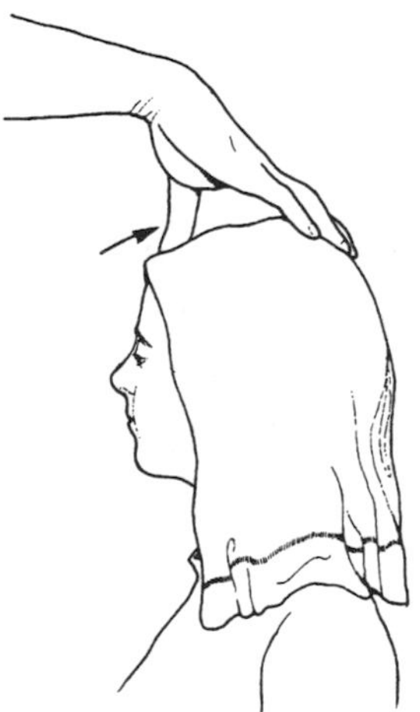

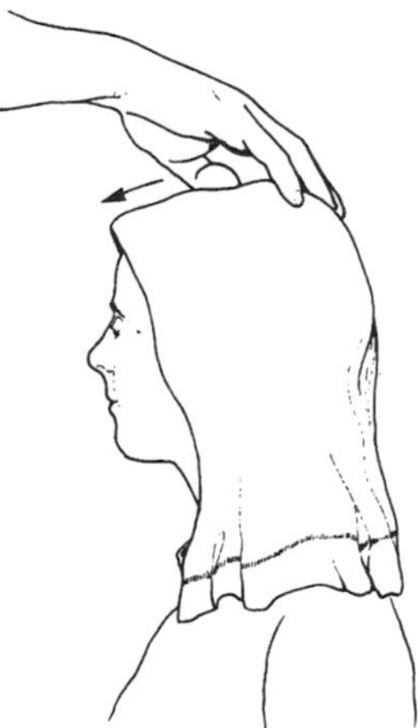

4. *Yintang* acupoint: a point situated between the eyebrows. See Diagram 58, p. 248.
5. *Zuanzhu* acupoint: a point located at the medial end of the eyebrow. See Diagram 59, p. 250
6. *Dazhui* acupoint: a point between the spinous process of the 7th cervical vertebra and that of the 1st thoracic vertebra. See Diagram 59, p. 250.

b) Side-of-the-thumb Push Method is also termed the "*shaoshang*[7] push method": This technique resembles the flat-thumb push. The only difference between them is that when pushing out, the force is applied with the lateral surface of the thumb (i.e., the *shaoshang* acupoint). This method of massage is often used on the *pitu*[8] line in the thumb and the *sanguan*[9] line of the forearm, and also on the head and limbs (when the extremities are in a state of paralysis).

c) The Thumb-Tip Push Method: This kind of manipulation is usually employed on an acupoint, or on the main site of pain in an illness. During the pushing, the tip of one thumb is used. It moves such a small amount, that it appears to have been attached to the acupoint. The wrist is bent and hangs downward. The joints of the thumb bend and extend quickly. Force is applied with both the wrist and the thumb, enough to reach into the tissues.

As a rule, this method is done with one hand, or with both hands alternately. Both hands can also be used simultaneously, as shown in Diagram 11. Enough force should be applied to reach down to the vital energy. Tapping the vital energy[10] is the main requirement for restoring a deficient, diseased body to health. Select the acupoints or pain sites to be massaged, establish their locations precisely, and then proceed to apply the thumb-tip push to them one by one in a definite order. The thumb-tip moves quickly, making a rotating motion at the same time. This method is, therefore, also called the "typing-up method." This kind of technique is widely used clinically, with considerable success in tapping vital energy.

7. *Shaoshang:* an acupoint on the outer side of the thumb, at the lower corner of the nail.
8. *Pitu:* a line along the base of the thumb. See Diagram 61, p. 255.
9. *Sanguan:* a line along the radial side of the forearm. See Diagram 61, p. 255.
10. Vital energy: *Qi (chi),* the life-giving energy believed in Chinese traditional medicine to flow through the body in a system similar to the circulatory and nervous systems. Disturbance of the flow causes disease, and is relieved by acupuncture or massage of the acupoints. Most acupoints are located on meridians of the life-energy system.

DIAGRAM 11 DIAGRAM 12

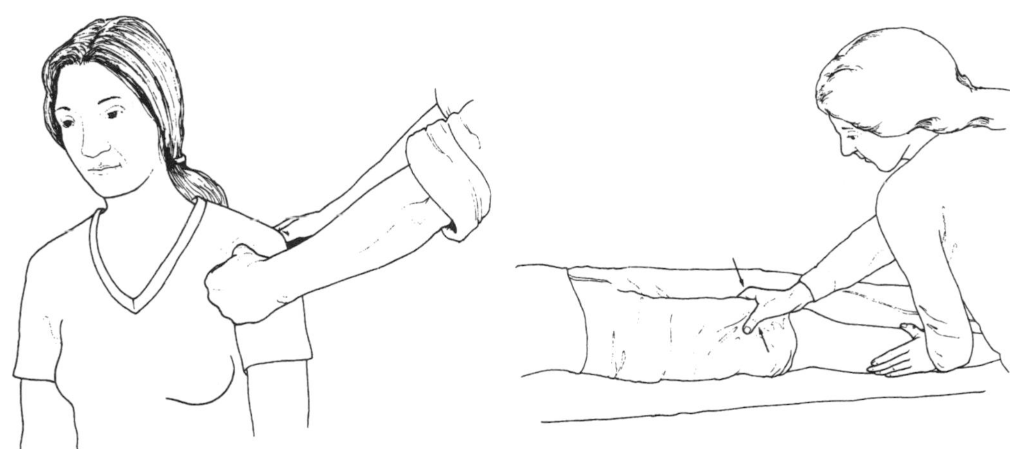

Flat-Palm Push Method: Push with the palm flat on the skin surface. The pushing is usually carried out from the farthest end of a limb towards the trunk. When administered on the chest or abdomen, it must follow the rise and fall of breathing. Generally this method is divided into two types: pushing with an expiration and pushing to cause expiration. Pushing with an expiration does not start until the patient starts to breathe out. Then at the end of the expiration, the hand is immediately released and drawn back, and pushing is discontinued until the next expiration. This is carried out again and again in a repeated sequence. In pushing to cause expiration, the patient's breathing follows the pushing action. Pushing forcefully causes expiration, and releasing and withdrawing causes inspiration. The latter technique works well to improve function of the respiratory system, and therefore is applicable to the patient affected with incapacity of function of the respiratory system.

Palm-Heel Push Method: Push forcefully on the skin, using the muscular pads on either side of the heel of the hand. In the course of pushing forward, these muscular pads are used to pinch the area gradually tighter and tighter. (See Diagram

12.) The pushing generally goes from the farthest end of a limb towards the trunk, returning to the original position after the action is completed to begin again.

This kind of massage is usually done on the limbs, and is divided into the slow push and smooth push, depending on the amount of force used and the speed of the pushing. When the slow push is used, the speed is slower and there is less force. In the smooth push the speed is faster and there is greater force: after a swift push, the hand is at once withdrawn from the limb, brought back to the starting point, and the push is repeated. This procedure is repeated over and over again. The smooth push method can effectively reach down into the muscles and enhance muscular stimulation.

4. Grasp Method

The grasp method is a type of massage that involves using the fingers to grasp and lift the muscle.

It is usually combined with acupoint massage. The grasping and lifting movements are done comparatively quickly. Applying the grasp to an area 2–3 times is usually sufficient. The amount of strength applied in grasping should result in the patient experiencing a feeling of soreness and swelling during massage, and after massage a loose, easy feeling. If pain is felt after the grasping, this shows that the force used was too great.

The grasping method is divided into three different types: the three-finger grasp, five-finger grasp, and shaking grasp.

Three-Finger Grasp Method: To grasp with the thumb, index, and third fingers is sufficient for small areas, such as the *jianjing*[11] point on the shoulder (see Diagram 13), the *weizhong*[12] point at the back of the knee, and the back of the neck.

11. *Jianjing:* an acupoint at the highest point on the shoulder. See Diagram 59, p. 250.
12. *Weizhong:* an acupoint in the back of the knee. See Diagram 60, p.252.

DIAGRAM 13

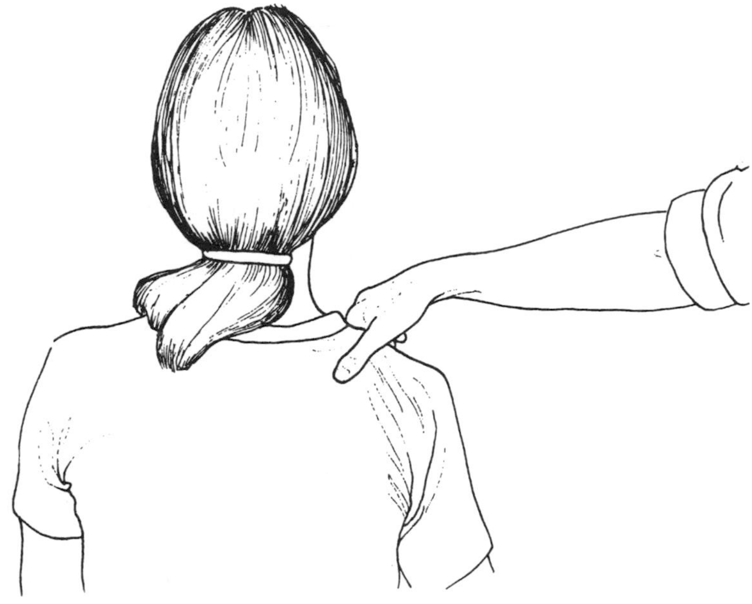

Five-Finger Grasp Method: This type of grasp uses the thumb and the four fingers, and is suitable for large, muscular areas, such as the front of the thigh (the musculus quadriceps femoris) and the back of the calf (the musculus gastrocnemius).

Shaking Grasp Method: After grasping with the fingers, do a light shaking, gradually allowing the fingers grasping the muscle to loosen. This is suitable for massage of the abdominal region.

Muscle-snapping method: This is a special type of massage technique. It is similar to the grasp method, but the manipulation is much stronger, and the degree of stimulation is greater. It is used with muscles such as the biceps and triceps of the arm and the outer hamstrings. With the thumb, index, and middle fingers, grasp the muscle by the intermuscular septum, either at its thickest point or near the muscle tendon, and draw it to one side. Having drawn it to a certain point, let it slip from between the fingers, like drawing a bow and shooting arrows. A snapping sound will then be heard and the patient will have a strong feeling of soreness and swelling, which is soon converted to a light, loose sensation.

The method can only be used on one muscle 1–2 times. It should be followed by some other methods of massage to relieve the strong stimulation and produce relaxation.

This method is suitable for injuries to the soft tissues and for rheumatic disorders, especially for muscular strains, rheumatic muscle pains, etc.

5. Roll Method

The roll method is a form of massage where the back of the hand is rolled over the body. It can be done with one hand, with both hands alternately, or with both hands simultaneously. With the hand in a loose fist, use the side of the hypothenar pad along with the upper part of the fifth metacarpal joint to contact the area to be massaged. Press down with some force, while making a vigorous backward motion. At this moment the fingers should quickly be slightly spread apart to add force to the movement. The points of force must all lie in the metacarpal joints of the back of the hand. In this method many back-and-forth rolling movements are made, and the application of force must be even and rhythmic. The rolling hand should seem attached to the patient's body; it should not jump around or strike the patient.

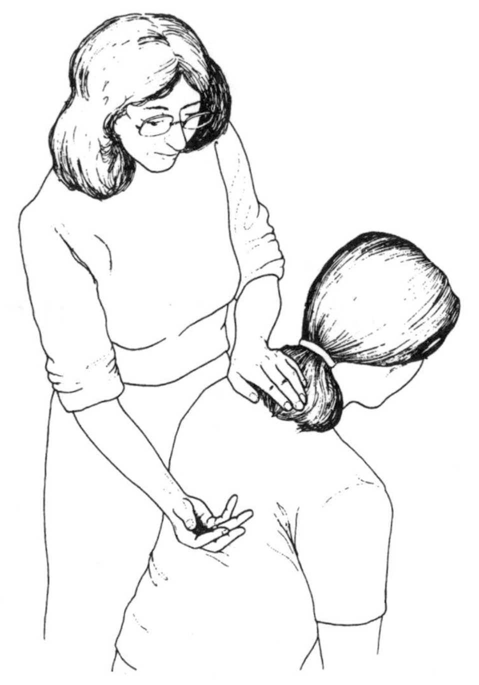

DIAGRAM 14

During the rolling the hand should gradually keep moving forward, as shown in Diagram 14. This method is properly applied to larger areas, such as the back, hip, leg, and shoulder, etc. Since the force applied goes so deep, it is best used on the spots where the muscle and soft tissues are thick. Though this method can be used independently, it is generally combined with other techniques. For example, at the very beginning of the massage, the rub and the knead methods may be used, and the roll method can follow them.

6. Dig Method

The dig method of massage involves a finger or fingers deeply digging into a certain part of the body or into a meridian point. It is also called the "finger-needle method." In massage therapy it is both unique and one of the most commonly used techniques. Where the dig method is performed, the practitioner has to trim his fingernails. The dig should be strong enough to result in the patient's feeling a sore, swelling sensation.

The dig method is divided into the single-finger dig, bent-finger dig, and finger-cut methods.

Single Finger Dig Method: The tip of the thumb or middle finger is used to press into the patient's flesh. When the middle finger is used, it is extended straight out and held tightly between the thumb and the index finger. The tip of the finger digs into a selected acupoint, most often one in the head or neck area, such as the *fengchi*[13] point at the back of the neck. (See Diagram 15.) When the thumb is used, the interphalangeal joint of

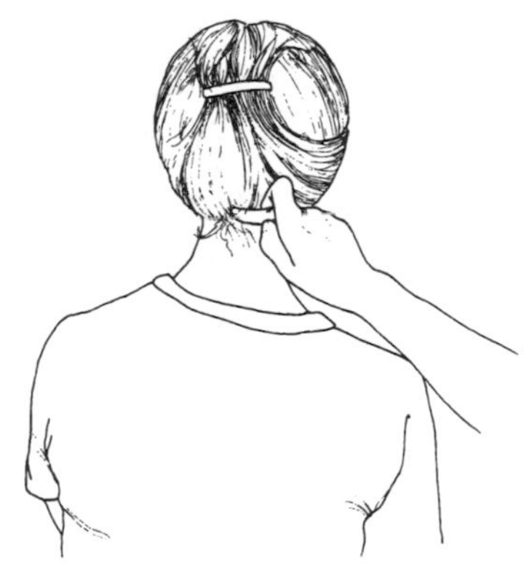

DIAGRAM 15

13. *Fengchi:* acupoints located at the base of the skull, behind the ears. See Diagrams 57 and 59, pp. 246 and 250.

the thumb is half bent, and the fingers are also bent to add strength to the dig. The thumb tip digs into a selected acupoint. This method is often used on the limbs, at acupoints such as *hegu*[14], *neiguan*[15] and *chu san li* or *zusanli*[16]. In children, dig massage is applied at *neilaogong*[17], *yiwofeng*[18] and the greater and lesser *hengwen*[19].

No matter what kind of a single-finger dig is applied, force must be exerted gradually, making the finger-tip press in, but avoiding any sudden force. After the dig has reached the vital energy, that is, when a flow of energy can be felt, continue to press for ½–1 minute. Vibration can be applied at the same time to intensify the stimulation. Then gradually relax the pressure and use the kneading method to soften the reaction resulting from the stimulation.

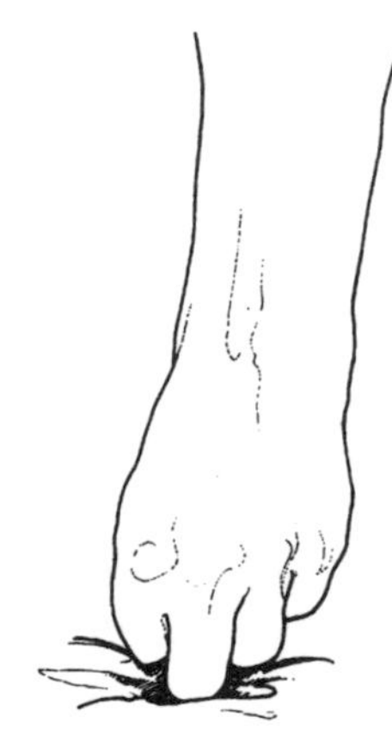

DIAGRAM 16

Bent-Finger Dig Method: First, the middle finger is bent. Then the first knuckle above the hand is used to press into the body. (See Diagram 16.) During this procedure the thumb has to press against the last knuckle of the middle finger. The index and the fourth fingers are also bent, and the bent middle finger is pinched firmly into place, as shown in Diagram 16. The force of this dig method is very great, and it digs quite deeply. It is suitable for places where the muscle is comparatively thick. When the single-finger method fails to obtain a reaction, this method is usually

14. *Hegu:* an acupoint on the back of the hand, between the bones of the thumb and index finger. See Diagrams 57 and 59, pp.246 and 250.
15. *Neiguan:* an acupoint on the underside of the forearm, above the wrist. See Diagrams 57 and 58, pp. 246 and 248.
16. *Zusanli* or *Chu san li:* an acupoint on the outer edge of the tibia, below the knee. See Diagram 60, p. 252.
17. *Neilaogong:* an acupoint on the middle of the palm. See Diagram 61, p255.
18. *Yiwofeng:* an acupoint on the back of the wrist. See Diagram 61, p. 255.
19. Greater *hengwen,* lesser *hengwen:* acupoints in the fold of the wrist (greater) and in the folds at the bases of the fingers (lesser). See Diagram 61, p255.

found effective; for instance at such acupoints as *huantiao,*[20] *geshu,*[21] *ganshu,*[22] *pishu,*[23] and *weishu.*[24]

Finger-Cut method: Use the end of the thumb to lightly and dexterously push along the skin in a dense pattern of strokes. (See Diagram 17.) As a rule this method is used only where the tissues are swollen. Since the swelling is pushed ahead of the finger, the movement must be toward the heart. Where a sprained joint is accompanied by swelling, this method can often cause the swelling to immediately disappear. The amount of force used must be small and the speed of stroke slow. Especially with any tender pressure point, be certain to avoid increasing the pain at the injured site.

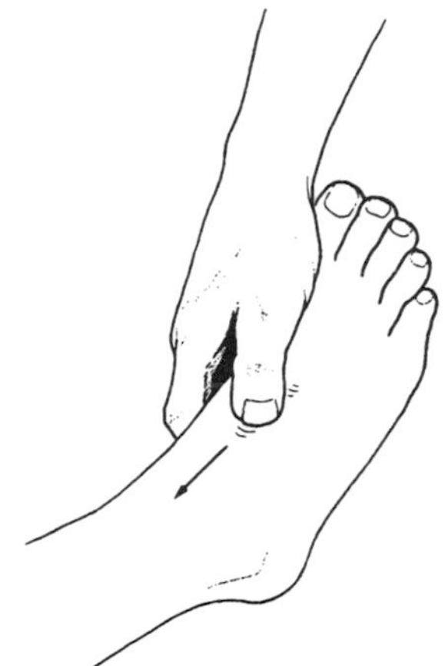

DIAGRAM 17

7. Pluck Method

The pluck method is a type of massage which uses the hand to pluck at the muscles. It is also called the "pull method." This method is usually applied with one hand, using the side of the thumb and the tips of the index and third fingers to grasp the muscle at its tendinous portion and pluck with the appropriate

20. *Huantiao:* an acupoint on the buttocks. See Diagram 59, p. 250.
21. *Geshu:* an acupoint on the back, beside the lower end of the spinous process of the 7th thoracic vertebra. See Diagram 59, p. 250.
22. *Ganshu:* near the 9th thoracic vertebra. See Diagram 59, p. 250.
23. *Pishu:* near the 11th thoracic vertebra. See Diagram 59, p. 250.
24. *Weishu:* near the 12th thoracic vertebra. See Diagram 59, p250.

amount of force. (See Diagram 18.) For instance, at the long and short origins of the biceps muscle of the arm, or the muscle on the inside edge of the scapula, this massage-method is applied 1–3 times, to the degree that the patient feels as much of a sore, swollen sensation as he or she can stand. This will produce a definite effect of relaxing muscle tension or freeing adhesion. There is also another type of pluck method, called the energy-system pluck method, which is very similar to this one.

DIAGRAM 18

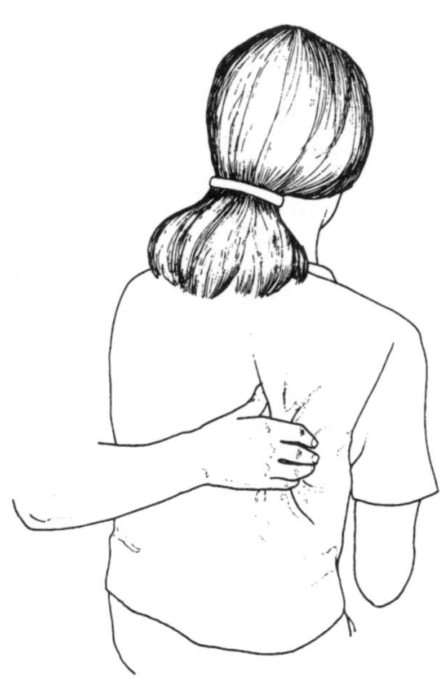

8. Kneading Method

The kneading method is a type of massage which involves making a kneading motion on the skin with the fingers or the palm. The palm and fingers are never withdrawn from contact with the skin, and the subcutaneous tissue in the area is allowed to slide along with them. Normally, this method is applied with one hand. The force used is relatively light, reaching only to the subcutaneous tissue. It has the effect of releasing the stimulation produced by stronger manipulations and of allaying pain. It is classified into the thumb kneading and palm kneading methods.

Thumb Kneading Method: The palmar surface of the thumb is pressed tightly against the skin and moved with a circular kneading motion. This method is suitable for restricted areas and acupoints. It is used in conjunction with the single-finger dig massage to relieve the sore, swelling reaction that method gives rise to. The force used in kneading should be increased from light to heavy, and then decreased from heavy to light again.

Palm Kneading Method: With the heel of the palm, or the whole palm, pressing closely against the skin, knead with a rotating motion, going either clockwise or counterclockwise. This is appropriate for larger areas, such as the abdominal region (see Diagram 19), or the back. In the course of palm kneading, though the palm does not shift position, the range of the sliding movement of the subcutaneous tissue is allowed to become wider and wider. Also the force applied gradually becomes heavier and heavier. The rate of frequency in the palm kneading method is generally slow, about 50–60 times per minute.

DIAGRAM 19

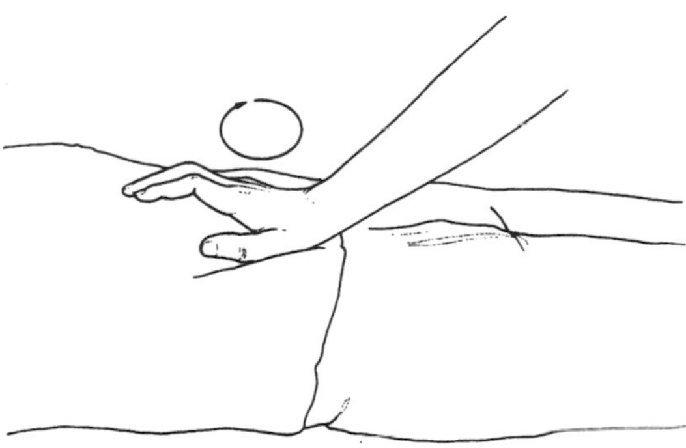

9. Vibrate Method

This method uses a fingertip, or the palm, to apply vibration to a part of the body or to an acupoint. In this method, the practitioner's arm, especially the muscles of forearm and hand, must exert a strong static force that becomes concentrated at the fingertip, or in the palm, making the massaged area vibrate. It is important that the vibration rate be high, and that the force used be great. Most often, one hand is used, but two hands can also be used simultaneously. This method comprises the finger and palm vibrate techniques.

Finger Vibrate Method: Vibration is applied with the thumb or the middle finger to the tissue in the area to be massaged. The posture of the hand is similar to the one used in the single-finger dig method. This method is often used following the single-finger dig. It is employed to step up stimulation after the sore, swelling reaction produced by the dig method. Continue vibration for about ½–1 minute. The finger vibrate method is also applied to such acupoints as *hegu*[25] (see Diagram 20), *neiguan*[26] and *chu san li* or *zusanli*[27]. It is also used on acupoints in the abdominal region, but here it must always follow the rise and fall of breathing. Apply the pressure with expiration; release the pressure with inspiration.

DIAGRAM 20

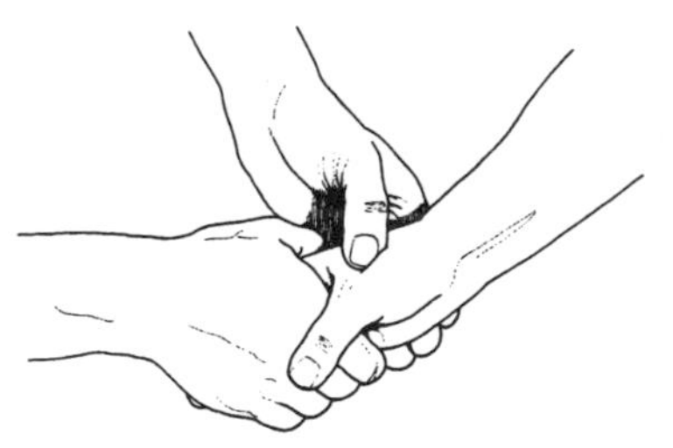

Palm Vibrate Method: The vibration is applied with the flat surface of the palm pressed against the skin. This method is appropriate for larger areas such as the thigh, lower back, etc. It can bring about muscle-relaxation and relieve pain.

Electric Vibrate Method: As it is necessary to apply a prolonged static force, vibration involves great physical effort by the therapist. To ease this burden, an electric vibratory apparatus may be used instead of the hand.

25. *Hegu:* an acupoint on the back of the hand between the thumb and index finger. See Diagrams 57 and 59, pp. 246 and 250.
26. *Neiguan:* an acupoint on the underside of the forearm, two inches above the crease of the wrist in the mid-line. See Diagrams 57 and 58, pp. 246 and 248.
27. *Zusanli* or *chu san li:* an acupoint just below the knee. See Diagram 60, p. 252.

10. Drag Method

The drag method involves pressing down on the skin with the fingers and then drawing them to one side with steady pressure. It is generally done with the flats of both thumbs simultaneously. The special characteristic of this method is the use of even, sustained pressure and a slow, gradual movement.

For headache, this method can be combined with other massage methods. The thumbs are dragged apart from the *yintang*[28] acupoint between the eyebrows toward the *taiyang*[29] acupoints in the temples. (See Diagram 21.) Then they are either dragged along both sides of the head back to the *fengchi*[30] acupoints on either side of the base of the skull or to the *tinggong*[31] acupoints in front of the ears. Repeat 2–3 times. The patient usually feels his head and eyes become lighter and clearer than before. This method can also be used to reduce swelling.

DIAGRAM 21

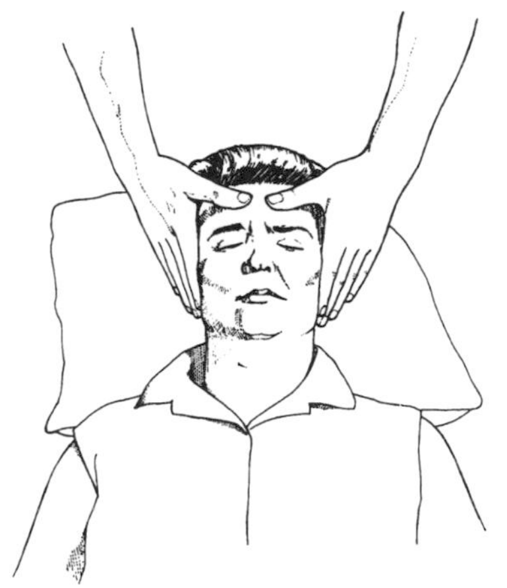

Muscle-Straightening Method: This massage technique is similar to the drag method. The only difference between them is that the muscle-straightening method is done more forcefully, to reach down into the muscle. The flat of one or both thumbs (or of the thumb and index finger, or of the middle finger) is used. With an even and continuous pressure, follow the muscle direction from up to down, or from up diagonally down. The

28. *Yintang:* See Diagram 58, p. 248.
29. *Taiyang:* See Diagram 57, p. 246.
30. *Fengchi:* See Diagrams 57 and 59, pp. 246 and 248.
31. *Tinggong:* See Diagram 57, p. 246.

force exerted by the fingers must be steady and their movement slow, and their force must not be relaxed during the movement. A tense muscle can be brought to complete relaxation by going down the muscle fibers several times.

11. Chafe Method

The chafe method is a type of massage which produces friction on the skin, using the fingers or the palm. The force used in this method must depend upon the reaction of the patient's skin. It is not desirable to exert too heavy a force. The purpose is just to reach as far as the skin and the subcutaneous tissue. The rate of speed of the movements is generally more than 100 times a minute. It is done with only one hand, and can be divided into two types, the finger chafe method and the palm-edge chafe method:

Finger Chafe Method: This method involves rubbing the skin with the fingers. It is particularly useful for a paralyzed limb. When the finger chafe method is applied to a paralyzed finger or toe, the practitioner holds the limb firmly in place with his left hand, fits the three middle fingers of his right hand around the affected finger or toe and chafes back and forth. In this way, the three sides of the finger can be rubbed simultaneously, as shown in Diagram 22.

DIAGRAM 22

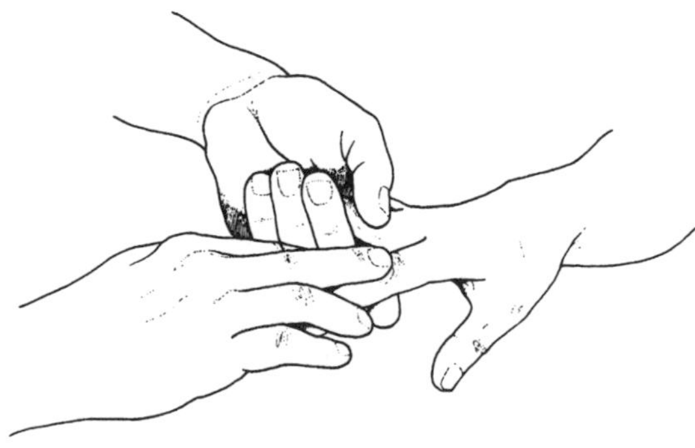

Palm-Edge Chafe Method: The outer edge of the palm is used to chafe the skin. This method is often applied on either side of the back in cases of common cold, rheumatic pain, and gastroenteric disorders. The patient takes a sitting position, while the practitioner stands in front. This massage can be applied directly on the skin or through the clothing. Go up and down along both sides of the back with a fast sawing motion, continuing until the patient's skin becomes red. (See Diagram 23.)

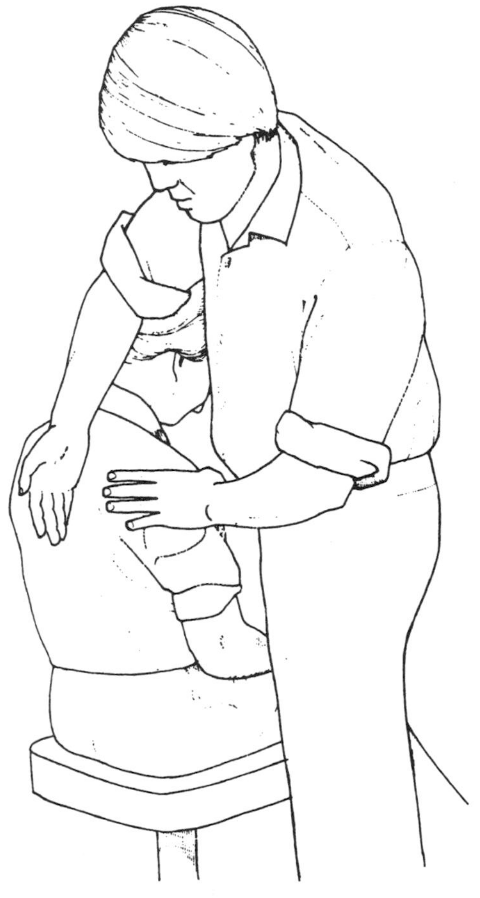

DIAGRAM 23

12. Rub-Roll Method

The rub-roll method is a form of massage where the affected limb of the patient is taken between the two hands and rubbed with a rolling motion. It is suitable only for the limbs. The action of this massage can reach as far as the subcutaneous tissue, the muscle, and even the bones. During the course of massage, increase speed from slow to fast, then decrease it from fast to slow again. The method is divided into the palm rub-roll and palm-edge rub-roll methods:

Palm Rub-Roll Method: The left and right palms are placed on either side of the affected limb and rubbed back and forth. If the upper limb is to be rubbed, the patient should be seated, and the arm will naturally hang downward, as shown in

Diagram 24. Or else, if sitting opposite the practitioner, the patient can rest the arm upon the practitioner's shoulder.

DIAGRAM 24

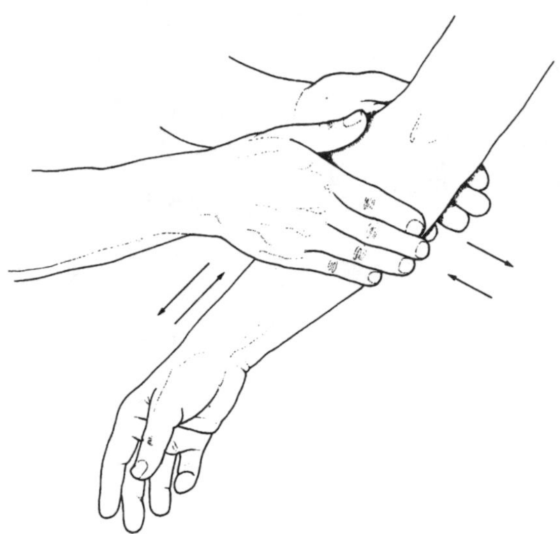

When the lower limb is to be rubbed, have the patient take a half-seated position and bend the knee. Or if the patient is lying on a bed, have the patient's leg rest on the practitioner's shoulder. In the case of the arm, the rub-rolling goes back and forth from shoulder to elbow and elbow to shoulder. With the lower limb the motion goes from knee to hip and hip to knee.

b) Palm-edge Rub-Roll Method: Apply the rub-roll with the outer edges of the palms on either side of the limb to be massaged. The body positions of both patient and therapist are similar to those in the palm rub-roll method. The effects of the palm-edge rub-roll can reach deeper into muscle, and the patient will experience a sore, swelling sensation.

13. Pinch Method

The pinch method is a type of massage employing the fingers to squeeze and pinch muscle and ligamentous tissue. Pinch the flesh with the thumb on top and the rest of the fingers below and then roll the thumb and fingers over one another while moving forward, following the outline of the muscle. The right and left hands can be used alternately or simultaneously. The pinch method is divided into the three-finger pinch and the five-finger pinch.

Three-Finger Pinch Method: The thumb, forefinger, and middle finger are used. Pinch the muscle between the flats of the thumb and fingers and then use wrist-action to pinch and roll forward at the same time. This method is suitable for smaller areas, such as the fingers, palm, and forearm. (See Diagram 25.) In comparatively confined areas, the fingertips should be used to dig deep enough into the tissues for the massage to be effective.

DIAGRAM 25

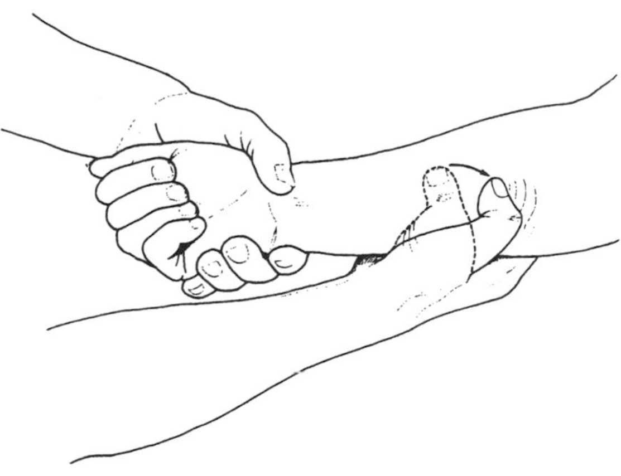

Five-Finger Pinch: This process is performed with all five fingers. The method is similar to that of the three-finger pinch. It is best suited to larger areas such as the thigh, leg, shoulder, etc.

Spinal Pinch Method: This method is often used with children. With the thumbs and forefingers of both hands, pinch the skin and subcutaneous tissues on either side of the spinal column. Release the skin and subcutaneous tissues as you move upward, alternating hands. Go from the buttocks up to the shoulder and neck areas.

14. Tweak Method

The tweak method, also called the "twist method," is a form of massage using the thumb and index finger to pull up a part of the skin and subcutaneous tissues, and then quickly release them. In the course of this maneuver the hand holding the pinched tissue is made to turn slightly backwards, pulling the pinched tissues to one side, before quickly releasing them. (See Diagram 26.) At this moment a snapping sound is often heard. Continue tweaking the same skin in the same direction until redness appears. In severe cases the skin can be tweaked until it develops red blotches.

DIAGRAM 26

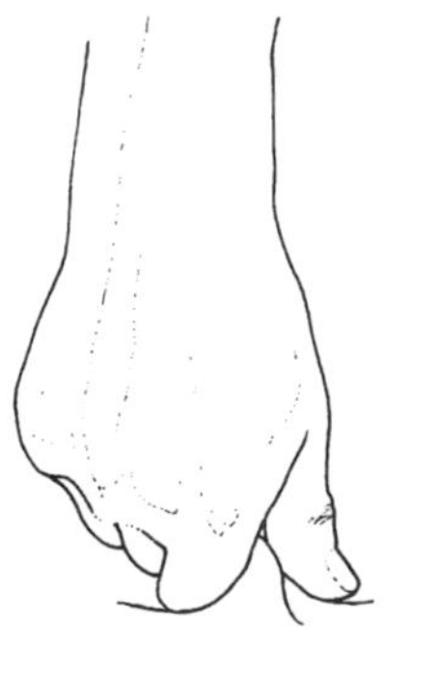

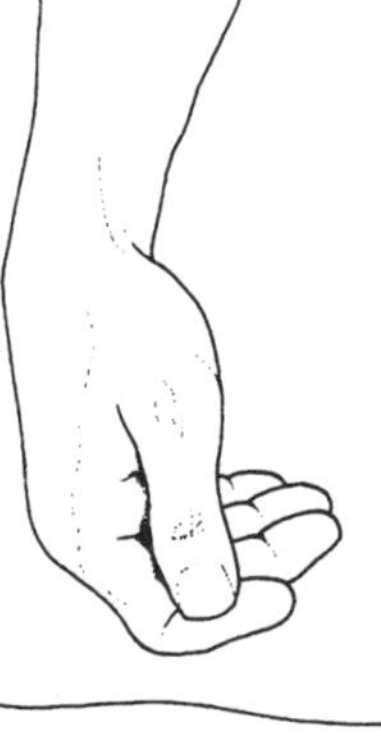

Tweaking with one hand is suitable for the back, neck, and abdominal areas. This method is widespread among the Chinese people and has been transmitted from generation to generation. The common cold, headache, and gastro-intestinal upset all respond well to it. It can also be used in some pediatric diseases, such as normal common colds and fever, disturbed digestion, etc.

When the tweak method is applied to children, generally both hands are used, and the palmar surfaces of the thumb and forefinger are held together like pincers. After the skin is pinched and twisted, it is immediately and smoothly released. In this way the two hands tweak and release alternately until the skin begins to show redness.

15. Flick Method

The flick method is performed by using a finger to flick against the body. The index finger is bent against the thumb or middle finger, and then flicked forcefully against the body. The strength of the spring-like strikes should go from light to heavy, but never to a degree that would give rise to any pain. It can suitably to be applied to any joint, flicking the soft tissue around the joint. (See Diagram 27.) It can be used to treat aching joints.

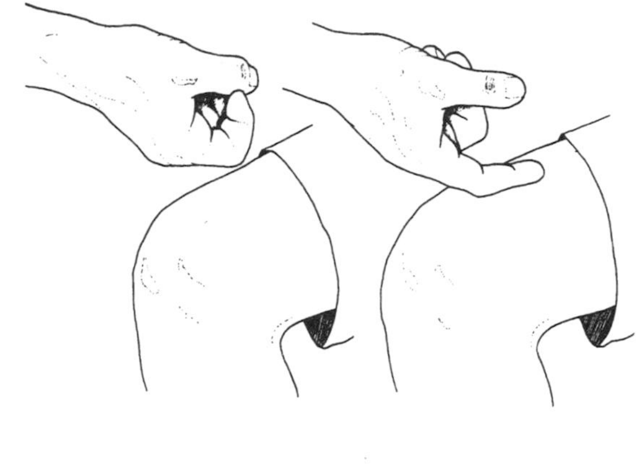

DIAGRAM 27

16. Knock Method

The knock method is a form of massage involving knocking on the tissue with the tips of the fingers. Force must be applied with both the wrist and the fingertips. The knocking must be dexterous, forceful, and elastic, and at the same time a conscious rhythm must be maintained. The knocking method gives rise to an oscillating force that can reach down to the bone. It is divided into the middle-finger knock and five-finger knock method:

Middle-Finger Knock Method: For this method the middle finger is half-bent, and the wrist is relaxed. The knocking then proceeds with a bend-extend motion. This method is appropriate for use all around the scalp area.

Five-Finger Knock Method: In this method the five fingers are drawn close to one another, the fingertips are held even with each other, and the wrist is relaxed. In order to carry out the knocking the fingers are repeatedly bent and extended. They strike the body in the same way that a chicken pecks grain. For this reason it is also called "the peck method." It is appropriate for use on all parts of the forehead. (Diagram 28.)

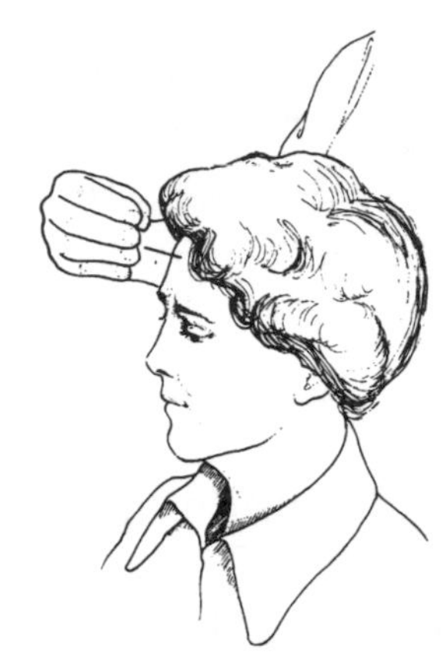

DIAGRAM 28

17. Pat Method

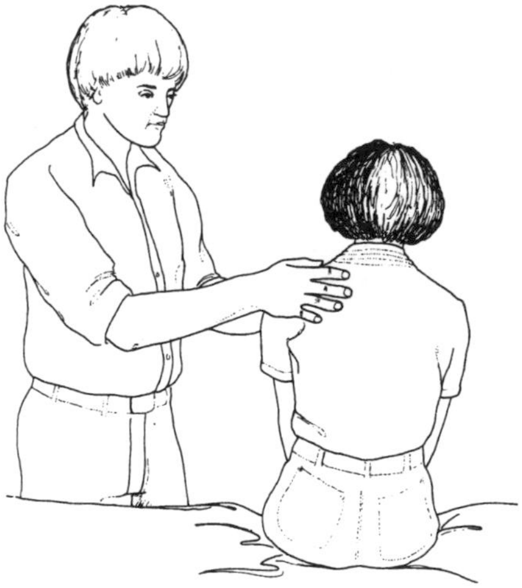

The pat method uses the fingers or the palm to lightly pat the body. It can be done with one hand or with both hands. The movement has to be dexterous and elastic. For this reason it requires that the wrist be exceptionally supple. When both hands are used, their movements must be coordinated. This method is classified into the finger pat, back-of-the-fingers pat, and palm pat methods.

Finger Pat Method: In this method, the fingers and thumb are spread wide apart. The fingers are slightly bent, and the palmar surfaces of the fingers and thumb are employed to lightly pat on the patient's body. (See Diagram 29.) It is appropriate for use on the back and chest areas, and is often used in the massage of children.

DIAGRAM 29

Back-of-the-Fingers Pat Method: Here the fingers are slightly spread apart, and the finger joints are slightly bent. The index, middle, ring, and little fingers are used to vigorously pat the body, as shown in Diagram 30. This method is suitable for the limbs and can also be used on the chest and back areas.

DIAGRAM 30

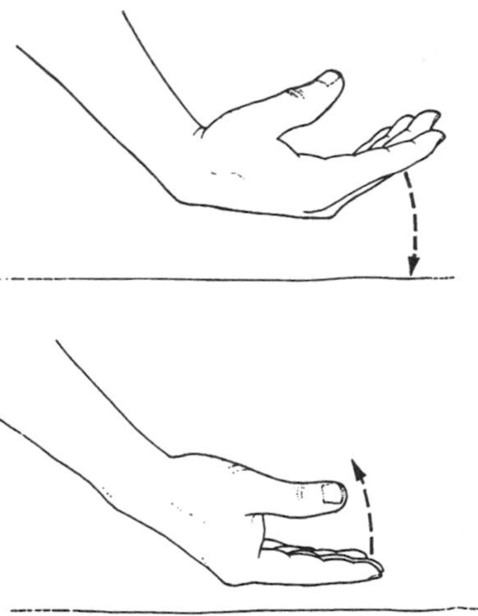

Palm Pat Method: Here the center of the palm has to be raised by flexing the metacarpal joints, and the fingers drawn close together, leaving a hollow in the palm with which to pat the body. This method is suitable for the back area.

18. Hammer Method

This is a type of massage which uses the fist to hammer on the body. The force used is heavier than that of the pat method and goes deeper into the muscles, joints, and bones. In this method the principal force comes from the wrist. Coordination and dexterity are required. The force used should be increased from light to heavy, while at the same time the blows remain elastic. The rate of speed is increased from slow to fast, or alternates between periods of slow and fast strokes. As a rule both hands are used simultaneously. This method is divided into the prone-fist hammer, upright-fist hammer, and palm-edge hammer methods, as follows.

Prone-Fist Hammer Method: Here both hands are held in loosely clenched fists. The second knuckles of the four fingers are all held even with each other, and used to exert a hammering force on the body. This method is appropriate for areas where there is fleshy, thick muscle, such as the thigh areas.

Upright-Fist Hammer Method: Here both hands are formed into clenched fists, with the fingers slightly spread apart. The thumb is bent and wrapped in the fist, or nests between the index and middle fingers. The fist is turned thumb upward, and the body is hammered with the fleshy part of the fist on the outer side of the palm. (See Diagram 31.) This method is suitable for the joint areas.

DIAGRAM 31 DIAGRAM 32

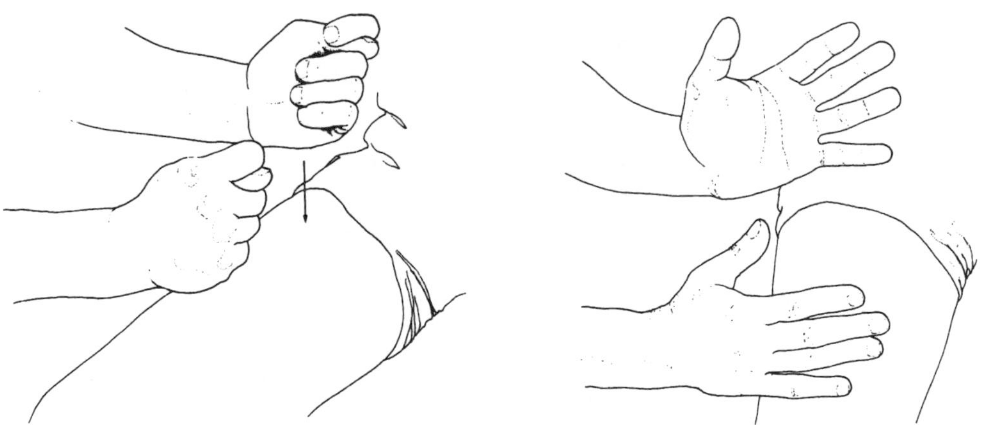

Palm-Edge Hammer Method: Here the fingers of both hands are extended and spread apart. The hammer massage is applied with the outer edge of the hand, as shown in Diagram 32. The method is appropriate for fleshy, muscular areas such as the thigh or the back.

Note: In order both to avoid tiring the therapist and to make the massage more comfortable for the patient, the hammering can be carried out with a mallet made from a piece of sponge rubber attached to a bamboo stick. Use two of these mallets, one in each hand.

19. Extension Method

The extension method is a form of massage which helps a malfunctioning joint to regain its normal extension. This technique can be classified as a form of passive manipulation. In this method the extent to which the affected joint can be moved must first be carefully tested. Then a slow, even, continuous force is applied to bring about the appropriate amount of extension. In general, this should not cause the patient any pain. A sudden force or violent extension must never be used. Before each treatment the amount of increased movement that is possible for the affected joint must be carefully estimated. The range of extension is gradually increased. For the manipulation, the practitioner and the patient must be properly and securely positioned. The most frequently used techniques are the shoulder-extension and elbow-extension methods.

Shoulder-Extension Method: In this method the patient takes a sitting position, while the practitioner stands in a half-crouch in front of him, with legs astride in the rider's position.[32] The affected limb rests on the back of the practitioner's neck, with the elbow resting on the practitioner's shoulder. The practitioner's hands are cupped over the patient's shoulder. (See Diagram 33 on next page.) The practitioner then slowly stands up, causing the patient's shoulder to abduct and bend forward to the appropriate extent. Maintain a fixed height for about 2–3 minutes before allowing the patient's shoulder to fall back. After a short pause the extension is repeated. The height of the second stretch may be slightly increased, but this must not be forced. The process should be repeated 3–5 times.

32. Rider's position (or stride stance): legs apart and crouching slightly, as if riding a horse.

DIAGRAM 33

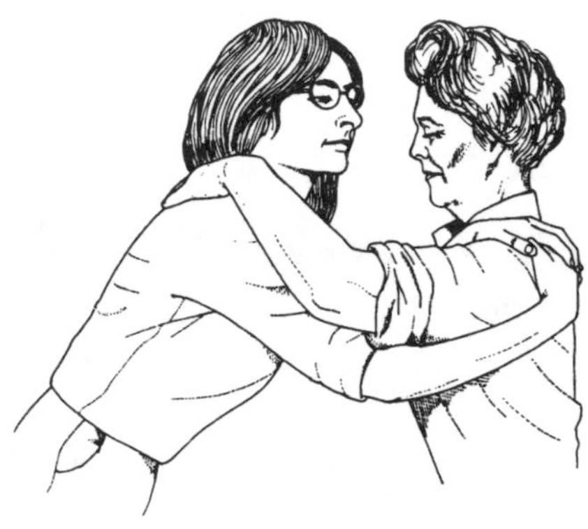

Elbow-Extension Method: In this method the patient sits opposite the practitioner. The practitioner cups the elbow of the affected arm, while the hand of the affected arm is pinned in the practitioner's armpit. The practitioner's other hand is placed on top of the affected shoulder. (See Diagram 34.) Then while pushing on the shoulder, the practitioner lifts up the patient's elbow, extending the joint. The degree of force used and amount of extension will depend upon the individual case, but violent force must be avoided.

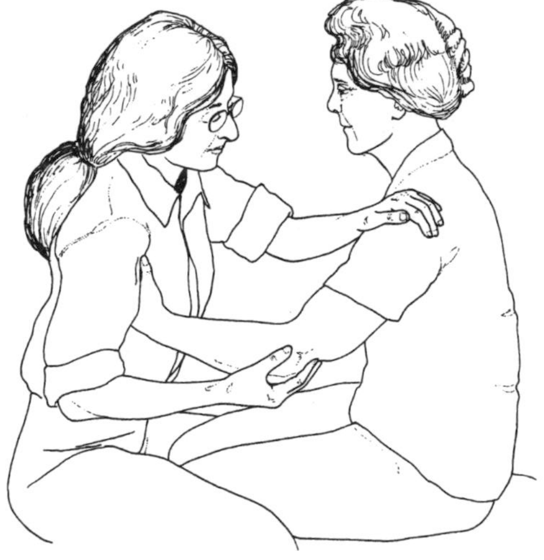

DIAGRAM 34

20. Bend Method

The bend method is a form of massage which helps a joint with impeded mobility to bend. It can be classified as a form of passive manipulation. In this method, force has to be applied with skill and restraint. It is usually applied to the lower extremities, such as the calf and hip.

Calf-Bend Method: Here the patient lies face down, and the practitioner stands beside him, on the side of the affected limb. The practitioner grasps the affected calf with one hand, while the other holds the sole of the patient's foot. Then the knee joint is gradually bent. (See Diagram 35.) The movements begin slowly, but gradually become faster. The extent of the bending must correspond with the degree of movement possible for the joint.

Hip-Bend Method: Here the patient lies on his/her back, while the practitioner stands beside the affected limb. One hand holds the patient's kneecap, while the other grasps the

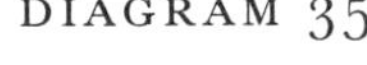

DIAGRAM 35

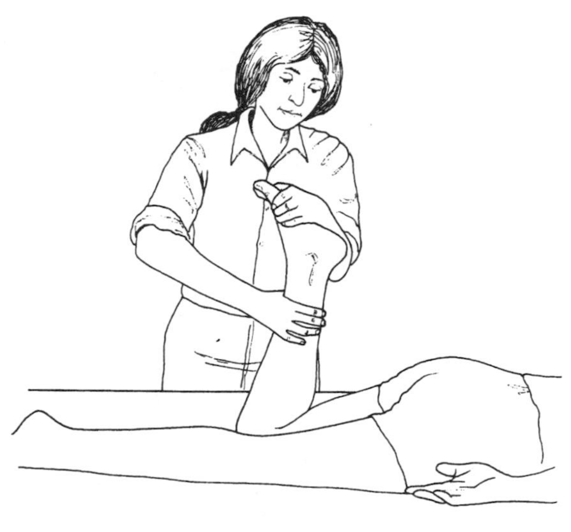

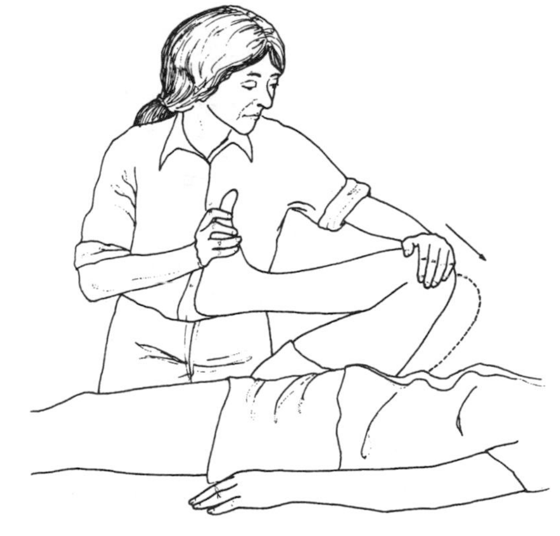

DIAGRAM 36

sole of the foot, and the hip, knee, and ankle are all made to bend at the same time. The practitioner then exerts a downward force to help the bending, the patient also tending actively to bend the limb. The thigh should be brought as close to the body as possible. (See Diagram 36.) The extent of the bending must correspond with the degree of movement possible for the joint.

Two-hip Bend Method: In this method the patient lies on his or her back, while the practitioner grasps the soles of the patient's feet with one hand, and with the other

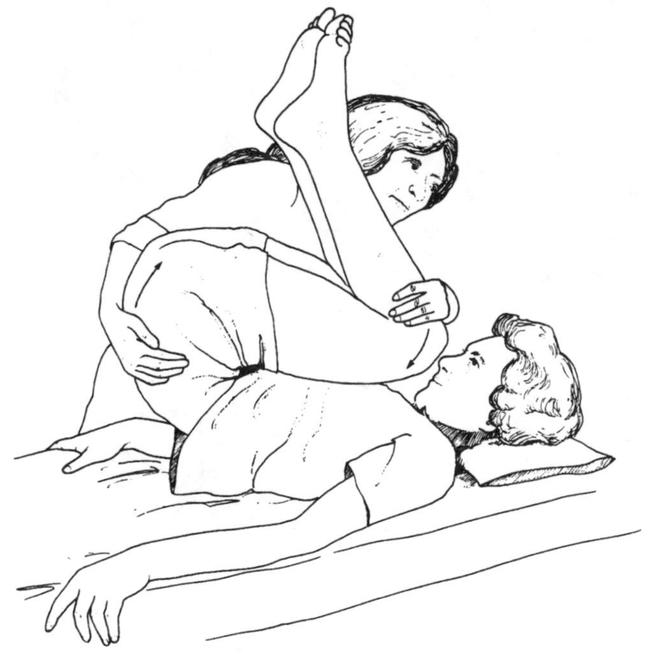

DIAGRAM 37

holds the kneecap area. The practitioner bends the knees and hips to a certain limit, and then elastically and rhythmically pushes forward. The extent to which the hips are bent may gradually be enlarged, bringing the thigh close to the abdominal wall. Next, the hand holding the feet is switched to the buttocks, and the whole body is bent. (Diagram 37.) Care must be taken to progress gradually and in the correct sequence, in accordance with the patient's potential mobility. As the hips are bent further, the amount of force used should gradually be increased. This manipulation not only promotes the mobility of the hip joint but also improves the ability of the spinal column to bend forward. Because of this, the method is appropriate in some cases of chronic low back pain and arthritic stiffness. In addition, it can be selectively applied in the case of protrusion of a lumbar intervertebral disk, where it can promote its return to its proper position.

21. Rotation Method

The rotation method is a form of massage involving rotation of a joint. It can be classified as a passive manipulation. It is often used to prevent and to treat functional disturbances of the rotatory movement of a joint. This method is applied to joints of all sizes from the knuckle joints to those as large as the joints in the lumbar and hip areas. Before applying this procedure, it is necessary to be familiar with the range of physiological movement in each joint and to observe in detail the state of joint mobility resulting from a disease. The direction of rotation is generally clockwise, and the speed should be slow rather than fast. The procedure for rotating the small joints in the hand, etc., is relatively simple. But when applying rotation to large joints, the patient has to be placed in a specific position.

The method is divided into the neck rotation, shoulder rotation, hip rotation , and lumbar rotation methods.

Neck Rotation Method: The patient takes a sitting position and the therapist stands behind him. The practitioner places one hand under the patient's jaw and the other on the top of his head, slowly swinging the neck from one side to the other with her hands. When the muscles are relaxed, and the neck is turned completely to one side, the therapist takes advantage of its tendency to turn back in the opposite direction and gives it a sudden and forceful twist in that opposite direction, though not more than 90° in extent (See Diagram 38.) This method should be applied only once at a time, and not repeated. After the neck has been twisted, the patient usually feels it suddenly more flexible and comfortable. This method is always used in torticollis (stiff neck).

DIAGRAM 38

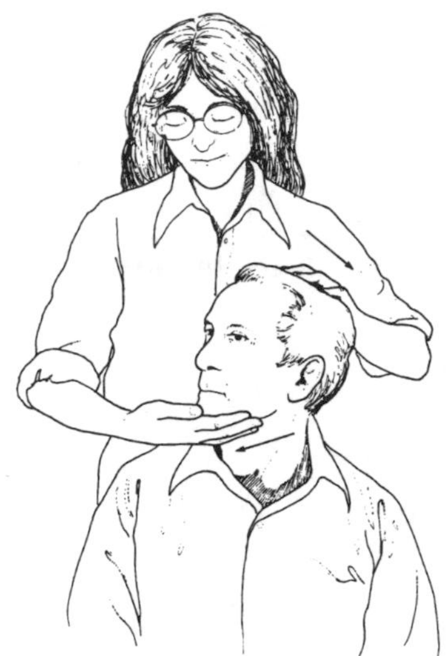

Shoulder Rotation Method, #1: The patient takes a sitting position. The practitioner stands firmly beside him with legs spread apart in the archer's position.[33] She grasps the patient's palm with one hand and holds his wrist with the other. First the patient's upper arm is pulled straight, then it is rotated. In the course of this rotation, the practitioner's hands must alternate with each other in holding the wrist area, never letting go. (See Diagram 39.)

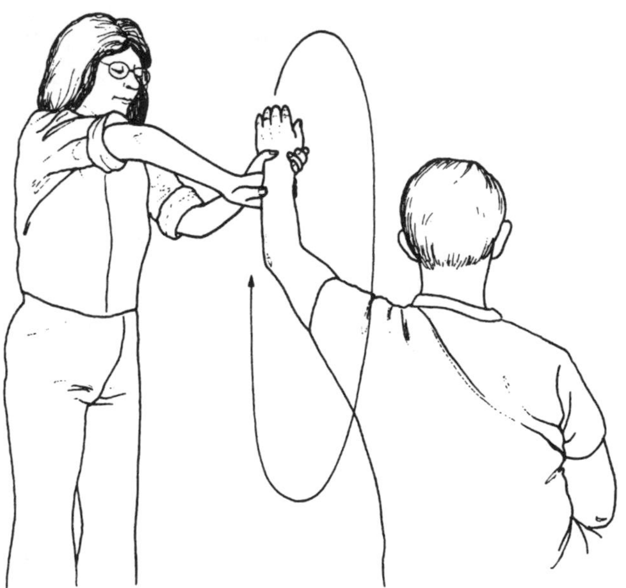

DIAGRAM 39

33. Archer's position: legs spread apart, one forward and one back, as if about to shoot with a bow and arrow.

DIAGRAM 40

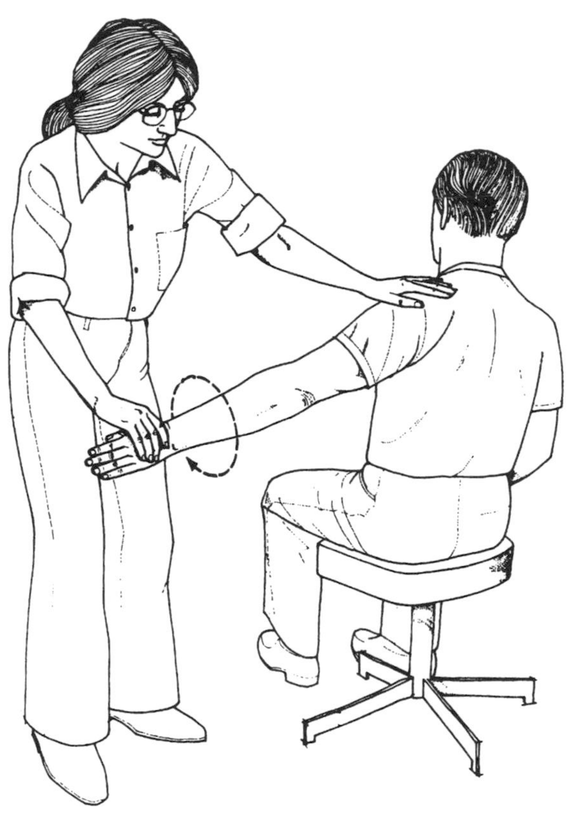

Shoulder Rotation Method, # 2: The patient sits with the elbow of the affected limb bent. The practitioner uses her own forearm and hand to support and hold the forearm of the affected arm, while her other hand presses on the patient's shoulder. She then rotates the shoulder clockwise and counterclockwise.

Shoulder Rotation Method, #3: The patient is seated with the affected arm relaxed and held out to one side. The practitioner grasps the hand of the affected arm with her own hand on the same side (i.e. her right hand for the patient's left hand, or vice versa). She then turns the arm clockwise and counterclockwise. (See Diagram 40.) The rotation should be deft and vigorous like spinning cotton into yarn.

Hip Rotation Method: The patient lies on his back, with the therapist standing beside him. With one hand the therapist supports the patient's kneecap, and with the other grasps his calf, a third of the way up from the ankle. The hip and knee joints are half bent, and then the hip joint is rotated alternately clockwise and counterclockwise. (See Diagram 41 on the following page.)

DIAGRAM 41

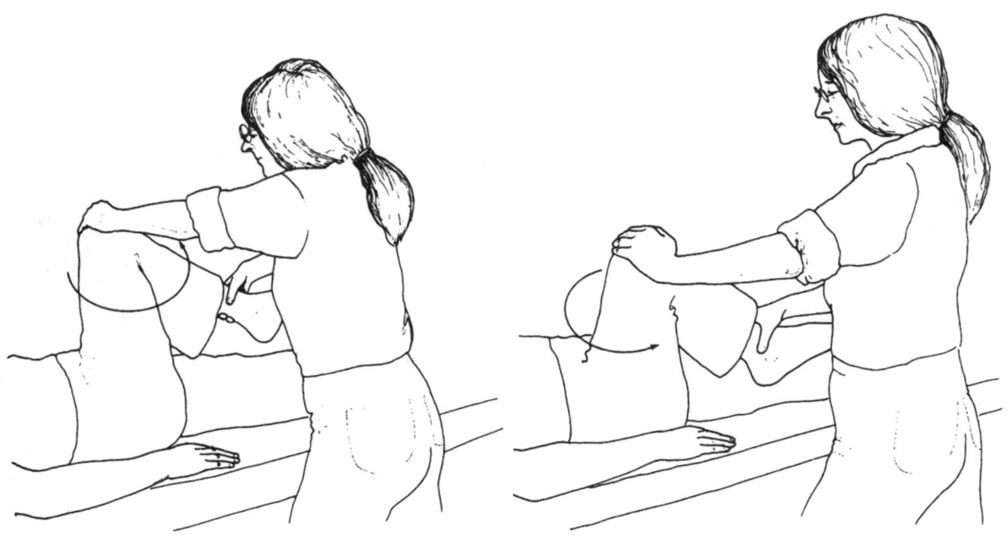

Lumbar Rotation Method: In lumbar rotation, the therapist must stand firmly, shifting her center of gravity to follow the direction of the rotation. She must also be quite strong. If the therapist is not strong, the range of the rotation she applies should not be too great, or she may lose her balance and fall.

Lumbar Rotation Method, #1: The patient is seated while the therapist stands beside him with her legs apart, or in front of him with her legs astride. One hand is passed under the patient's armpit and grasps the opposite shoulder; the other reaches across the abdomen to hold the farther side of the waist. Then the patient is told to relax his whole body and the spine is rotated. (See Diagram 42.)

DIAGRAM 42

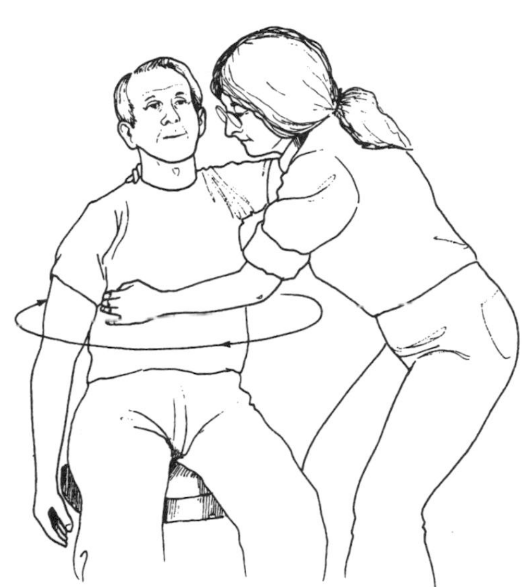

Lumbar Rotation Method, #2: The patient is told to stand facing a crossbar, or the back of a steady chair. He grasps the crossbar with both hands and bends his body slightly forward. The therapist stands behind him, legs astride, and tightly holds his waist with both hands. She tells the patient to relax his whole body and, with the vertical axis of the patient's body as center of rotation, she rotates the patient's spinal column.

22. Shake Method

This method is a form of massage that involves shaking the limbs, and can be classified as a passive manipulation. It is applied only to the upper and lower limbs. The practitioner holds the end of the patient's limb and shakes it gently like a rope, making it rise and fall in waves. The method is classified into two types, the upper-limb shake and lower-limb shake methods.

Upper-Limb Shake Method, #1: The patient has to be seated, while the practitioner stands on one side of him. Using both hands to hold the five fingers of the affected limb and pull the limb tight, the practitioner moves the limb with a shaking motion. The range of the shaking is increased from small to large, so that waves are transmitted all the way to the shoulder. This shaking movement is performed 3–5 times.

Upper-Limb Shake Method, #2: The patient is in either a sitting or a standing position, while the therapist stands beside him. The patient's shoulder is held firmly with one hand and the hand of the affected limb is grasped with the other. The affected limb is then pulled out tight and shaken up and down or left and right. (See Diagram 43.)

DIAGRAM 43

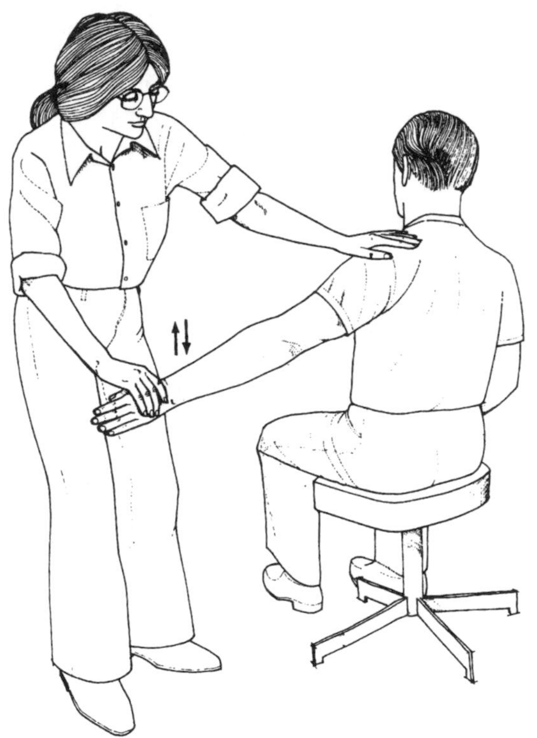

Lower-Limb Shake Method: The patient lies on his side and the therapist stands behind his feet. The therapist grasps the toes and back of the foot of the affected leg with her two hands, lifts the leg and shakes it. This is repeated 3–5 times.

23. Stretch Method

The stretch method is a type of massage which stretches the joints. It is a special form of passive manipulation. The pulling motion must be dexterous but forceful. The method has the functions of stretching contracted muscles and helping to restore a joint to its proper position. It may be divided into the following forms.

a) Lumbar Stretch Method, #1: The patient lies on his side, affected side upward, and the practitioner stands behind his back. The thumb of one hand is used to press on the painful part of the lumbus, while the other forearm supports the calf of the affected leg, with the hand cupping the kneecap. After bending the thigh upward toward the abdomen a few times, deftly and forcefully pull the leg out backwards. At the same time, the thumb pushing against the aching area exerts a little extra pressure. (See Diagram 44.) This process is repeated 5–6 times. This method is suitable in cases of slipped lumbar intervertebral disk, helping to restore the normal position. It is also used for other chronic lumbar pains.

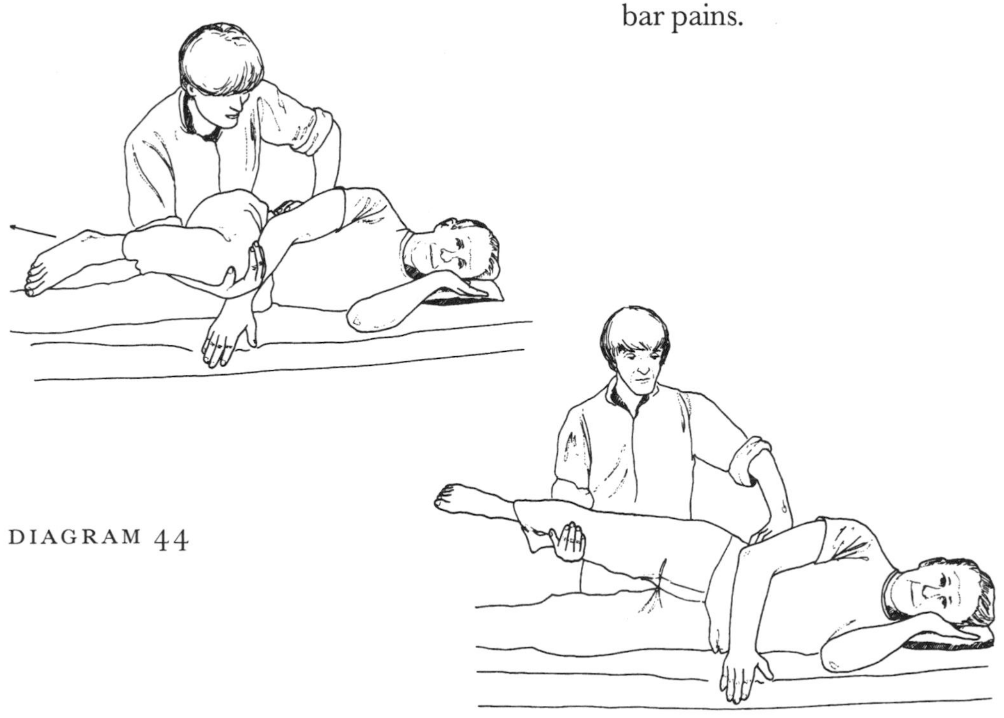

DIAGRAM 44

Lumbar Stretch Method, #2: Practitioner and patient stand back to back. The practitioner uses his elbows to hook the patient's arms and lifts the patient up so that the practitioner's buttocks are somewhat lower than the patient's. Then the patient is told to relax his whole body. The practitioner bends and straightens his knees repeatedly, forcefully shaking the patient with his buttocks, thereby stretching the patient's spinal column. (See Diagram 45 on the following page.) To finish up, the practitioner can swing the patient's body from side to side several times.

DIAGRAM 45

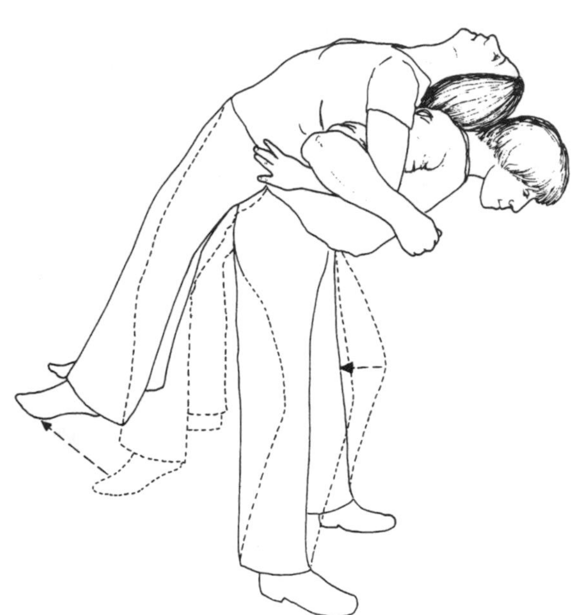

Lumbar Stretch Method, #3: Here the patient lies face down. The practitioner first uses the kneading and rub methods to relax the muscles of the lumbar area. Then he places his forearm under the patient's kneecaps and lifts the lower half of the patient's body so that only the chest is touching the bed. He places his other hand on the patient's lower lumbar region and presses and releases several times in a rhythmic and elastic manner. When the patient's muscles have become quite relaxed, the practitioner suddenly uses his forearm to press down hard on the patient's lumbar area. Simultaneously, the forearm which is supporting the patient's knees is raised upward with force, causing the patient's lumbar area to extend backward. (See Diagram 46.) After the patient's legs have been let down, the lumbar area is again given a short kneading massage.

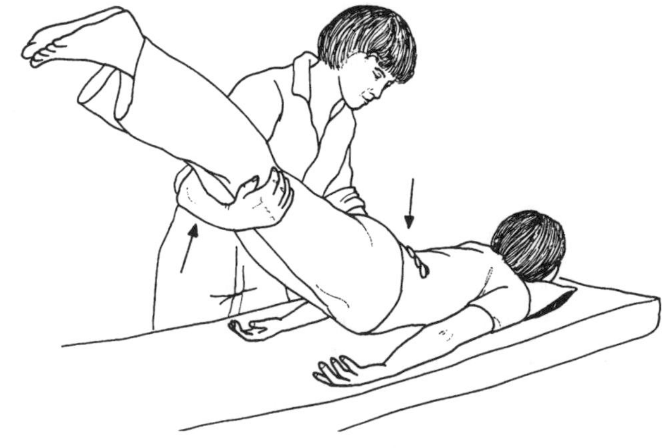

DIAGRAM 46

Lumbar Stretch Method, #4: Here the patient lies on his side with the affected side upward. The practitioner grasps the ankle of the leg on the affected side with his hands, and pulls the leg backward. At the same time he lifts his leg and places the sole of his foot tightly against the small of the patient's back, simultaneously pulling with his hands and pushing with his foot. First, the practitioner should push lightly several times until he feels the patient's lumbar area has become comparatively relaxed. Then the combined pushing and pulling movement is performed with a sudden, powerful force, causing the patient's lumbar region to extend backwards. (See Diagram 47.) Providing that an effective amount of strength is used, one such action is generally enough.

DIAGRAM 47

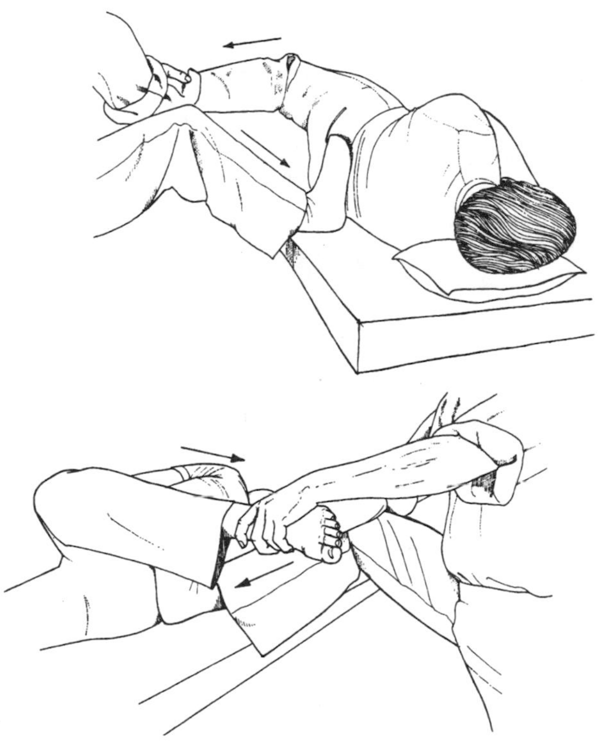

Upper-Limb Stretch Method: The patient sits on a low stool and the therapist stands facing him, a little towards the affected side. The affected arm is held out with the back of the hand toward the therapist, who grasps the fingers in two groups with his two hands. He rotates the arm in a circle from top inside to top outside, down and around again, several times. When the muscles of the affected limb feel as if they have relaxed, and the limb moves freely, the therapist suddenly and forcefully lifts it upward. (See Diagram 48.) This method has been found effective in treating patients with soreness in the upper limb or shoulder, but where movement of the joints is not greatly impeded. It is generally applied following the application of other methods of massage, and is used only once or twice at a time.

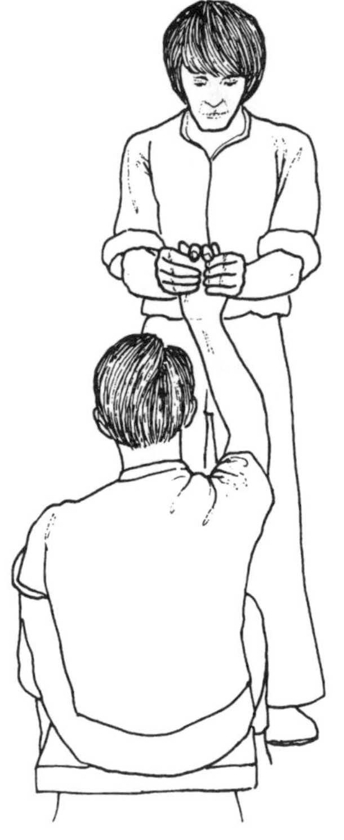

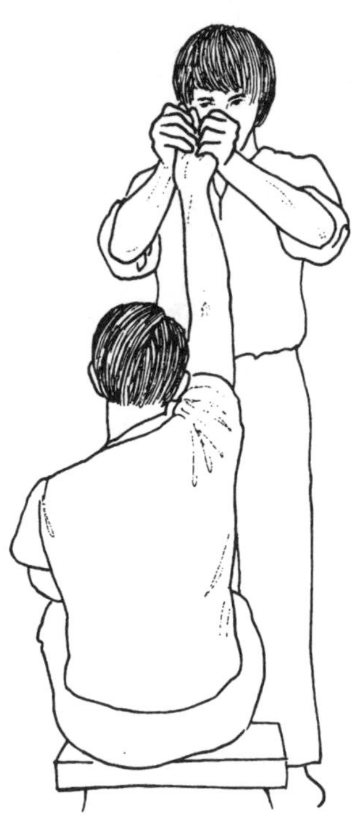

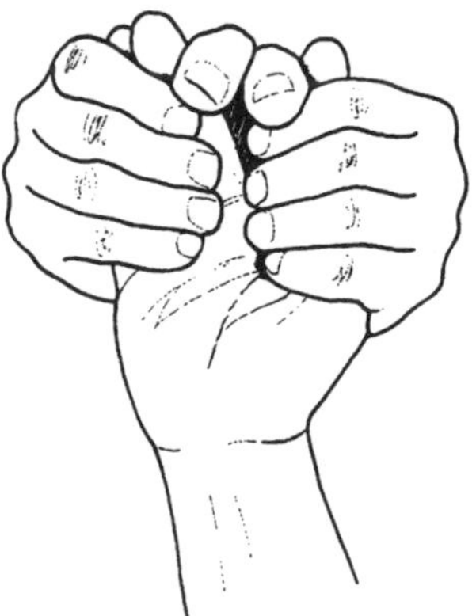

DIAGRAM 48

Lower-Limb Stretch Method: This method is also called moving the leg. The patient lies on his back. The practitioner supports the calf of the affected leg with one arm and hand, pressing the kneecap with the other hand. First the hip and knee joints are bent, and a slight amount of force is used to press the thigh downward. As soon as the thigh comes close to the abdominal area, the affected limb is dexterously and forcefully pulled out straight. At this point, with the hip joint half bent and the knee joint completely extended, the patient is told to kick his leg up and forward. (See Diagram 49.) The degree of bending of the hip joint must correspond with the height that the patient can raise a straight leg and the degree of elevation should gradually be increased. The movement is done 10–20 times during each session.

DIAGRAM 49

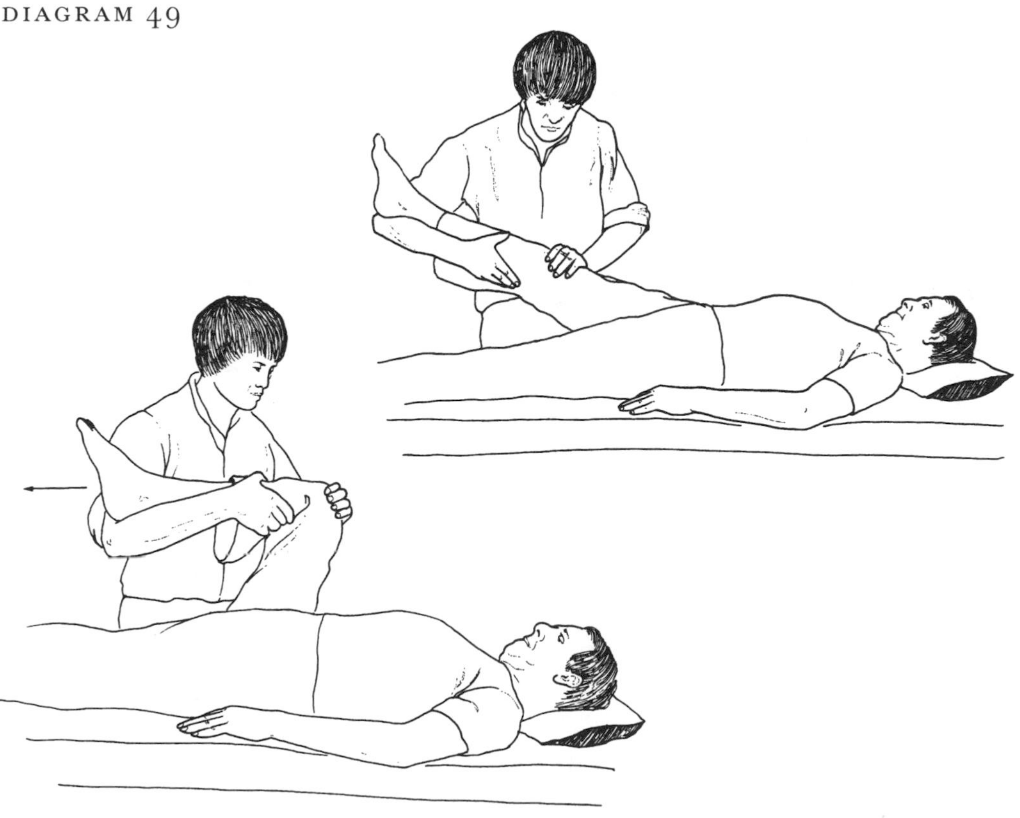

24. Tread Method

The tread method is a form of massage involving treading on the patient's body. It is often applied to the lumbar area. The patient lies face down on a rather short massage bed. The pectoral area and the thighs each are cushioned with a pillow about 12 inches (30 cm) high, so that the lumbar region itself rests over empty space. The practitioner hangs tightly with his hands onto a sturdy bar fixed above the patient's bed. He lightly steps down on the lumbar-sacral area with one foot, first applying light pressure several times, then gradually increasing the force. He rhythmically alternates stepping down on the spine and releasing the pressure, rising and falling like the carrying-pole of someone carrying heavy loads on each shoulder. (See Diagram 50.) The patient is told to keep his mouth open and breathe in and out with the rhythm. The force of the treading is increased from light to heavy until an effective strength is reached. The treading is repeated about 20 times, then a rest, then treading again. Three to four bouts of treading can be done at one session. This method has the effect of hastening the restoration of a protruding intervertebral disk to its proper position.

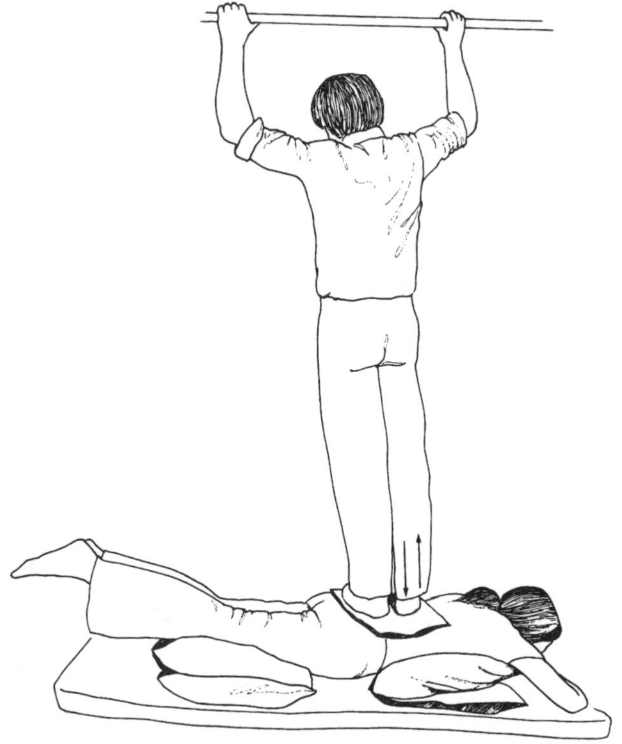

DIAGRAM 50

Section 2: Practicing Massage Techniques

Well-practiced technique, agile and flexible joints, and strong fingers are all necessary for massage therapy. The therapist's movements must be smooth, dexterous, and gentle, and he or she must be able to keep them up over long periods of time. Only under all these conditions can a good therapeutic effect be obtained. Consequently, it is necessary that the therapist undertake continuous training, building up strength and practicing the massage techniques, in order to serve people better. Basically, training is divided into two parts: general physical training and practicing the finger techniques.

1. Physical Training

Massage therapy calls for great physical strength, and especially for stamina. At the same time the practitioner must be able to maintain definite positions for long periods of time, such as standing with the legs spread apart in the rider's (or stride) position or the archer's position. (See Diagram 53, following.) All this demands that the practitioner regularly engage in a good exercise program. The following introduces several exercises aimed at developing the strength of the limbs and the lumbar area.

Exercise 1: Stand with the feet shoulder width apart. Hold the body erect, with the head slightly bent and the eyes looking straight ahead. Press the tongue against the upper palate and breathe through the nose. Then evenly raise both hands with the palms facing downward. After a deep breath, the palms are brought together and held in front of the chest, the fingertips of the joined hands gradually turning towards the chest, and the elbows being brought level with the shoulders. At the same time, flex the knees slightly, half squatting into the rider's position, with the body's gravity centered. (See Diagram 51 on the following page.) Continue to breathe deeply and easily. This position should be held for 1–3 minutes or even longer, the time being gradually extended with practice.

DIAGRAM 51 DIAGRAM 52

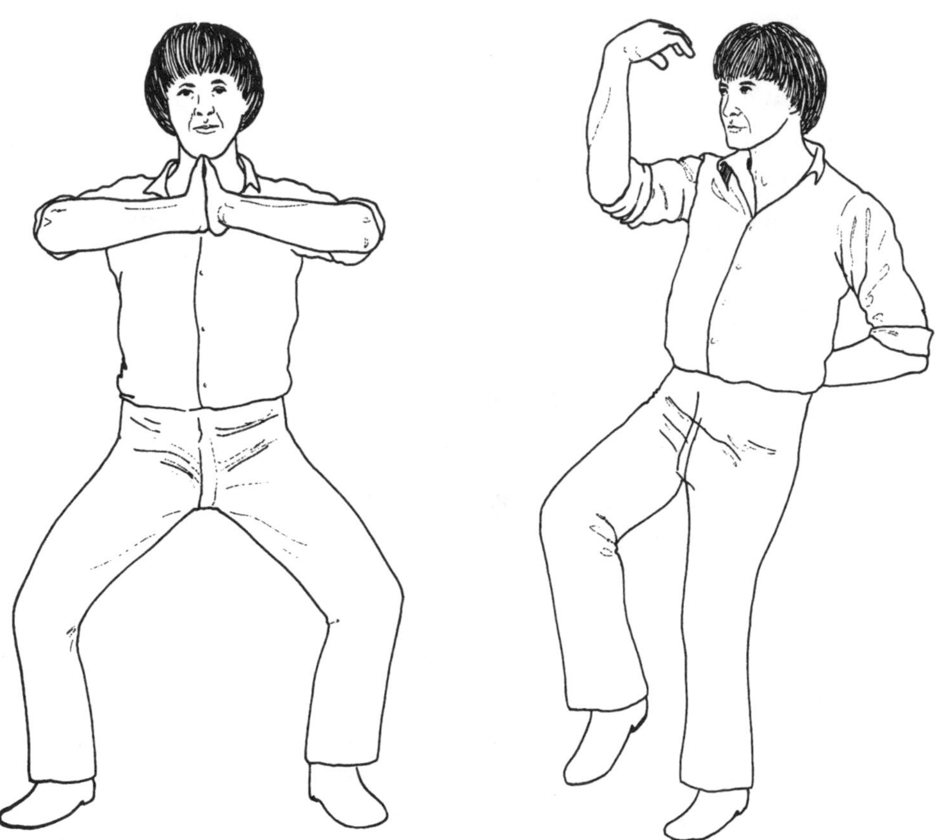

Exercise 2: After the first exercise has been completed, revert to a natural position and rest for a moment, then do Exercise 2. Take a half step forward with right foot and bend the left knee slightly, going into a half-crouch. The tip of the right foot touches the ground, and the heel is raised; the weight of the body is placed on the left leg. At the same time form the left hand into a loose fist and, with the center of the fist facing outward, place it behind the back. The five fingers of the right hand are extended straight and held closely together; the wrist is fully bent and rotated inward as far as it will go. The elbow forms a 90° angle and

the upper arm is extended forward, level with the shoulder. (See Diagram 52.) Fix your eyes on your right hand, compose yourself, and breathe deeply. Hold this position for 1–3 minutes. Alternate the positions of the left and right hands and feet. In succeeding sessions, gradually increase the amount of time for which the position is held.

Exercise 3: After completing Exercise 2, relax and move freely, then do Exercise 3. Put the right foot forward in the archer's position, with the toes pointing forward. (See Diagram 53.) The left leg is extended backward, with the foot pointing to the side. The heels must be flat on the ground and planted firmly and the body erect, with its weight centered. A fist is made with the right hand and the wrist is bent and rotated inward as much as possible. The elbow area is bent at an obtuse angle and the upper arm held level with the shoulder. Then, form the left hand into a fist, with the wrist bent. The elbow is slightly bent and the arm extended out behind the back. The head turns somewhat to the right, with the eyes on the right hand. Pull tightly with the right hand, like a rider holding a tight lead on a horse. Then take a deep, easy breath. This posture should be held for 1–3 minutes. The process is alternated, left and right, and the length of time for which it is held is gradually increased, with increasing ability.

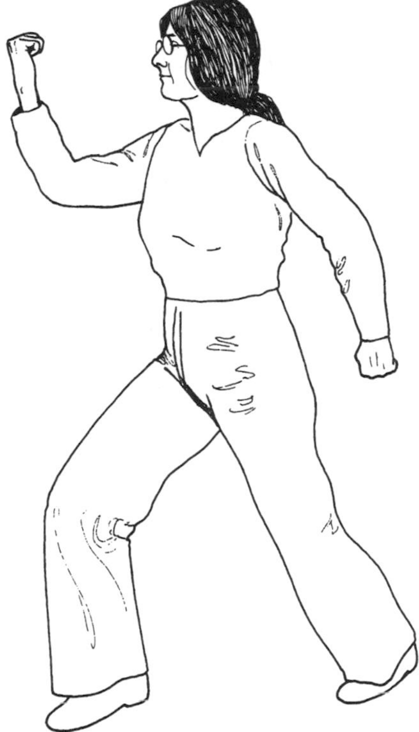

DIAGRAM 53

Exercise 4: After completing Exercise 3, rest a while, then do Exercise 4. Set the legs shoulder width apart, and gradually squat down until the knees are bent to about 90 degrees. Rest the hands on the legs above the kneecaps, with the thumbs on the upper thigh, so that the arms form a rough circle. Hold the chest area upright, and keep the weight of the body centered. (See Diagram 54.) Then, with the eyes looking straight ahead, do a deep-breathing exercise. This posture should be held for as long a period of time as possible, the longer the better.

After completing these four exercises, do some movements to relax.

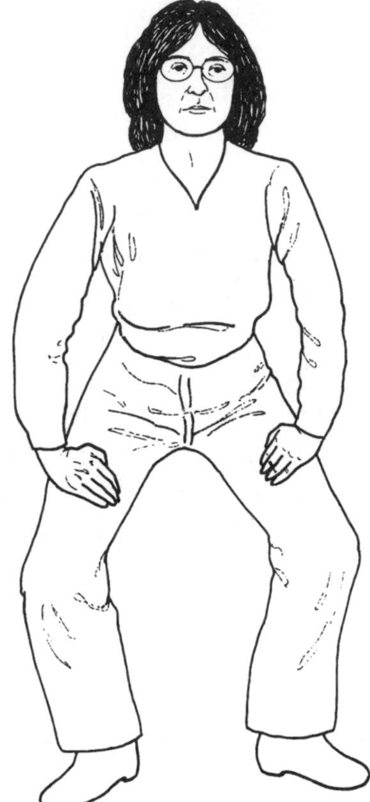

DIAGRAM 54

2. Practicing the Techniques

Massage therapy is applied chiefly with the hands. Therefore, the hands must be trained to be strong, gentle, dexterous, well-coordinated, and untiring. The hand exercises are in two stages. The first stage involves practicing on a bag filled with sand. After becoming skillful with practice on the sandbag, then practice on the human body (two people can practice on each other). The sandbag may be sewn out of white linen or cotton cloth. The specifications for the sandbag are: one foot (30 cm) long, one foot (30 cm) wide, 2 inches (5 cm) high, and filled with cleanly washed sand. The most commonly used massage techniques and the most important aspects of the practice are introduced on the following pages:

Thumb Push Method: The thumb push is divided into three types: the flat-thumb push, side-of-the-thumb push, and thumb-tip push. However, the main aspects of practicing all of these are identical. In practicing the push method, a standing position is normal but a sitting position can also be used. Concentrate your thoughts; let the shoulders sink and the elbows hang down; flex the elbow; bend the wrist and let the hand hang down. The hand is held in a partial fist, with the fingers not allowed to go beyond the center of the palm. The thumb is extended and rests on the second knuckle joint of the index finger, covering the eye of the fist.[34] Now, with the tip of the thumb against the sandbag, swing from the wrist and move the thumb back and forth rhythmically so that the thumb is pushed out forward and then drawn back. (See Diagram 55.) In pushing out about two-thirds of one's strength is used, and in drawing back about one-third. When pushing forward, do not let the thumb jump, and in drawing back, do not let the bent phalangeal joint touch the surface of the sandbag. The thumb should push forward along a straight, and not an oblique line.

DIAGRAM 55

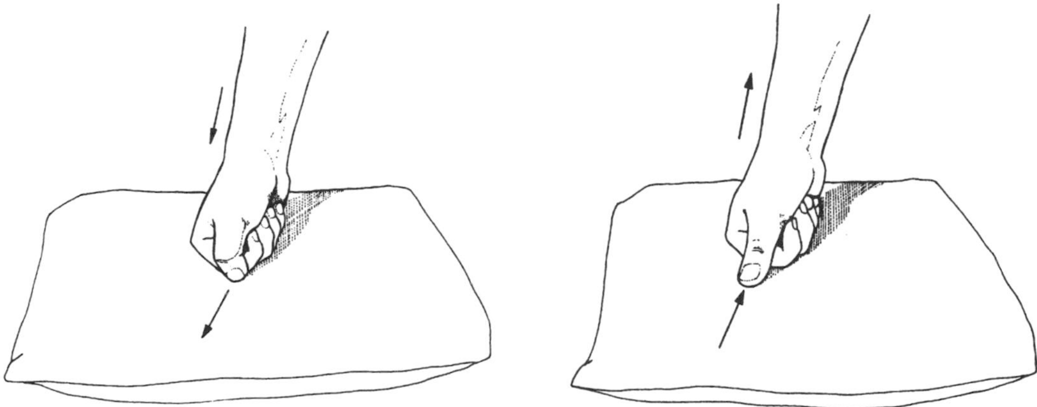

34. Eye of the fist: the index-finger end of a fist; the space in the crook of the finger is like an eye.

The wrist should be completely relaxed. The rate of pushing is maintained at 120–160 times a minute. When this technique is perfected, the thumb will seem to be attached to the surface of the sandbag, attaining the requirement of: "Heavy but not rigid, light but not floating." It is best to perfect the use of both right and left hands, so that one hand can alternate with the other when this method is used clinically.

Roll Method: Take a standing position; allow the shoulders to sink, and the elbows to hang down. One elbow is bent and the wrist relaxed; the hand is formed into a loose fist, with the center of the palm turned upward. The fingers and thumb are somewhat bent, but not stiff; the index and middle fingers are extended freely. With the back of the fifth finger, together with the hypothenar pad, against the sandbag, make a backward-rolling motion with the wrist. Repeat this rolling exercise over and over again. (See Diagram 56.) Be careful to avoid making jumping movements, or any scraping, in order to prevent damage to the skin. Both hands must be trained to do the rolling smoothly, with deep-reaching force and unflagging rhythm, so that the hands can be alternated.

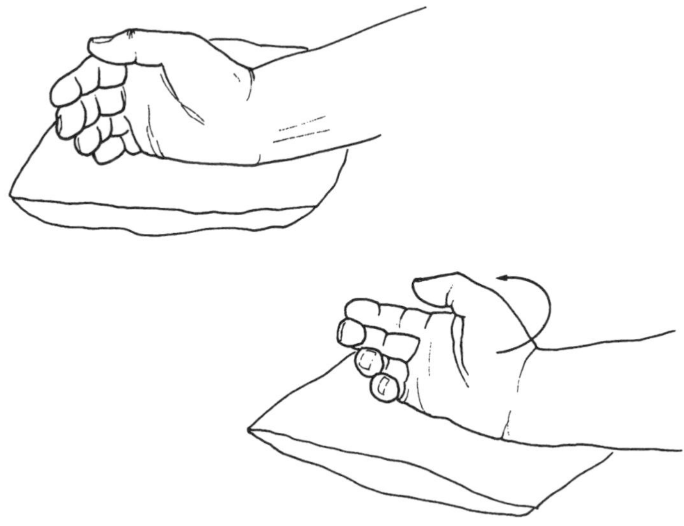

DIAGRAM 56

Finger Vibrate Method: The finger-vibrate method is applied with either the middle finger or the thumb, and generally with the right hand. In practicing the middle-finger vibration, the thumb and the index finger are used to hold the middle finger, and the tip of the middle finger is placed against the sandbag. In the thumb vibration, the outer edge of the thumb-tip contacts the sandbag. The wrist area is bent slightly toward the palm. Both the hand and the forearm muscles exert a static, tense force to produce a vibrating motion. It is possible that when one starts to practice, one may not be able to produce any vibration, or to sustain vibration for any length of time. But after some practice, vibration will be produced. The vibration should be slight and even, with the force coming from the tip of the finger. One should be able to sustain vibration for over a minute.

Pinch Method: The pinch method most often uses the thumb, index, and middle fingers and is usually done with one hand. It can be practiced along the edge of the sandbag. The thumb, index, and middle fingers pinch together on the edge of the sandbag with a relatively strong force. At the same time the thumb moves clockwise with a rolling, rubbing, pinching motion. The index and middle fingers make a similar motion in the opposite direction. In the course of this rolling, rubbing, pinching motion, the fingers should gradually move forward. This technique calls for coordination, smoothness, sensitivity, and control of the amount of force imparted by the fingertips. One must be able to sustain it for over ten minutes at a time.

Hammer and Pat Methods: Here both hands are usually used simultaneously. Whether the flats of the fingers are used for patting or the fist is used to hammer, the main aspects of the practice are the same. The surface of the hand used in hammering or patting must always make a flat contact. In patting, the flat of the fingers is used, and in hammering, a loose fist must be used. In patting the fingers are slightly bent and spread apart. In both hammering and patting, most of the movement should come from the wrist being swung up and down. The wrists should be trained to the point that they move smoothly and dexterously, but with strength. They should rise and fall in coordination, with an even rhythm. You should be able to change the rate of movement and sustain it for more than ten minutes at a time.

Practicing is often quite boring, especially at the beginning when you are likely to experience soreness, swelling, and fatigue. For this reason, your attitude must be serious, and you must be persevering and not lax. Moreover, as this sort of practice is also a form of physical exercise, it should be carried out according to the general rules of physical exercise. The following points are set forth for reference:

- Practice is best carried out early in the morning, soon after getting up, and in an open yard, or park.
- During practice wear loose clothes and a loose belt. Do not wear clothing that is either too tight or too heavy.
- Do not begin practicing when you are too full or too hungry. Generally, practice should not be done within 1 ½ hours after a meal.
- Before the practice do some preparatory exercises: move your hands and your feet, and take a few deep breaths before beginning the practice session. Before practicing finger techniques, all the joints of the fingers should be flexed a bit.
- After the practice session, do some settling-down movements and deep breathing. If you have perspired, immediately rub yourself dry, and put on all your clothing.
- During practice you have to concentrate your thoughts, in order to develop the good habit of devoting all your attention to carrying out the treatment. In this way, the practice sessions will achieve a greater effect and value, and you will be less likely to injure yourself.
- In practicing the techniques, be aware of cleanliness and avoid scrapes and scratches. If the skin reacts sensitively, practice should be suspended.

CHAPTER XXII

Acupoints Commonly Used in Massage Therapy

Acupoints for Adults

Baihui: (acupoint on the governor vessel meridian) located on the midline at the top of the skull where it intersects with a line drawn connecting the tips of the left and right ears.

Changshan: (foot greater *yang,* bladder meridian) a point on the back of the leg in the middle of the gastrocnemius muscle 7 *cun* below the crease at the back of the knee.

Chengfu: (foot greater *yang,* bladder meridian) on the posterior surface of each thigh, on the midpoint of the crease below the buttock.

Chize: (hand greater *yang,* lung meridian) a point in the depression on the line of flexure of the elbow, outside the tendon of the biceps. Find the point with the elbow half bent.

Chongyang: (foot bright *yang,* stomach meridian) at the highest point of the instep at the articular junction of the 2nd and 3rd tarsal bones with the 2nd and 3rd metatarsal bones on the medial margin of the extensor digitorum longus muscle.

Dachangshu: (foot greater *yang,* bladder meridian) 2 ½ *cun* from the midline at the level of the depression between the 4th and 5th lumbar vertebrae.

Daling: (hand absolute *yin,* pericardium meridian) in a depression in the middle of the crease line on the front of the wrist (between the tendons of the palmaris longus and flexor carpi radialis muscles.)

Danshu: (foot greater *yang,* bladder meridian) on the back, 2 *cun* from the midline, at the height of the depression between the spinous processes of the 10th and 11th thoracic vertebrae.

Dazhui: (governor vessel meridian) in the depression below the spinous process of the 7th cervical vertebra.

1. *Taiyang*
2. *Zanshu*
3. *Jingmang*
4. *Sibai*
5. *Renzhong*
6. *Chize*
7. *Shaohai*
8. *Neiguan*
9. *Lieguan*
10. *Taiyuan*
11. *Daling*
12. *Shenmen*
13. *Baihui*
14. *Tinggong*
15. *Tinghui*
16. *Fengchi*
17. *Jianyu*
18. *Quchi*
19. *Shousanli*
20. *Yangxi*
21. *Hegu*
22. *Yifeng*
23. *Yingxiang*
24. *Tianting*

DIAGRAM 57

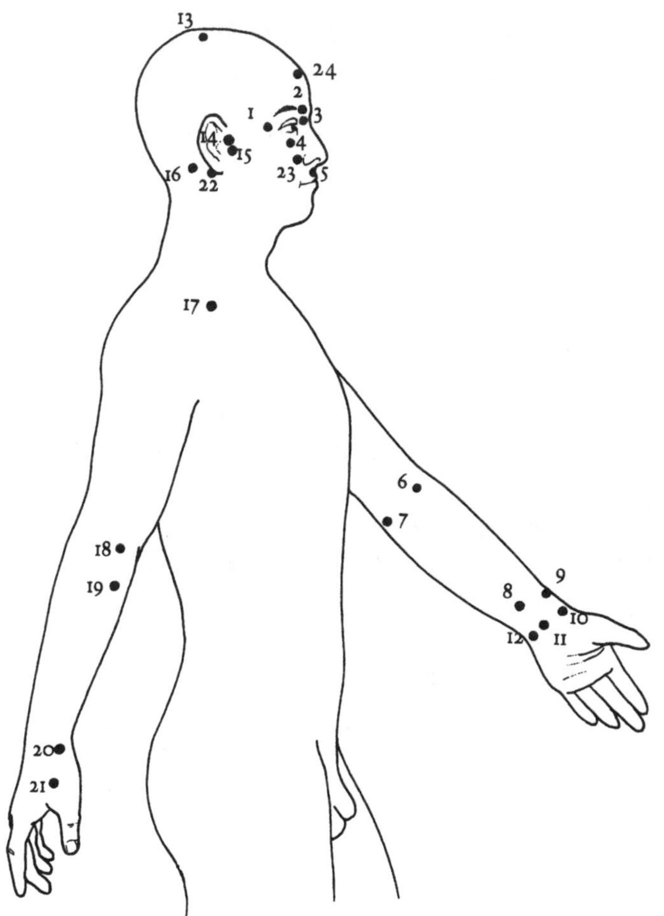

Feishu: (foot greater *yang,* bladder meridian) on the back, 2 *cun* from the midline, at the height of the depression between the spinous processes of the 3rd and 4th vertebrae. *Fengchi:* (foot lesser *yang,* gallbladder meridian) points on either side of the *fengfu* acupoint, at the lower margin of the occipital bone, in the depression between where the trapezius muscle and the sternocleidomastoid muscle have their origins.

Fengfu: (governor vessel meridian) in the exact center of the space between the occipital bone and the first cervical vertebra.

Fengmen: (foot greater *yang,* bladder meridian) bilateral points 2 *cun* to each side of the space between the 2nd and 3rd thoracic vertebrae.

Ganshu: (foot greater *yang,* bladder meridian) on the back, 2 *cun* from the midline, at the height of the depression between the spinous processes of the 9th and 10th thoracic vertebrae.

Gaohuang: (foot greater *yang,* gallbladder meridian) on the back, 4 *cun* from the midline at the height of the depression between the spinous processes of the 4th and 5th thoracic vertebrae.

Geshu: (foot greater *yang,* bladder meridian) on the back, 2 *cun* from the midline, at the height of the depression between the spinous processes of the 7th and 8th thoracic vertebrae.

Guanyuan: (conception vessel meridian) 3 *cun* below the navel.

Hegu: (hand bright *yang,* large intestine meridian) in the depression between the 1st and 2nd metacarpal bones, near the angle formed where they meet.

Huantiao: (foot lesser *yang,* gallbladder meridian) located on the hip behind the greater trochanter, in a depression formed in the muscle when the buttocks are tensed.

Jianjing: (foot lesser *yang,* gallbladder meridian) in the depression right between the *dazhui* and *jianyu* acupoints (see above) on the front edge of the trapezius.

Jianliao: (hand lesser *yang,* triple warmer meridian) in the depression behind and below the acromion, about 1 *cun* behind the *jianyu* acupoint (see above).

Jianyu: (hand bright *yang,* large intestine meridian) a depression between the outer edge of the acromion and the trochanter major of the humerus. Find the point when the upper arm is abducted.

Jianzhen: (hand greater *yang,* small intestine meridian) in a depression on the posterior surface of the shoulder just above the crease of the armpit.

Jiexi: (foot bright *yang,* stomach meridian) located on the upper part of the instep, in the center of the anterior crease of the ankle, between 2 tendons. The point is located with the knee slightly bent.

Jingming: (foot greater *yang,* bladder meridian) in the depression *fen*[1] inside and above the inner canthus of the eye.

1. *fen:* 1/10 of a *cun,* which is a unit of measurement equal to the inside length of the 2nd section of the patient's own middle finger. The *cun* is measured between the ends of the creases formed when the finger is bent.

DIAGRAM 58

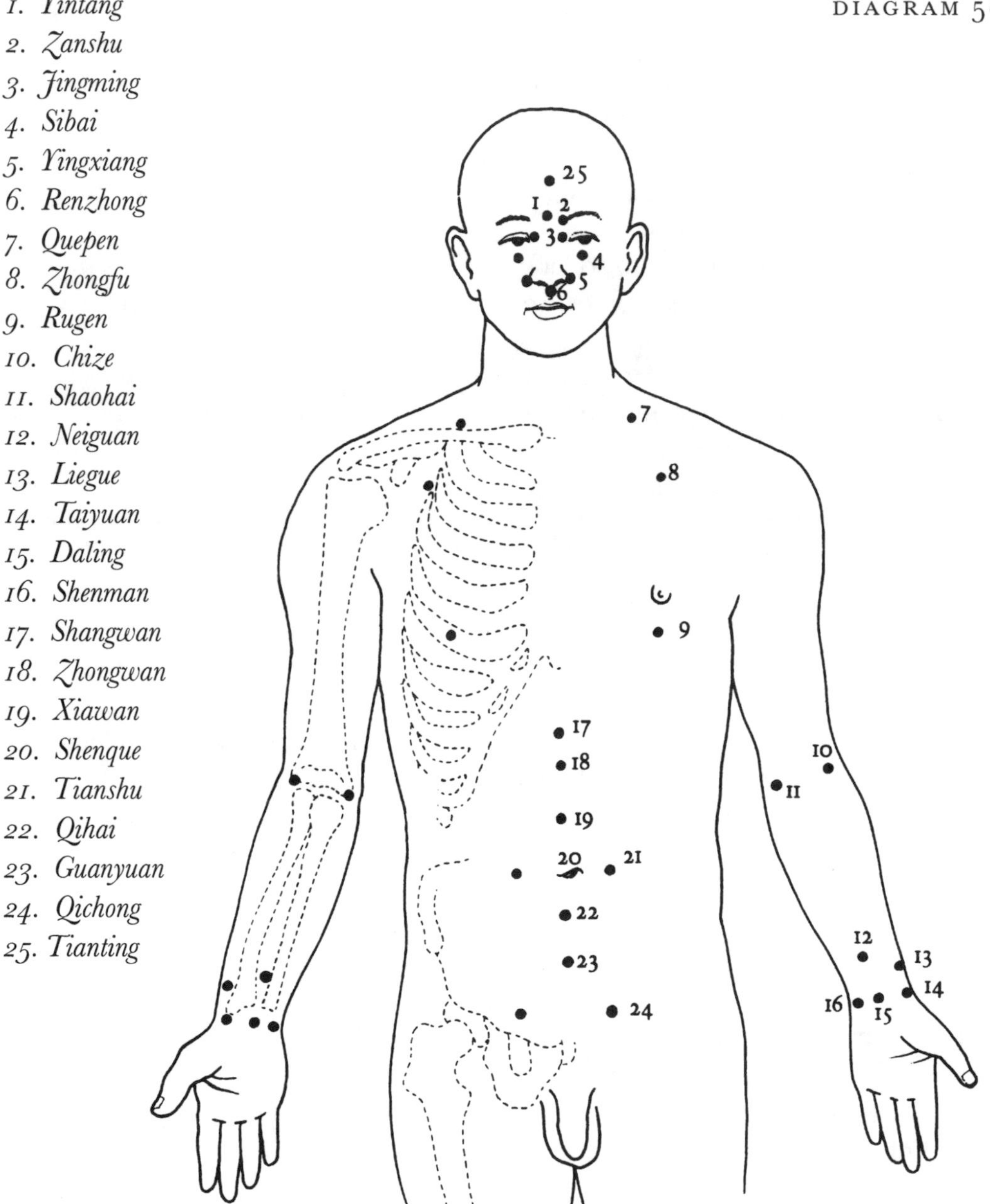
1. *Yintang*
2. *Zanshu*
3. *Jingming*
4. *Sibai*
5. *Yingxiang*
6. *Renzhong*
7. *Quepen*
8. *Zhongfu*
9. *Rugen*
10. *Chize*
11. *Shaohai*
12. *Neiguan*
13. *Liegue*
14. *Taiyuan*
15. *Daling*
16. *Shenman*
17. *Shangwan*
18. *Zhongwan*
19. *Xiawan*
20. *Shenque*
21. *Tianshu*
22. *Qihai*
23. *Guanyuan*
24. *Qichong*
25. *Tianting*
25
1
2
3
4
5
6
7
8
9
10
11
12
13
14
15
16
17
18
19
20
21
22
23
24

Juegu: (foot lesser *yang,* gall bladder meridian) 3 *cun* above the lateral malleolus, between the fibula and the tibia.

Kunlun: (foot greater yang, bladder meridian) in a depression between the highest point of the lateral malleolus and the Achilles tendon.

Liegue: (hand greater *yang,* lung meridian) upon the anterior surface of the forearm, 1.5 *cun* above the crease of the wrist, just to the outer side of the radial artery.

Mingmen: (governor vessel meridian) in the depression below the spinal process of the 2nd lumbar vertebra.

Neiguan: (hand absolute *yin,* pericardium meridian) in a depression 2 *cun* above the crease on the front of the wrist, between the 2 tendons (those of the palmaris longus and flexor carpi radialis muscles).

Pishu: (foot greater *yang,* bladder meridian) on the back, 2 *cun* from the midline, at the height of the depression between the spinous processes of the 11th and 12th thoracic vertebrae.

Pucan: (foot greater *yang,* bladder meridian) 2 *cun* straight below the *kunlun* acupoint, on the outer side of the heel bone.

Qichong: (foot bright *yang,* stomach meridian) points 2 *cun* to either side of the top of the pubic bone.

Qihai: (conception vessel meridian) 1.5 *cun* below the navel. (The distance from the navel to the pubic bone is 5 *cun.*)

Quchi: (hand bright *yang,* large intestine meridian) between the lateral end of the elbow crease, when the elbow is bent at a right angle, and the outer protuberance of the humerus.

Quepen: (foot bright *yang,* stomach meridian) a depression above the clavicle, directly above the nipple.

Renzhong: (governor vessel meridian) a point midway in the groove between the bottom of the nose and the upper lip.

Rugen: (foot bright *yang,* stomach meridian) 1.6 *cun* below the nipple at the 5th intercostal space.

Sanyinjiao: (foot greater *yang,* spleen meridian) 3 *cun* above the top of the medial malleolus, in a depression behind the tibia.

Shangliao, ciliao, zhongliao, xialiao: (foot greater *yang,* bladder meridian) *Shangliao* is situated in the 1st posterior sacral foramen, about midway between the postero-superior iliac spine and the median line. *Ciliao* is in the 2nd posterior sacral foramen,

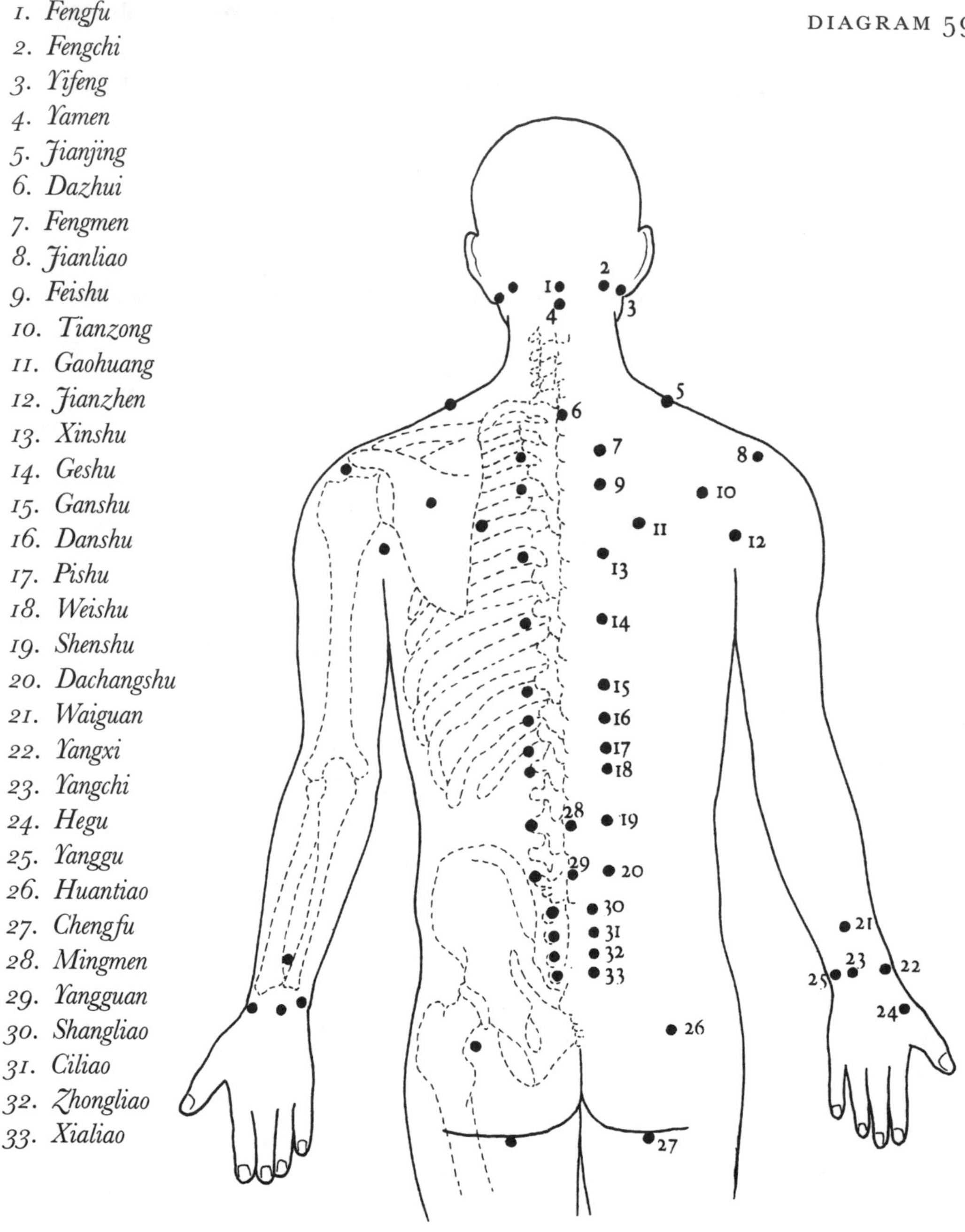
DIAGRAM 59
1. Fengfu
2. Fengchi
3. Yifeng
4. Yamen
5. Jianjing
6. Dazhui
7. Fengmen
8. Jianliao
9. Feishu
10. Tianzong
11. Gaohuang
12. Jianzhen
13. Xinshu
14. Geshu
15. Ganshu
16. Danshu
17. Pishu
18. Weishu
19. Shenshu
20. Dachangshu
21. Waiguan
22. Yangxi
23. Yangchi
24. Hegu
25. Yanggu
26. Huantiao
27. Chengfu
28. Mingmen
29. Yangguan
30. Shangliao
31. Ciliao
32. Zhongliao
33. Xialiao

zhongliao in the 3rd and *xialiao* in the 4th. Left and right together, there is a total of 8 *liao* acupoints.

Shangwan: (conception vessel meridian) 5 *cun* above the navel. (The distance from the depression at the lower end of the sternum to the navel is 8 *cun.*

Shaohai: (hand lesser *yin,* heart meridian) close to the inner end of the elbow crease when the elbow is slightly flexed; about halfway between the inner protuberance of the elbow and the tendon of the biceps.

Shenmen: (hand lesser *yin,* heart meridian) in a depression between the pisiform bone and the ulna on the inner (medial) side of the crease on the front of the wrist.

Shenque: (conception vessel meridian) the navel itself.

Shenshu or *Shen shu:* (foot greater *yang,* bladder meridian) on the back 2 ½ *cun* from the midline, at the level of the depression between the 2nd and 3rd lumbar vertebrae.

Shousanli: (hand bright *yang,* large intestine meridian) a point about 2 *cun* below the bend of the elbow on the radial side, between the musculus extensor carpi radialis longus and the musculus extensor carpi radialis brevis.

Sibai: (foot bright *yang,* stomach meridian) in the depression just above the infraorbital foramen, 3 *fen* below the lower edge of the bony orbit.

Taichong: (foot absolute *yin,* liver meridian) located on the top of the foot, in the angle between the 1st and 2nd metatarsal bones.

Taixi: (foot lesser *yin,* kidney meridian) in a depression between the Achilles tendon and the top of the medical malleolus, opposite *kunlun.*

Taiyang: (irregular acupoint not on a meridian) in the depression about a finger's width outside a point between the outer canthus of the eye and the tip of the eyebrow.

Taiyuan: (hand greater *yang,* lung meridian) in a depression on the outer side of the radial artery, at the outer end of the crease line on the front of the wrist.

Ten xuan: (irregular acupoints not on a meridian) on the tips of each of the ten fingers, 1 *fen* from the nail.

Tianshu: (foot bright *yang,* stomach meridian) points 2 *cun* to either side of the navel.

Tianting: (irregular acupoint not on a meridian) 1 ½–2 *cun* directly above *Yintang* on forehead.

Tianzong: (hand greater *yang,* small intestine meridian) in a depression below the midpoint of the spine of the shoulder blade.

Tinggong: (hand greater *yang,* small intestine meridian) in a depression in front of the tragus of the ear. Find the point when the mouth is open.

DIAGRAM 60

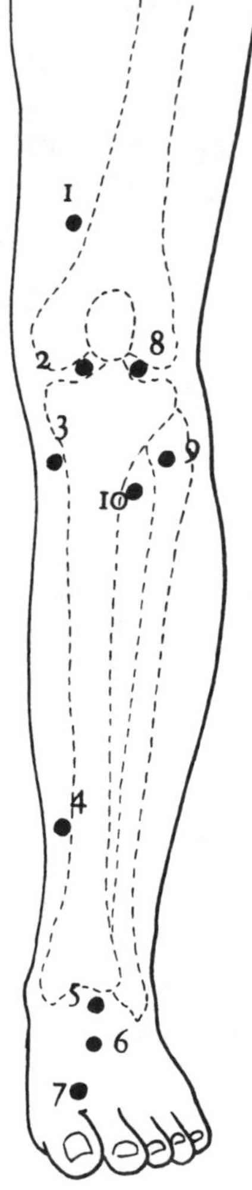

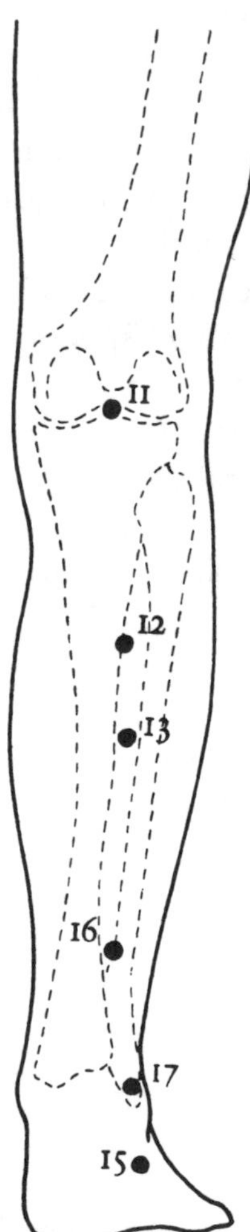

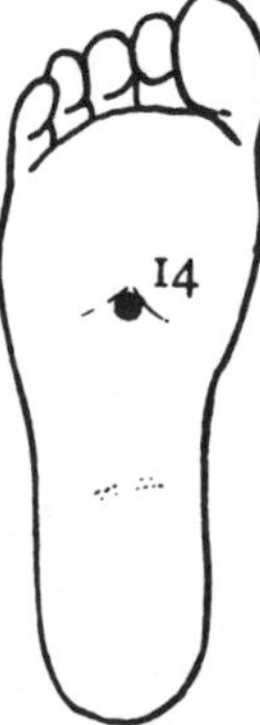

1. *Xuehai*
2. *Neixiyan* (Inner *xiyan*)
3. *Yinlingquan*
4. *Sanyinjiao*
5. *Jiexo*
6. *Chongyang*
7. *Taichong*
8. *Waixiyian* (Outer *xiyan*)
9. *Yanglingquan*
10. *Zusanli* *(or chu san li)*
11. *Weizhong*
12. *Chengjin*
13. *Chengshan*
14. *Yongquan* *(or yung chuan)*
15. *Pucan*
16. *Juegu*
17. *Kunlun*

Tinghui: (foot lesser *yang,* gallbladder meridian) in a depression in front of the intertragic notch. Find the point when the mouth is open.

Waiguan: (hand lesser *yang,* triple warmer meridian) a point 2 *cun* above the skin crease on the back of the wrist, directly opposite *neiguan.*

Weishu: (foot greater *yang,* bladder meridian) on the back, 2 *cun* from the midline, at the height of the depression between the spinous processes of the 12th thoracic and the 1st lumbar vertebrae.

Weizhong: (foot greater *yang,* bladder meridian) a point at the mid-point of the crease at the back of the knee located when the knee is slightly bent.

Xiawan: (conception vessel meridian) 2 *cun* above the navel.

Xinshu: (foot greater *yang,* bladder meridian) on the back, 2 *cun* from the midline, at the height of the depression between the spinous processes of the 5th and 6th thoracic vertebrae.

Xiyan: (irregular points not on a meridian) in the depressions on either side of the ligament below the patella; known as the inner and outer *xiyan.* Locate with the knee bent.

Xuehai: (foot greater *yin,* spleen meridian) on the anterior medial surface of the thigh, 3 *cun* above the crease of the knee in the bulge of the vastus medialis muscle.

Yamen: (governor vessel meridian) 5 *fen* below the fengfu acupoint.

Yangchi: (hand lesser *yang,* triple warmer meridian) in a depression on the back of the wrist below the base of the 4th metacarpal bone.

Yanggu: (hand greater *yang,* small intestine meridian) in a depression on the inner side of the wrist in the hollow between the tip of the ulna and the carpal bones.

Yangguan: (governor vessel meridian) in the depression below the spinal process of the 4th lumbar vertebra.

Yanglinquan: (foot lesser *yang,* gall bladder meridian) in a depression on the side of the leg, below the head of the fibula, between the 2 muscles.

Yangxi: (hand bright *yang,* large intestine meridian) in the "anatomical snuffbox" formed by 2 tendons when the thumb is extended, on the outer side of the wrist.

Yifeng: (hand lesser *yang,* triple warmer meridian) in a depression behind the earlobe in front of the point of the mastoid bone.

Yingxiang: (hand bright *yang,* large intestine meridian) in the depression on the ala nasi sulcus just above the edge of the nostril.

Yinlingquan: (foot greater *yin,* spleen meridian) in a depression below the lower margin of the medial condyle of the tibia, level with the tibial tuberosity.

Yintang: (irregular acupoint not on a meridian) between the inner ends of the eyebrows, at the most prominent point of the frontal bone.

Yongquan or *Yung Chuan:* (foot lesser *yin,* kidney meridian) in a depression between the anterior ⅓ and the posterior ⅔ of the sole of the foot, located when the toes are flexed.

Zanzhu: (foot greater *yang,* bladder meridian) in the depression at the inner end of the eyebrow, 1 *cun* from the median line.

Zhongfu: (hand greater *yang,* lung meridian) on a level with the second rib about 1 *cun* below the depression below the clavicle and medial to the coracoid process.

Zhongwan: (conception vessel meridian) 4 *cun* above the navel.

Zusanli or *chu san li:* (foot bright *yang,* stomach meridian) located on the front of the leg, 3 *cun* below the patella just 1 *cun* lateral to the edge of the tibia.

Acupoints for Children

In pediatric massage, besides the meridians and acupoints used for adults, there are some special acupoints, of which the most commonly used are these:

Dujiao: points on either side of the navel.

Errenshangma: in a depression on the back of the hand between the 4th and 5th metacarpal bones.

Fanmen: in the upper part of the fleshy pad at the base of the thumb.

Five *zhijie:* points at the proximal interphalangeal joints on the back of the hand. The 5th is on the interphalangeal joint of the thumb.

Four *hengwen:* the 4 points on the palm side of the proximal interphalangeal joints.

Greater *hengwen:* at the base of the palm of the hand, on the crease of the wrist.

Guiwei: at the tip of the coccyx.

Lesser *hengwen:* points on the 4 creases where the fingers meet the palm.

Liufu: a line along the inner side of the front of the forearm from the elbow crease to the wrist.

Neilaogong: a point in the middle of the palm.

Pitu: a line at the base of the thumb from a point on the fleshy eminence to a point on the crease of the wrist.

Sanguan: a line along the outer side of the front of the forearm from the wrist to the *quchi* point at the outer end of the elbow crease (see above).

Two *shanmen:* in depressions on either side of the 3rd metacarpal bone on the back of the hand.

Tianheshui: a line along the middle of the front surface of the forearm, from the wrist to the elbow crease.

Yiwofeng: a point in the middle of the crease of the back of the wrist.

Waijianshi: a point on the back of the forearm, above the *waiguan* point and between the ulna and the radius.

DIAGRAM 61

1. *Liufu*
2. *Neilaogong*
3. Four *hengwen* (*Sihengwen*)
4. *Tianheshui*
5. *Sanguan*
6. Greater *hengwen* (*Dahengwen*)
7. *Pitu*
8. *Fanmen*
9. Lesser *hengwen* (*Xiaohengwen*)
10. *Waijianshi*
11. *Yiwofeng*
12. Two *shanmen* (*Ershanmen*)
13. *Errenshangma*
14. Five *zhijie* (*Wuzhjie*)

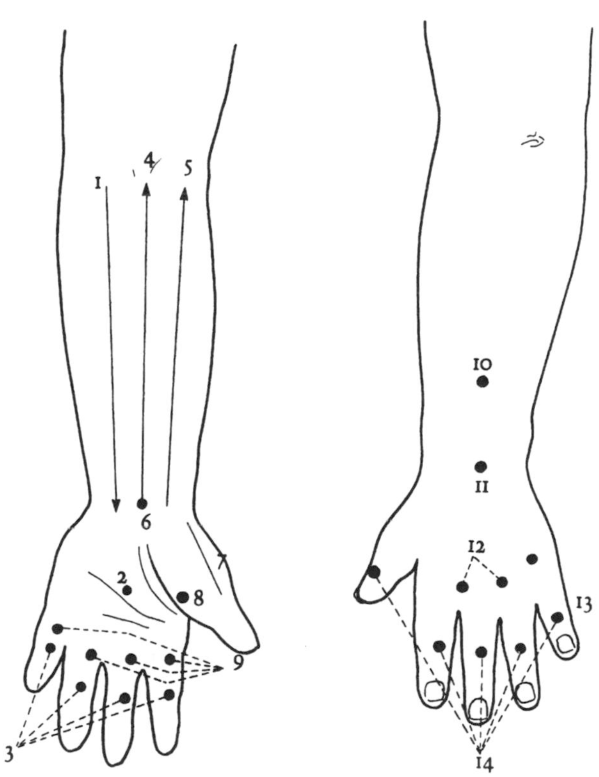

CHAPTER XXIII

How to Use Massage Therapy

Massage therapy is different from any other form of therapy, because the practitioner has to expend considerable physical strength in doing it, and the success of the treatment is exactly equal to the amount of effort that goes into it. This means that in the course of treatment, if you do not expend enough physical strength on a massage, you will not attain the required standard for effective treatment. On that account the therapist must work hard and not be afraid of fatigue, or of pain. You must make every effort to improve your technique. This will require much painstaking drilling. In actual clinical practice, we must continuously evaluate all our past experiences, in order to break new ground and create new methods. In this way, massage therapy will continue to be developed and brought to a still higher level.

It is necessary to tell the patient about massage therapy, to let him know that during the course of treatment some discomfort of pain may appear, and that sometimes a large number of sessions may be necessary before the treatment takes effect. Encourage patients to make up their minds not to be afraid of difficulties, and to be full of confidence that they can overcome their condition. Particularly encourage those patients with stubborn, chronic conditions to combat them with a strong will.

Section I: Actual Practice

1. Amount of Massage

It is very important that neither too much nor too little massage be given. Generally, the amount of massage will depend upon the number of massages daily, the length of time required for each massage, the intensity and the number of repetitions of each kind of manipulation, and observation of local reactions. The number of massages is determined by the requirements of different conditions. Generally, massage is applied once a day. But for some ailments, massage every other day or at a two-day interval is more appropriate. Some conditions can be treated twice a day. The duration of each massage treatment also varies. For example, where there is a sprain at a joint, localized massage and acupoint massage at the injured joint are all that is required. Generally, 15 minutes will be quite sufficient. There are some internal diseases, however, for which massage is applied to the head, the back, the limbs, and even over the whole body. Normally, this will take 30 minutes or so. This describes the general situation, but treatment must be based upon the individual case.

In children's massage, the number of times each massage is repeated during one session is generally determined by what is required for each site. Different regions of China have developed different approaches. In some provinces, massage is applied several tens of times, in others several hundred times, and in still others even as many as 2,000–3,000 times. Usually, we ourselves massage a site 200–300 times, which takes about 15–25 minutes in all. For children, the amount of massage is also determined by the amount of reddening of the skin. This is a criterion that is relatively easy to weigh. For adult massage, in the case of some techniques, the amount of time required is also determined by the number of repetitions. (See details given in the treatment sections for each disease.)

2. The Degree of Force to Use in Massage

The degree of force used in massage is directly related to the amount of massage. Whether the degree of force is adequate will greatly affect the result of the treatment.

Proper sequence and gradual progress: Both in each massage session and in the whole course of treatment, the massage must be light at the beginning, becoming gradually heavier. The amount of force should be increased, but not so abruptly as to be unbearable to the patient.

When the dig method is applied to an acupoint: The dig method should reach down to a point where the vital energy *(chi* or *qi)* appears, producing an aching, swelling reaction like a pin prick, or sometimes a shooting, painful, numb sensation. The strength of these sensations is determined by the intensity of the finger-digs, and this intensity must be under skillful control. The vibrate and kneading methods can be used in coordination with the dig method in order to intensify or lessen these sensations.

During massage on the head and back: Here no pain should be allowed to occur, nor should the skin be damaged. Rather, the massage should give the patient a sensation of warmth, and make him or her feel relaxed and comfortable.

When massage therapy is applied to a wounded patient: In this case the pain in the area of the wound should be added to as little as possible. When various kinds of passive manipulation are used, the range of the passive movement, and the amount of force to be used in stretching a limb should be fully estimated at the outset, and the amount of force gradually increased to the maximum possible.

The strength of the manipulation: This will have a definite relation to the amount of time for which it is applied. When great force is used, a massage should be applied somewhat fewer times in a session; when little force is used, the massage should be applied somewhat more times.

3. Treat Each Case Individually

Every patient has his or her own individual characteristics. There are the obvious differences of sex, age, and physical constitution. But there are also marked differences between different diseases and different phases of the same disease. Hence, in applying the various massage therapy manipulations, amount of force and length of time are adjusted to the individual patient. Some patients are relatively sensitive, and even though only a light manipulation is used, the patient feels a strong reaction. In such a case both the amount of massage and the degree of force used should be reduced. Conversely, there is often little reaction in the patient with a strong constitution, and the degree of force used should be increased.

In summary, each case must be dealt with individually. Especially with a new patient, the amount of massage and degree of force used must first be tested out, and the patient's reactions observed. Then, gradually, a suitable procedure can be established.

4. Important Considerations

- Receive the patient warmly and diagnose his/her condition in detail.
- Before beginning, place the patient in a suitable position, such as sitting, lying, or with the affected limb raised, in order to relax the muscles and to facilitate massage.
- The therapist should always be aware of his own position, so that it will help produce the correct force, and will also save his own energy. In general, the therapist can stand beside, behind, or facing the patient. A sitting position generally involves sitting face to face. In the standing position, the archer's and the rider's (stride) positions are both sometimes used.
- While he is applying the massage the practitioner has to devote his entire attention to it, comfortably adjusting his breathing and carrying out the treatment whole-heartedly. In this manner, the goal of the treatment can be reached, and injury can be avoided.
- The hands of the therapist should be kept warm and clean, and the fingernails must be trimmed often.
- In massage sessions where no exhaustive diagnosis is to be made prior to treatment, any circumstance that may contraindicate massage must still be noted. The progress of the disease must also be discerned, the patient's reactions noted and an explanation given.
- When massaging, be sure to proceed from site to site in the proper sequence, going from the distant points toward the center of the body. Make skillful use of the various techniques, applying them with appropriate degrees of force and in appropriate amounts.
- If the patient is very full or very hungry, it is inadvisable to carry out the mas-

sage. Generally, it is best not to proceed with massage during the period from ½ hour before to 1 ½ hours after a meal.

Section II: Media Used in Massage

During massage, therapists often put some liquid or powder on their hands to reduce friction and increase lubrication, or to gain the additional benefit of a medication. These liquids or powders are called the "media" for use in massage. There are numerous kinds of media, including liquids, tinctures, oils, and powders. The most common media are these:

Fresh ginger juice: Pound fresh ginger into a mud-like consistency and put it in a container. Dip the fingers into the juice exuded by the ginger, using it as a medium for massage. This is one of the most frequently used media, and is almost always used in massage of children. Because children have soft, tender skin and because the ginger juice is very slippery, the skin is unlikely to be abraded during massage. At the same time, the ginger juice produces a radiating warmth and helps to dispel harmful external influences.[1]

Cold water: If ginger juice is not available, substitute clean, cold tap water. Especially when a child has a fever, cold water is often used as a medium.

Shavings water: Soak wood shavings in water, and use the resulting liquid as a medium. Shavings water is very slippery and is therefore also very suitable for massage of children.

Egg white: Make a small hole in an egg shell, extract the egg white from the shell, and use it as a medium. The egg white can also be mixed with flour to make a dough-ball. The practitioner holds the dough-ball in his hand and applies the rub-roll, the rub, and the roll methods on a child's chest, abdomen, and back areas. This medium is often used in the folk treatment of children's influenza, "food build-up"[2] and other illnesses.

1. This refers to a concept of Chinese medicine whereby diseases can be caused by certain external factors, the most important of which are heat, cold, wind, moisture, and warmth.
2. Food build-up: a condition described by Chinese medicine in which the patient eats too much and undigested food builds up inside.

Songhua powder: Pulverize Songhua into a fine powder. Use this powder as a medium by dipping the fingers into it or by applying it directly with a powder-puff to the site to be massaged. It acts to absorb moisture and increase lubrication. In summer, when the skin perspires easily, use of this powder is especially appropriate.

Talcum powder: Generally, talcum powder is used medically chiefly for its lubricating effect.

Medicinal liquor for external use: Soak various Chinese medicinal herbs in strong liquor. After a few days, you can use the resulting liquid as a medium. The generally used Chinese medicinal herbs all belong to the group of drugs used for moving the vital energy and invigorating the blood. Several frequently-used prescriptions follow.[3] (See Appendix 3, Table of Weights and Measures.)

(1) *Ruxiang*	Boswellia glabra (frankincense)	1 *qian*
Moyao	Commiphora myrrha Engler (myrrh)	1 *qian*
Shenshanqi	Rhus verniciflua Stokes	1 *qian*
Tibetan *honghua*	Carthamus tinctorius (safflower)	1 *qian*
(Szechuan *honghua* may be used instead)		
Meibingpian	Dryobalanops camphora Coleb. (borneol)	2 *fen*
Guangmuxiang	Saussurea lappa Clarke (costusroot)	3 *fen*
Zhangnao	Camphor	2 *qian*
Xuejie	Daemonorops draco Blume (dragon's blood, a bright red gum exuding from a kind of palm fruit)	3 *qian*

The above herbs are soaked in 2 *catties* of strong liquor for a period of two weeks. The mixture is appropriate for acute and chronic injuries.

(2) *Honghua*	Carthamus tinctorius L. (safflower)
Chuanwu	Aconitum carmichaeli Debx. (prepared root)

3. Chinese medicinal herbs are available in cities with large Chinese populations, in herbal medicine shops, and some Chinese grocery stores.

Caowu	Aconitum chinense Pext. (root)
Guiwei	Angelica sinensis (root ends)
Taoren	Prunus persica (peach kernel)
Gancao (fresh)	Licorice-root
Jiang (fresh)	Ginger-root
Mahuang	Ephedra vulgaris
Duanzirantong	Native copper
Maqianzi	Strychnos nux vomica L. (nut)
Guizhi	Cinnamomum cassia Blume (sticks)
Ruxiang	Boswellia glabra (frankincense)
Moyao	Commiphora myrrha Engler (myrrh)

Soak 1 *liang* of each of the above thirteen herbs in 3 *catties* of strong liquor for two weeks. The mixture is suitable for general injuries, and is especially effective in the treatment of acute and chronic injuries of bone or cartilage.

(3)	*Mahuang* (fresh)	Ephedra vulgaris	7 *qian*
	Sangzhi	Morus alba L. (mulberry twigs)	3 *qian*
	Fangfeng	Saposhnikovia divaricata (root)	3 *qian*
	Wushaoshe	Zaocys dhumnades (snake)	4 *qian*
	Tianchong	Dried silkworm	1 *qian*
	Honghua	Carthamus tinctorius L. (safflower)	5 *qian*
	Chuanwu (fresh)	Aconitum carmichaeli Debx. (root)	3 *qian*
	Baizhi	Angelica anomala (root)	2 *qian*
	Qianghuo	Notopterygium incisum Ting. (root)	1 *qian*
	Duhuo	Angelica pubescens Maxim. (root)	1 *qian*
	Baixianpi	Dictamnus dasycarpus (root bark)	2 *qian*
	Xixiancao	Siegesbeckie orientalis var. pubescens (leaves)	

The above twelve kinds of herb soaked in 3 *catties* of *Gaoliang* (sorghum) liquor for two weeks are suitable for poliomyelitis, and child pneumonia.

1. 1 catty = 10 *Liang* = 17.6 ounces (1.1 lbs) = 500 g.

(4) Fresh green onion and ginger in equal amounts, soaked in 95% alcohol for two weeks is suitable for children with the common cold.

Yushushenyou (cajuputi oleum): This is a synthesized Chinese medicine that acts as a resolvent and an analgesic. It is often used as a medium in massage of wounds.

Sesame oil: This has the chief effect of increasing lubrication. It is often used as a medium in the "scraping" and "twist" methods of Chinese folk medicine.

Chuandaoyou ("conduction oil"): This is a medium first used in Shanghai. It is composed of cajuputi oil (see 8 above), glycerin, turpentine, alcohol, and distilled water. It can reduce swelling, kill pain, and dispel the effects of wind and cold.

Cinnamon oil: Cinnamon is fragrant and promotes warmth. It is used as a medium in deficiency ailments caused by cold.

Zhanjindan[5] "Muscle-stretching powder," also called "kneading medication": Grind the following seven herbs into a fine powder and pack in a sealed bottle for later use. *Zhanjindan* acts as a resolvent and an analgesic and is mostly used as a medium for massage when there has been an injury.

Ruxiang	Boswellia glabra (frankincense)	2 *qian*
Moyao	Commiphora myrrha Engler (myrrh)	2 *qian*
Tibetan *honghua*	Carthamus tinctorius L. (safflower)	1 *qian*
Shexiang	Musk	5 *fen*
Bingpian	Dryobalanops camphora (borneol)	5 *fen*
Zhangnao	Camphor	5 *fen*
Xuejie	Daemonorops draco Blume (dragon's blood, bright red gum exuding from a kind of palm fruit)	5 *qian*

5. *"Dan"* has many different meanings. Here it refers to a pulvis of dried herbs, triturated and mixed in the amounts specified. The word can also refer to a pill, troche or magna, to cinnabar, to alchemy or to a panacea.

CHAPTER XXIV

Clinical Applications of Massage Therapy

1. Lumbar Strain

Lumbar strain is a chronic type of condition frequently seen among working people, especially those engaged in heavy labor requiring bending of the lumbar area or carrying heavy loads. For example many foundry-workers suffer from this problem.

Etiology

The ligaments and muscles around the lumbar vertebrae have not healed completely, or are continually being injured; there is no history of acute injuries, but the general constitution is comparatively weak. There are also those individuals engaged in heavy physical labor who cannot compensate for abnormalities originally existing in the spinal column. All these conditions can result in lumbar strain.

However, there are some patients with good constitutions and no acute traumatic history in whom this condition sets in gradually due to long-term overbending of the lower back, or the carrying of heavy loads on the back. This is also known as "occupational strain."

Symptoms

Pain in the lower back is the essential symptom of this disease. It mostly happens in the middle of the lower lumbar spinal column. It can also often produce aching on either side of the spinal column and on the iliac crest. Sometimes the pain is intense, at other times it is light. Generally, the pain is light in the morning and heavy in the evening. It is aggravated by long sitting, by overtiredness, or by damp weather. When the symptoms are severe, the patient has difficulty doing any labor, and even sitting up or turning over in bed may be difficult. Sleep and appetite are also affected.

Treatment

Massage:

(1) The patient lies prone; his hands are placed on either side of his body. One or more pillows are placed under his abdomen, and all muscles are allowed to relax. First, the palm rub method is applied, starting from the pain-free part of the back and gradually progressing to the painful area. The manipulations should be applied lightly, so as not to cause pain, but to make the massaged area comfortable.

(2) Next, the palm-heel kneading method or the roll method is employed, with a gradual increase of intensity, on either side of the spinal column, going up or down several times.

(3) Third, with the thumb, deep kneading is applied to the main site of pain. It can simultaneously be combined with other methods such as the finger dig, the finger vibrate and the thumb kneading methods. Using all these methods, massage can be applied to such acupoints as *shenshu, mingmen,* and the eight *liao* (*shangliao, zhongliao,* etc.). The thumb-tip push method is also used. Also, acupoint massage can be applied to the principal pressure pain sites.

(4) Finally, at the conclusion of the massage, the kneading and the roll methods are again applied. At the same time the rotation and bend methods for the lower limbs can be performed lightly.

Methods for specific applications:

(1) When the disease is caused by a chronic lesion of the interspinous ligaments, the pain is often confined to a certain spinous process or intervertebral space right in the middle of the spine. The pain occurs with the forward bending, or backward extending of the spine and there is a fixed local tender point. Stress should be placed on the thumb kneading and thumb-tip push methods, which are applied to the immediate painful area. The force of the thumb should gradually penetrate deeply into the painful area and from there one should push outward into the surrounding area.

(2) If the condition is the result of a chronic lesion of the lumbar muscles, most of the pain will be in the lower part of the muscles at the sacral vertebrae or in the upper attachments of the lumbar muscles. Muscle tension on one or both sides is often hyperactively great. There is pain when the spine is bent forward and the sides of the body are moved. A swollen mass or hard lump can sometimes be

found in the soft tissues. When massaging the muscles, the kneading and roll methods should be used most. The thumb kneading method is employed on the site of the pain or the swollen mass. At a later stage, the energy-system pluck method can also be used. The kneading and rolling should be combined with rotation and stretching of the lower limbs.

(3) If there is no history of external injury, and the strain of the lumbar muscles is due only to spinal deformity or overtiredness in the lumbar region, and if the patient's lumbar muscles show the pathological changes associated with fasciitis, there will usually be obvious soreness in the lumbar area, as well as high muscle tension and pressure pain over a comparatively large area. Massage should be light. In the local area, the rub, kneading, and roll methods are used. Acupoint massage is also important. Besides the *jianyu, mingmen,* and eight *liao* acupoints, distant acupoints on the lower limbs, such as *chengfu, weizhong, chengshan,* and *taixi* can be used.

Therapeutic effect

The therapeutic effect of massage therapy on lumbar strain will be greatly affected by the pathological process by which the strain was formed, and the duration of the condition. Generally speaking, massage therapy is effective in treating this condition. (For treatment by massage therapy of lumbar strains ensuing from bone injuries or spinal deformity, see the section on Chronic Lumbar Pain following.) Some patients may suffer recurrences which must be guarded against. This is especially so in the case of occupational lumbar strain. Preventive measures are discussed below.

2. Chronic Lumbar Pain

Lumbar pain is an extremely common symptom. It can be symptomatic of a wide variety of conditions. In addition to protrusion of a lumbar intervertebral disk, lumbar strain and rheumatoid spondylitis, there are other causes of chronic lumbar pain such as obsolete and compressive fracture, and lumbo-sacralized or sacro-lumbarized megalo-spondylitis. Massage therapy has definite therapeutic effects in all of these. Because the massage therapy methods indicated are for the most part similar, these diseases are all described together below.

Etiology

In compressive fracture of the spine, there is generally a history of acute lesion. In the other diseases there is usually no obvious traumatic history, but just a slow development of the disease. The diseases are chiefly due to changes in the vertebral power line that cause retrogressive changes of a differing degree in the vertebral column. These affect normal physiological function, giving rise to lumbar pain.

Symptoms

The symptom common to these various conditions is chronic lumbar pain. It is often a persistent aching pain that occasionally becomes excruciating. Generally, the pain becomes more severe because of overwork or on gloomy, rainy days. It is usually located in the lumbar region, but some pains are referred to the back and some even appear in one or both of the sciatic nerves, leading to weakness in the lower limbs and numbness in the calf, etc. A protracted illness can affect systemic function as well as the ability to work.

Treatment

Massage:

(1) The patient is in a prone position. The chest and abdominal areas are padded with pillows. Apply the rub, kneading, and roll methods to relax the paravertebral muscles.

(2) The thumb push and roll methods are used in deep massage, concentrating on the aching areas. The thumb push, finger dig, and finger vibrate methods are applied to the acupoints that correspond to the aching areas and at the site of the pain.

(3) Passive movement of the lumbar area: As a rule, a forceful backward-extension is used (see Diagram 46, p. 232). No great force is needed, but the extension should be repeated about 10 to 20 times. If there are symptoms of sciatica, then the slanting backward-extension method may be added. This procedure is repeated 5 or 6 times, using somewhat greater force for the last extension.

Other Treatment: Other physical therapies may be used in conjunction with the massage therapy. The number of massage therapy sessions need not be many—

Medical Exercise

(1) *Backward extension of both legs:* The patient is in a prone position. The legs are drawn tightly together and extended straight. Try to keep the knees as straight as possible. Slowly lift both legs, the higher the better, and maintain them at their highest point for 30–60 seconds. The lumbar muscle will feel very tense and full of force. When this position can no longer be sustained, slowly lower the legs and rest for a while. Repeat a total of 5–10 times. (See Diagram 62).

(2) *Lumbar stretch:* The patient is in a standing position, with legs set shoulder-width apart and both hands supporting the lumbar area. With a gentle bouncing motion extend the waist forward and flatten the abdomen, repeating 30–60 times and gradually increasing the amount of extension.

(3) *Lumbar suspension:* With both hands, grasp a horizontal bar, such as the top of a door-frame, set just high enough that the toes can still touch the ground (see Diagram 63). Hanging half-suspended, swing the lower back loosely and naturally forward and backward, and from side to side. The breadth of the swing can gradually be increased to a point where the lumbar vertebrae can rotate. Persist until the arms can no longer hang on, rest for a while and then repeat several times.

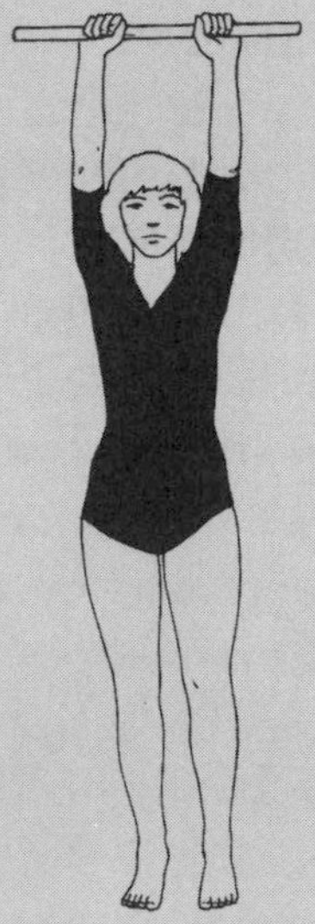

DIAGRAM 63

DIAGRAM 62

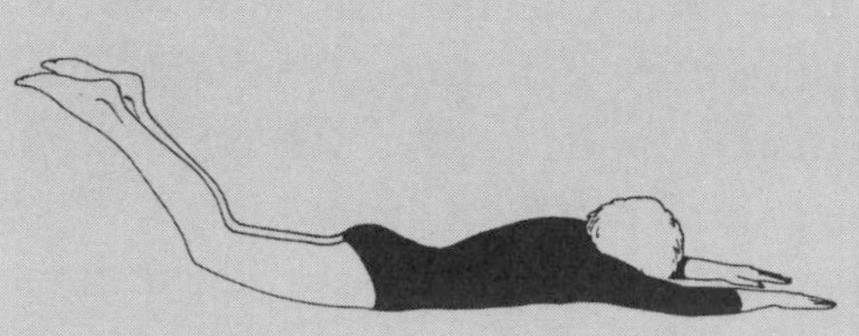

about 10–15. When the pain has lessened or disappeared, encourage the patient to undertake a long-term program of medical exercise lasting at least 3 to 6 months, to correct the shape of the spine and strengthen the paravertebral muscles.

Therapeutic Effect

At the beginning of the therapy and medical exercises there may be severe lumbar pain. This is normal before treatment. Long-term medical exercise is important to consolidate and heighten the therapeutic effect.

3. Sprains

Massage therapy has a beneficial effect on soft tissue and this is especially apparent with sprains. There is a wide variety of sprains, including all acute disorders that result from a sudden wrenching or twisting. A description follows of the common sprains in the sites with soft tissues, particularly involving a sudden overstretching of the ligament, or injury due to wrenching.

SPRAIN OF THE ANKLE JOINT

The sprain of the ankle joint is seen frequently. Usually when referring to an ankle sprain the true meaning is an injury to the lateral malleolar ligament. It seldom occurs in the medial malleolar joint. The injury occurs because of an overstretching of the ankle joint that suddenly bends outward or inward beyond the physiological scope of the articular movement, thereby causing injury to the lateral malleolar ligament. The injuries associated with differing degrees of sprain can be divided into the overtension of the ligament, and its partial or complete tearing away.

Etiology

This kind of injury most often occurs while walking on uneven ground, or jumping down from a height. Injury results from the foot suddenly bending outward or inward.

Symptoms

Aching pains: When an injury occurs pain suddenly appears in the lateral (or medial) part of the ankle, becoming more severe while moving about, or carrying a heavy load.

Swelling: Because of localized hemorrhage and the effusion of tissue fluid, the injury at once results in swelling. Swelling is usually confined to the antero-inferior part of the ankle.

Hematomatic area under the skin (bruising): This is caused by the localized rupture of a small blood vessel with the blood collecting under the skin. In more serious cases of sprain the hematomatic spot and the bluish-purple discoloration of the skin are usually present in the antero-inferior part of the ankle.

Crippling: Generally a crippling reaction appears right after the injury with the patient unable to bear weight on the ankle.

Treatment

In accordance with the principle of accelerating the removal of the hematoma, generating new blood, and facilitating the flow of vital energy and blood, massage therapy is best applied at the acute stage of sprain.

Massage:

(1) Apply a light push or a light rub massage around the sprained area.

(2) Apply a heavy stimulating manipulation like the finger dig method, or the finger vibrate method, on the *juegu* acupoint (the space between the tibia and fibula) of the affected limb, and continue manipulating this area for one minute. This is called the pain-removing method.

(3) The push, rub, and kneading methods are applied around the sprained area along the direction of the vein and lymphatic returns.

(4) Adopt the light to gradually heavier push and rub massage techniques, moving gradually from the circumference to the center of the injured area. If swelling and circumscribed bruising are present, use the thumb to apply, alternately, the finger-cut and push methods lightly and smoothly and with a dense pattern of strokes to the swollen area where blood has accumulated (the bruised area). Push upward from the lower part of the ankle to the cruciate ligament, continuing until the swelling disappears.

(5) Immediately thereafter apply the finger dig and finger vibrate methods to massage points in the area of the injury, such as *juegu, chengshan, kunlun, taixi, jiexi, pushen* (below the lateral malleoleus, about 2 *cun* directly beneath the *kunlun* cavity, the depression beside the calcaneus bone) and *rangu* (in the depression in front of the medial malleoleus and below the sphenoid bone). *Note:* When the finger dig method is applied, go from shallow to deep until a reaction is produced, then add the vibrate method and go from deep to shallow.

Massage once a day for 10–15 minutes until all the symptoms are gone.

LUMBAR SPRAIN

Sprain in the lumbar region is seen frequently. It can be caused by several different types of injuries:

- When the waist bends forward to the lumbar point at which the lumbar spine is completely bent, the muscle-contraction that protects the ligament is no longer possible. So when the upper body bears a weight, the ligament to the lumbar region is susceptible to injury.
- When the lower limbs are in the extended position, i.e. when the pelvis is fixed, and an excessive tractive force is suddenly applied to the lumbar region, injury to the ligament results.
- A blow to the lumbar region and a sudden twisting when lifting a heavy object are factors that can produce lumbar sprain directly. In addition to injury of the ligament, injury of the lumbar muscles is also likely to occur.

Etiology

Lumbar sprain can be brought on by working with a bent back, by falling while doing heavy physical labor, and especially by a sudden twist while lifting a heavy object up off the floor.

Symptoms

There is pain on one or both sides of the lumbar region, which can neither bend forward nor backward, nor turn left or right. In serious cases, the patient needs someone to support him while he walks, and the pain becomes worse when he takes a deep breath or coughs. Swelling is often not manifest.

During examination let the patient lie prone with several pillows under his abdomen. Then, with light and careful finger pressure, a local pressure point can be discovered on lumbar spine 4 or 5, or in the space between lumbar spine 5 and sacrum 1. Sometimes, when the tender area is extensive, simultaneous injury to the muscle should be considered.

Treatment

Massage:

(1) The affected person is in a prone position. The light rub method or the thumb push method is first applied to the lumbar region to relax the lumbar muscles and reduce the pain.

(2) Apply the roll method to both sides of the lumbar area. The massage should be light. Then the thumb, or the palm and outside edge of the hand, is employed to knead around the circumference of the injury, after a while working gradually in toward the middle. Slowly move from light kneading to deep kneading, in order to relax the muscles and enliven the blood, clearing away the accumulated blood and producing new blood. This procedure is repeated several times.

(3) Acupoint massage. Use the kneading and dig techniques on sites in the lumbar region, and the *shenshu, mingmen, shangliao, ciliao, huantiao, chengfu,* and *weizhong* acupoints.

(4) Press on the lumbar spine and shift the pelvis. With his right hand, the therapist lightly presses on the lumbar region and with his left hand he moves the right side of the pelvis upward. Go from top to bottom, coordinating each pressure on the lumbus with a shift of the pelvis.

(5) Strike the lumbar region with the palm. With a concave palm, slap the lumbar region 10 times, or more.

(6) With the patient on his feet, apply the kneading and lumbar stretch methods to the lumbar region. For more detailed information on the lumbar stretch method, see page 230–33. Massage once daily for 20–25 minutes until all the symptoms disappear.

Therapeutic Effect

If the treatment for sprain is applied immediately after an injury occurs, then its therapeutic effect is greater, and the time required for treatment is shorter. The longer the time that elapses after injury, the poorer the therapeutic effect and the more treatments required. The effect of the treatment is related directly to the severity of the injury. The results of massage-therapy on a sprain involving partial laceration of the ligament are good. But massage therapy on a completely lacerated ligament will be insufficient, possibly requiring surgical intervention. An uninterrupted course of treatments is very important. During the treatment period, proper rest should be taken as an unhealed acute sprain is easily re-injured.

4. Bruises

Bruises are a commonly seen injury to soft tissue. They occur in the limbs and also in internal organs. Here we chiefly deal with the bruising of the limbs.

Etiology

A bruise is chiefly an injury to the soft tissue (including the skin, the subcutaneous tissue, the muscles, the nerves, the blood vessels, the lymphatic vessels, etc.) caused by an obtuse force. At the time of injury there may occur exudations of both lymph and blood, swelling, pain, and abnormality in sensation. Massage therapy treatment of this condition acts chiefly to disperse the accumulated blood and to improve the flow of vital energy and blood. It can help in absorbing the exudations and in improving the local nourishment of the tissues, and so is favorable to restoring the tissues to a healthy condition.

Symptoms

The local contused area immediately produces a swelling. Hemorrhage and a hematomatic mass may develop under the skin and there are sensations of pain or numbness in the swollen area. Bruises to the limbs produce differing degrees of disordered movement. A serious bruise, because of the rupture of the blood vessels and the lymphatic vessels, may produce a disturbance in the return of lymph and/or blood. Therefore it may leave a long-term swelling of the tissue and even the deposition of its exudate, together with adhesion and contracture, which make the limb difficult to move.

Treatment

In massage treatment of contusion, methods vary with the stage at which the injury is treated.

Massage Treatment for Contusion—acute stage:

(1) When acute symptoms are extremely obvious, place the limb in a comfortable raised position before proceeding with massage.

(2) First, take a commonly used acupoint near the site of the injury and apply the finger dig and finger vibrate methods until there is quite a strong reaction of soreness and swelling, about 1 minute.

(3) Then, also in the area of the injury, apply the push, rub, kneading, and divergent push methods for about 2 minutes, going up and down and side to side until the accumulation dissipates and blood circulation around the site of the injury is improved.

(4) Next, knead very lightly with the flat of the thumb or with the center of the palm for about 1 minute at the site of the injury, kneading just lightly enough not to cause any increase in pain. Then massage around the circumference of the injury as in (3) above for about 10–15 minutes.

Massage Treatment for Contusion—later stage: This refers to the period 2 or 3 days after the injury, when pain and swelling have begun to improve; or to an even later period, where swelling and impeded mobility remain.

(1) First find a commonly used acupoint in the neighborhood of the injured area. Then apply the finger dig and finger vibrate methods until they produce a strong reaction of soreness and a swollen feeling. This should take about 1 minute.

(2) Use thumb or palm push methods to massage around the circumference of the injured area. In general, go from the furthest point and work in. For example, on a finger or toe start from the tip of the digit. On large areas, both hands can be used. The divergent push method can be used to do both sides of the injured site. Then push and knead on the injured site, lightly. Massage on and around the injury for about 10 minutes.

(3) If the swelling is still severe enough that pressing with a finger leaves a mark, then the finger-cut method may be applied, lightly and in a dense pattern of strokes. In the center of the injury or where pain is evident, movements should be light and slow. Continue until there is some reduction in the swelling.

(4) If there is adhesion, contracture and disordered mobility in a limb, apply passive manipulations such as rotation, extension, or bending to help restore mobility. Be sure to avoid overextension.

Therapeutic effect

At the acute stage of contusion, swelling and pain can be reduced immediately by massage. Generally, bruises that are not serious can be basically healed in about a week (6–7 massage sessions). Serious bruises take longer, but massage can greatly shorten the healing process here, too. At the same time it can prevent contracture, stiffening, and reduced function in the joint, and lessen the contusion's residual symptoms.

5. Torn Muscles (*Muscular Laceration*)

Muscle lacerations are also referred to as either "twisted" or "torn" muscles, depending on the severity of the laceration. In most cases the muscle fiber is partially torn; complete severance of the muscle bundle is rare.

Etiology

Muscle laceration is usually produced by a sharp, uncoordinated contraction of the muscle. It can also be the result of a sudden passive or active traction. The condition is most common among athletes and those engaged in heavy labor. Muscle tissues which have already undergone pathologic changes or whose function is comparatively weak are particularly susceptible.

Symptoms

At the time of the injury, the patient is often conscious of a tearing sensation. Then contraction pain occurs in the affected group of muscles. A swollen mass forms locally due to hemorrhage under the skin. The next day, small bruised spots in the skin may appear near the injury. Over the next several days, the sharp pain at the site and the pain of the muscle contraction gradually lessen. The bruised spots are also gradually absorbed, but the swelling at the injury gradually hardens into a swollen lump, sometimes called a "knot" of extravastated blood (blood that has been forced into surrounding tissue), and this does not easily disperse. The lump causes the symptoms of motion pain and local pressure pain to persist.

Treatment

Massage: Different manipulations should be applied at different stages. If the muscular laceration is accompanied by muscular calcification, then massage therapy must be temporarily delayed. However, at a later stage, when the ossification (hardening) has become stable, massage may be used with caution.

(1) At the time of the injury, or within 24 hours, do not use strong, deep massage. Lightly and slowly apply the palm rub method, starting at the circumference and moving gradually to the center of the injury. Do not continue for too long.

(2) After two or three days, hemorrhage will have ceased, and swelling and small bruised spots in the skin will appear. Then the flat-palm push method is applied above and below the injured area, pushing from the distal point toward the proximal. This process is repeated about 10 times. Then the base and the edge of the palm are employed for light kneading of the swollen area, going from the circumference to the center of the injury and then from the center to the circumference. Do not use enough force to cause pain. To the superficial bruises around the injury, apply the finger-cut method.

(3) If a hard swollen knot and motion pain remain in the late stage of the injury, but the complication of muscular calcification is not diagnosed, deep kneading can be applied locally, or the flat-thumb push or thumb-tip push method can be used. Then, while the push and kneading methods are being applied, add passive manipulations such as the rotation and stretch methods. Rotate and knead at the same time, with the amount of rotation or stretching not great enough to cause pain. Conclude with the shake method.

Other Treatment: Rest must be taken at the acute stage of a muscle laceration. External application of medication, under pressure, is extremely important. Various physical therapies can be used, in combination with medical exercise.

Therapeutic Effect

Massage applied to the muscle laceration at an early stage must be light. Massage applied to a case in its late stages has the effect of reducing the swelling, eliminating the superficial bruises, loosening the tendons and ligaments, killing pain and restoring mobility.

6. Flatfoot and Foot Strain

Etiology

This condition occurs mainly among working people who stand too much, or who work half-crouching, and among athletes, especially teenagers. Thus it may be called an occupational or athletic strain. The condition usually develops because the tissue structures in the area have not yet solidified, while body weight has developed more quickly, and the load placed on calf and foot in labor or sports exceeds the ability of the structures in the area to support it.

Strain of the foot area is very often accompanied by secondary sagging of the arch of the foot. This is because the body weight is too great, and the muscles and ligaments of the calf and foot that maintain the arch cannot support the load. As the muscles that maintain the arch, such as the anterior and posterior tibial muscles and the peroneus longus and brevis muscles, lose tension because of overexhaustion, the force of the body weight is all imposed upon the ligaments that support the arch. The ligaments are gradually pulled slack, resulting in the arched bone structure of the foot being unable to maintain itself, and the arch sags. Over a long period of time, this leads to strain and to a deformation that is not easily reversed.

Symptoms

At the onset there may only be symptoms such as weakness of the affected foot, easy tiring and inability to walk very far. In the early stages, there is the symptom of pain, usually pain in the sole, but sometimes a spasmodic pain in the gastrocnemius (calf muscle), or radiating pain in a certain muscle group. During examination, a pressure pain in a certain muscle group can often be found, too, and occasionally resistance pain can be discovered in the same muscle group. Generally, there is excessive tension in the muscles, and also tension and a pressure pain in the deep tissues and ligaments of the sole of the foot, as well as a mild limp.

In the late stage a slight club foot tendency appears. At that time the pain usually lessens. Generally the arch of the foot gradually becomes flatter, particularly as the scaphoid bone gradually collapses. In the knotted area of the scaphoid bone an obvious pressure pain appears, affecting labor and sports.

Treatment

Massage:

(1) First have the patient lie face down. The shin is supported with a pillow so that the leg rests comfortably. Apply the flat-thumb push method or the roll method from the back of the knee space downward; use the thumb push method on the popliteal space and on both sides of the Achilles tendon; and use the roll method on the gastrocnemius (or calf) muscle. Go back and forth several times. Apply the finger dig and thumb kneading methods to acupoints such as *weizhong*, *chengshan*, *taixi* and *kunlun*.

(2) Then have the patient turn over onto his or her back. Massage using the thumb push method or the roll method, going back and forth several times over the extensor muscle in front of the tibia, as far as the instep area. At the same time apply massage to acupoints such as *chu san li* or *zusanli*, *yanglingquan*, and *jiexi*.

(3) With one hand, firmly grasp the bottom of the patient's foot, and apply the pinch method to the instep of the foot. Start by pinching a wide area, then pinch along between each of the metatarsal bones. Finally, do a deep pinching along the flexor and extensor muscles of the calf and the muscle bundles of the peroneus longus and brevis. This should be done for about 5–10 minutes.

(4) Have the patient actively or passively shake his ankle. Then apply the rub-roll and the vibrate methods on the calf and the foot area to conclude the massage.

Therapeutic Effect

In early cases, the symptoms improve markedly after one massage session and are completely cured after several sessions. At a later stage, after the secondary strain of flatfoot has already appeared, results are poorer and the course of treatment required is longer. But in general, symptoms such as pain and tension can be gotten rid of, malformation can be improved, and athletic ability can be restored.

7. Frozen Shoulder (*Shoulder Pariarthritis*)

Shoulder periarthritis is also called "frozen shoulder," or "congealed shoulder." It is common among middle-aged and older people, and therefore is called "fifty-year-old's shoulder," as well. It usually develops on only one side.

Etiology

This condition consists essentially of inflammatory changes in the soft tissues around the shoulder joint. The cause of it is not yet completely understood. Certain cases may be related to trauma or chronic strain. Doctors of Chinese medicine consider it to be caused by wind, cold, and moisture attacking a shoulder that is vulnerable due to the weakness of old age, deficiencies of blood and vital energy, and nutritional imbalance. Today there are those who consider it a "collagen disease."

Symptoms

For no apparent reason, soreness, weakness, and impeded mobility gradually develop in the shoulder area. At the onset of the disease, pain is usually the main symptom. Soreness spreads through the shoulder area, and is often particularly noticeable at the front of the shoulder. It sometimes radiates into the forearm. Raising the arm from the side and rotating it outward increases the pain, so the affected shoulder is usually held in a fixed position. At the same time, the patient often feels weak, or unable to continue for very long, when he does activities such as carrying something on his shoulder.

When a later stage is reached, the aching symptoms are often gradually reduced, but the mobility of the shoulder joint is increasingly impeded. Especially difficult are abduction and outward rotation; adduction and forward flexing are also somewhat impeded. Therefore, not only is productive labor affected, but movements involved in writing, eating, combing the hair, and putting on clothes also become difficult. Whenever there is wet weather the local symptoms become more severe.

Treatment

Massage:

(1) Have the patient take a sitting position, with shoulders relaxed. First the thumb rub and the flat-thumb push methods are applied on the back and scapula areas of both shoulders. Then with the base of the palm apply the kneading and rub methods or the roll method to the scapulo-dorsal area of the affected shoulder. Go from light to heavy and shallow to deep, massaging for about 5–10 minutes, until the local area feels comfortable and warm, and the muscles are relaxed and soft.

(2) Slowly and dexterously apply the pinch method. You can go from the shoulder down to the upper arm, concentrating on the front of the shoulder. Repeat several times. Combine this with massage of such acupoints as *fengchi, jianjing, jianliao, jianyu, jianzhen,* and *hegu,* using the finger dig and finger vibrate methods or the thumb-tip push method.

(3) Then the light hammer method or the light pat method is applied on the shoulder area. At the same time the shake and rotation methods are also used. The range of the shaking and rotation should gradually be increased.

(4) Finally knead and rub the shoulder, neck, upper back, and arm on the affected side, and finish with a rub-roll massage of the arm.

Methods for specific situations:

(1) When the case is in its early stages, where pain is evident and the patient is weak, one should make more use of the push and roll methods, or else apply con-

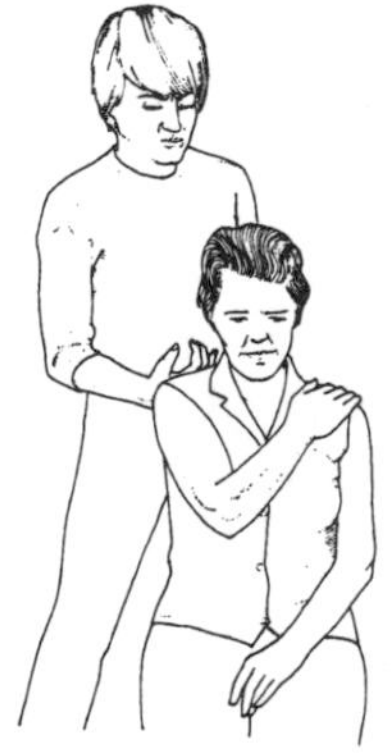

DIAGRAMS 64

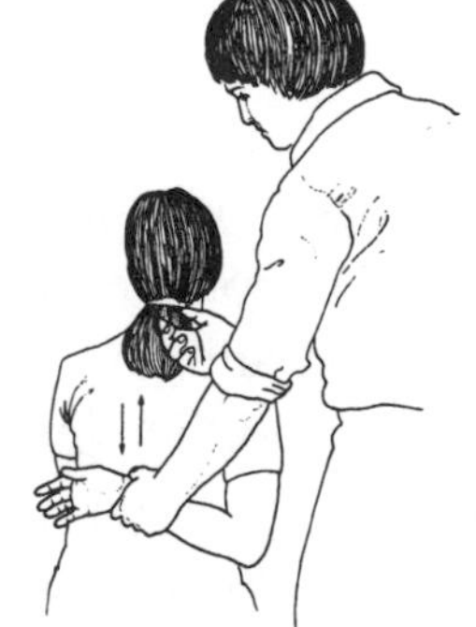

DIAGRAMS 65

Medical Exercise

Shoulder lift: Bend forward at the waist, let the arms hang down and clasp the hands. Swing the arms forward, gradually increasing the distance that they swing. See Diagram 66.

Shoulder abduction: Bend at the waist and let the upper limbs hang down. Swing them naturally left and right, gradually increasing the range of motion. See Diagram 67.

Shoulder back-extension: Stand with feet shoulder width apart and hands clasped palm-outward behind the back. Use the sound hand to stretch the affected hand as far out backwards as possible without bending the body forward. See Diagram 68.

Shoulder circles: Stand with feet set shoulder width apart and the arms held out straight to each side. Move the arms round and round, first forward and then backward, gradually increasing the size of the circles formed.

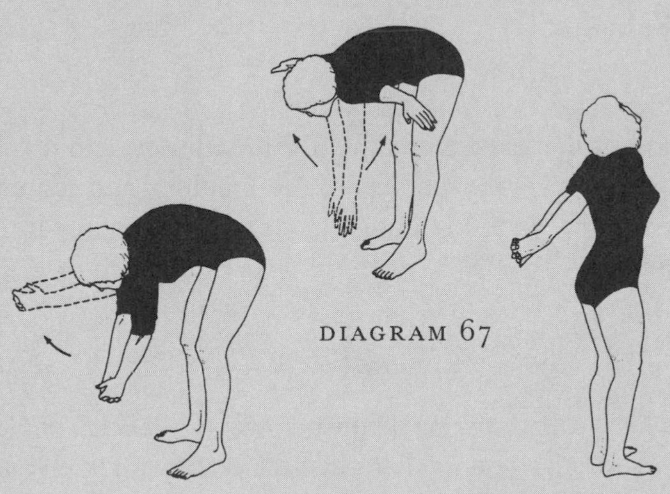

DIAGRAM 67

DIAGRAM 66

DIAGRAM 68

duction oil or medicinal liquor and use the chafe method. Make less use of the shake and rotation methods. If slight rotation immediately gives rise to severe pain, then do not use the rotation method at all for a while.

(ii) With a case in its later stages, when impeded mobility is the main symptom, and the patient's general condition is comparatively good, make moving the joint the main treatment. Do a passive movement of the shoulder with one hand, while with the other hand applying the knead, rub, and roll methods to the shoulder area, particularly any specific painful site. See Diagrams 64 and 65. Attention must be paid to gradually enlarging the range of movement. When the movement of the shoulder joint has been reasonably well restored, stretching of the limb should be combined with the other aspects of treatment.

(iii) In cases of long-term illness, particularly when movement disturbance is comparatively severe and restoration of mobility is not evident, the extend method and the grasp method may also be used on the shoulder. In some such cases, abduction, forward flexing and rotation, as well as the forward-rotated and back-extended positions, give particular difficulty. In these cases, the energy-system pluck method can often be effective, applied at the tendons of both the deltoid muscle and the biceps.

Therapeutic Effect

Massage is quite satisfactory for treating this condition. It not only relieves pain, but restores or improves the mobility of the shoulder, and restores the ability to work. However, the period required for treatment is comparatively long, usually about a month.

8. Stiff neck (*Torticollis*)

In China torticollis is called "falling off the pillow," "lost neck," or "lost pillow." This neck condition is noticed on waking when a sudden pain is felt and the head cannot be freely turned. Torticollis also occurs as a result of trauma. A minor case may last a few days and clear up spontaneously. A severe case may last for a long time, and the pain may become increasingly severe. The therapeutic effects of massage therapy on torticollis are quite good.

Etiology

Torticollis occurs either when one is extremely tired and sleeping exposed to a draft giving rise to muscle spasms or myofasciitis, or else when the synovial membrane of one of the small joints of the cervical vertebrae becomes inlaid, or there is a partial dislocation.

Symptoms

There is a severe pain in the neck that becomes worse when the neck is turned. These symptoms usually manifest themselves suddenly, after awakening from a sound sleep. This is the typical wryneck. The symptoms may also occur after a wrenching or twisting movement of the neck or under conditions where the head is held in a fixed position, while the body suddenly leans forward. However, the pain in the neck may occur suddenly without any of these histories. Sometimes there is just a pulling sensation in the neck, and the symptoms set in gradually, recurring often and becoming worse, especially when the neck is exposed to cold.

Treatment

Massage:

(1) The patient is seated, while the practitioner stands behind him or her and to one side. First, the flat-thumb push method is applied to the shoulders and the upper back, especially on the affected side. This will make the patient more comfortable and relaxed.

(2) With the thumb and index finger, continue by applying the knead and grasp massages to the muscle group at the back of the neck, starting from the *fengchi* acupoint down along the muscles and around to the *jianjing* acupoint on the affected side, grasping the acupoint 2–3 times, until the vital energy appears. In this manner knead and grasp repeatedly, until relaxation of the muscle group in the patient's neck area is achieved.

(3) Apply the neck rotation method. (See Diagram 38, p. 226.) Be quite certain to avoid producing any pain. The range of movement should be small. While you are turning the neck, ask the patient to relax the neck muscles. Wait till the neck muscles are completely relaxed, and no resistance to the rotation remains. Then sharply twist the neck. Finally, again knead and grasp the muscle group at the

back of the neck 2–3 times. Where synovial inlay is suspected, it is most appropriate to use the neck rotation method.

Special Procedures:

(1) When a semi-dislocated joint is suspected, the neck-rotation method is not advisable. After relaxation of the neck area by the normal massage, a neck-lifting manipulation can be used: Ask the patient to sit cross-legged on the ground. The practitioner stands behind the patient's back. With his two hands he supports the two sides of the patient's lower jaw and slowly lifts. Then he bends the patient's head back to face upward.

(2) When the patient has an obvious traumatic history, and the injury involved great force, it is inadvisable to twist the neck suddenly when applying the neck rotation method. Wait 2–3 days before using this part of the manipulation.

(3) When no traumatic history is evident, but the symptoms are aggravated by exposure to wind and cold, it is advisable to perform more of the push and grasp massages, to grasp deeply and to knead heavily.

Other Treatment: A typical case of torticollis will recover after 2–3 massage sessions. In general, there is no need of other treatment. Where there is a traumatic history, a longer course of disability, or continued exposure to wind and cold, massage can be combined with the application of physical therapy, Chinese herbal lotions, and local hot compresses.

9. Bedsores (*Decubitus Ulcer*)

Decubitus ulcer is a type of necrotic ulcer in the soft tissue. It is often seen in a bed-ridden patient with a weak constitution. Once bedsore is formed the ulcerated part heals extremely slowly. Serious decubitus ulcers can even bring about septicemia, causing death.

Etiology

The patient who is bed-ridden for long periods of time, especially one who is unable to change position, will develop bedsores due to local malnutrition when the weight of the body puts pressure on an area of skin, subcutaneous tissue, and other soft tissues, leading to poor blood circulation and impeded supply of nutrients.

Symptoms

In the early stages, there are usually no subjective symptoms. By the time the patient feels discomfort and sharp local pain, the ulcer has usually already formed.

Treatment

Massage: In massage treatment of decubitus ulcer, different conditions call for the adoption of different methods of massage, which are separately described below.

(1) Preventive measures: The patient who is bed-ridden for a long period of time, especially the paralytic patient, must start to receive prophylactic massage as early as possible. The massage is concentrated on the areas of the body that are under pressure, but general massage of the whole body is given as well. Normally, the palm-base circular-rub method is adopted, following the direction of the blood flow. The manipulation is increased from light to heavy. The effect of the massage will be improved by dipping the palm into medicinal liquor before massaging.

(2) Massage for bedsores in their early stages: Generally, the thumb or the fleshy pad at the base of the thumb can be employed to apply the circular rub method, rubbing from the center of the bedsore toward its circumference, so that the blood that has collected in the area is dispersed. This in turn promotes resupply with fresh, new blood, turning the skin from dark to red. At this point, although an ulcer has not yet formed, skin is poorly supplied with nutrients, and easily broken, so massage must be light and dexterous. General massage and passive manipulations of the limbs must also be intensified.

(3) Massage for bedsores in their later stages: Since an ulcer has already formed at this point, the effect of the massage is to accelerate the healing of the ulcer. Massage is applied mainly around the circumference of the ulcer. The rub and kneading methods are used. At the same time, apply the kneading, pinch, rub-roll, and vibrate methods to the limbs, with a view to improving blood circulation over the whole body.

Other Treatments: Medical exercise has great value in the prevention and treatment of bedsores. It is also very important to frequently change the position of the body, to keep bedding clean and unwrinkled, and to reduce the pressure on the supporting points of the body as much as possible.

10. Headache

Headache is only a symptom, and can occur in a great number of diseases. However, not all types of headache are suited to the application of massage therapy. For example, headaches resulting from contagious diseases, such as cerebrospinal meningitis, etc. are not suited to this type of treatment. Consequently, it is necessary to apply massage therapy selectively in the case of headache.

Etiology

Headache is associated with numerous diseases. In addition to occurring with some contagious diseases and with high fever, headache can occur with common cold, flu, and in certain eye and nose diseases. The patient with high blood pressure often has headache. Moreover, there are also certain chronic, recurring functional headaches, such as migraine and psychosomatic or tension headache.

Symptoms

The headache occurring in common cold and flu is likely to be in the form of an acute attack, with such accompanying symptoms as fever and runny nose. The headache resulting from eye and nose diseases may be manifested in subjective complaints or in objective symptoms of the eye and nose, and commonly is located in the forehead. Migraine and psychosomatic headache are presented as a chronic process or recur repeatedly, now light and now heavy. Migraine pains occur on one side of the head and are often accompanied by dizziness; psychosomatic or tension headache is felt in both temples, at the back of the head, or at the back of the neck. In the presence of intense headache, both appetite and sleep are affected.

Treatment

Massage therapy is most effective in functional headaches such as migraine, psychosomatic headache, etc. It is also effective in reducing headache symptoms caused by the common cold and flu. Temporary relief of headache resulting from some eye and nose diseases can also be obtained.

Massage:

(1) The patient usually takes a sitting position. If he cannot sit up, he may take a supine position. The practitioner stands at the patient's head, and the head is wrapped in a towel.

(2) With the left hand hold the patient's head in place; with the right hand apply a flat-thumb push to the head. First perform a light push massage over the entire head. Then push massage along the midline of the head, going from the hairline in front to the hairline at the rear. Do extra pushing at the *baihui* acupoint. First, go from light to heavy, then vice versa. Then the side-of-the-thumb push method can be used to push along both sides of the head, also starting from the front hairline and going to the back hairline. If the patient complains of more discomfort in a certain part of his head, do more pushing there. The above push methods should take about 10 minutes.

(3) With both thumbs, apply a push massage to the forehead, going from the *yintang* and *zanzhu* acupoints between the eyebrows to the *taiyang* acupoints in the temples. Or else use the drag method, dragging the thumbs apart from the *yintang* point to the *taiyang* points. At the *taiyang* points, the dig and vibrate methods can be added. After that, drag around the sides of the head to the *fengchi* points behind the ears. For aches in the forehead caused by some eye and nose diseases, even more of these push massages can be applied.

(4) With the two thumbs, rub and knead both of the *fengchi* acupoints. Then, with the thumb and the first two fingers apply a three-finger pinch going from the back of the head to the nape of the neck. Then use both hands to pinch both *jianjing* acupoints. This process should be repeated several times.

(5) Massage acupoints in the limbs, such as *neiguan, hegu, zusanli (*or *chu san li),* and *sanyinjiao.* The finger dig, finger vibrate, and thumb tip push methods may be used.

Therapeutic Effect

After massage the headache patient will feel relaxed and comfortable. After one or several massage sessions, the headache will subside or disappear.

Self-massage

(1) Knead the eye sockets: With the thumb, index, and middle fingers of both hands, knead around both eye sockets in a rotary motion, first turning outward, then inward, 7–8 times each.

(2) Knead the *taiyang* acupoints: With the tips of the middle fingers of both hands knead both *taiyang* points with a rotary kneading motion, first clockwise, then counter clockwise, for 7–8 rotations each.

(3) Drag across the forehead: With the tips of both middle fingers, wipe from between the eyebrows, to the *taiyang* acupoints in the temples, then along both sides of the head to the *fengchi* acupoints at the back hairline.

(4) Push along the head: With the edge or base of the palms of both hands, firmly press on either side of the head and push from the front hairline to the back hairline. Do this about 30 times.

(5) Pinch the nape of the neck: With the thumb, index, and middle fingers of the right hand pinch from the back of the head downward to the back of the neck. Repeat 5–6 times.

II. Treatments for Common Ailments

by A. R. Lade, Massage Therapist

11. Fatigue

Fatigue and general body exhaustion have become common symptoms for many people in our stressful modern society. Chinese massage therapy can be used to revitalize the system.

Etiology and Symptoms

Fatigue and exhaustion can be caused by many and varied factors. In an acute situation, fatigue is the result of hard or prolonged mental or physical activity, or of emotional stress. The body's energies can rapidly enter into a state of depletion, but with an individual's inherent strength, this period of depletion may last only a short while. On the other hand, in a chronic situation where the patient is in a prolonged state of exhaustion and fatigue, there may have been many precipitating factors, such as a long debilitating illness, malnutrition, severe emotional, physical, or mental stress, or even the side effects of some drugs. In this situation the body is weak and deficient to begin with, and its recuperative powers are low. In both chronic and acute cases, symptoms such as tiredness, muscular aching or cramps, dull pressure-type headaches, weak and sunken pulse, dizziness, lack of appetite, inability to concentrate, over thinking, and depression may appear.

Treatment

Have the patient lie down on his or her back with a pillow under the knees to support and flatten the lower back. A pillow under the head is unnecessary unless the patient feels uncomfortable; if so, use only a thin, firm pillow.

(1) First, standing on the right side of the patient, place your left palm on the forehead with the thumb resting on *yintang.* The right hand is placed on the abdomen between the navel and the point *guanyuan.* No pressure is applied; simply maintain a light touch for 3 minutes.

(2) Start on the same side on the lower leg, using the thumb rub method to massage the points *zusanli* (or *chu san li)* and *yanglingquan.* Then using palm rub method, work down in between these two points along the lateral side of the leg to the ankle. Repeat 3 times. Then use finger or thumb press method on the points *sanyinjiao, taixi* and *taichong.* Following this, move to the opposite side and repeat this step on the patient's left leg.

(3) Moving back over to the right side, thumb rub the point *quchi* at the elbow. Then use the palm rub method from this point along the lateral surface of the forearm to the wrist. Repeat 3 times. Follow with finger or thumb press method on the points *hegu, taiyuan, daling* and *shenmen* on the wrist and hand. Now switch over to the left arm and repeat this step.

(4) Standing above the patient's head, apply the three-finger grasp method to the area of *jianjing* on the shoulders. Then with bent fingers, press the point *feng fu* at the base of the skull. You may then finger press from *feng fu* laterally (one side at a time) along the occipital ridge towards the ears, massaging any sensitive spots found along the way. Following this, rub the area of *taiyang* on the temples with flat fingers or heel of palm.

(5) Finally, move to the side and repeat the first step for 3 minutes.

Note: This treatment can be given 2 to 4 times daily to refresh and tone the patient. A session should last approximately 15 minutes.

12. Motion Sickness

Motion sickness is a functional disorder caused by repetitive motion, primarily characterized by nausea and vomiting. Travel in cars, trains, on the sea, or in the air can all cause this unpleasant disorder.

Etiology and Symptoms

Excessive stimulation of the vestibular apparatus (in the inner ear) by motion is the primary cause. Emotional stress (such as fear or anxiety) and visual overstimulation are also contributing factors. Other factors, such as lack of sleep, or an empty or upset stomach, can make a person readily susceptible.

The main symptoms are nausea and vomiting, which may be preceded by hyperventilation, pallor, cold sweating, sleepiness, dizziness, headache, or fatigue. Once the main symptoms appear, the patient may feel unable to concentrate. Motion sickness can aggravate other diseases already present, such as heart or lung disease.

Prevention

Massage should be given as a preventive measure starting 1 week before beginning a journey as well as during and after an attack. Loose clothing should be worn, especially around the neck, and it is important to only eat easily digestible food 1 hour before beginning a trip.

Treatment

During an attack, allow the person to vomit if nauseated and loosen the clothing. It is best to have the patient lie on his or her back with a pillow under the knees. If necessary, this treatment can be done in the sitting position.

(1) First, the following points should be massaged by the finger or thumb press method: *baihui, fengchi, yifeng, renzhong,* as well as in the area directly behind the ear and parallel to the ear canal.

(2) Next, on the extremities, thumb rub the points *zusanli* (or *chu san li)* and *neiguan.*

Note: This treatment can be given once or twice a day, for 10 to 15 minutes a session, as a preventive measure.

13. Hemorrhoids

Congestion and clotting of the small blood vessels around the anus can lead to blood vessel swelling and possibly bleeding during defecation; this is commonly referred to as hemorrhoids or piles.

Etiology and Symptoms

Western and Chinese medicine have similar views on the causes of hemorrhoids, namely, irregular eating habits, overconsumption of spicy foods or alcohol, constipation, general weakness and deficiency of the body, and prolonged sitting and lying on cold, damp surfaces. Symptoms include bleeding on defecation (usually stopping after the bowel movement) and raised swelling in and around the anus with or without pain. Sometimes hemorrhoids may lead to anal prolapse which is a more severe problem. Another related problem is the extremely painful anal fissure which causes anal sphincter spasm.

Treatment

(1) First, the patient is asked to lie face down with a pillow placed under the lower legs and feet. (See illustration on p. 191.) Use the finger or thumb press or rub method on the following points in order: *baihui* (this is an important point for hemorrhoids and is usually very painful), *dazhui, mingmen,* and back *yangguan.*

(2) Using the thumb kneading method, work on the sacral *liao* points (Diagram 59, p. 250, points 30–33) until the skin becomes slightly red. Then, using the finger press or small circular finger rub method, work down both sides of the coccyx (tail bone) to the tip. Care should be taken to go gently in this area.

(3) Use the palm vibrate method over the point *chengshan* at the bank of the lower leg, increasing pressure according to the patient's tolerance.

14. Insomnia

Insomnia is defined as the inability to obtain a proper amount or quality of sleep.

Etiology and Symptoms

The causative factors for insomnia can be many, although the prime cause is usually psychological, such as stress, anxiety, worry, and depression, which may be aggravated by external factors such as noise. However, disturbances of the autonomic nervous system, anemia, high blood pressure, gastrointestinal disorders, consumption of coffee or caffeine products (especially before bedtime), and respiratory difficulties can all bring about disturbance in the sleep pattern. The main symptoms are inability to fall asleep or maintain sleep, dream-disturbed sleep, irritability, and a feeling of tiredness upon waking up.

Prevention

For lasting relief, the causes must be dealt with. Care should be taken to ensure a pleasant sleeping environment with fresh air, humidity, and a moderate temperature. Also, taking time to relax before going to bed is most helpful.

Treatment

(1) Begin with the patient lying down on his or her stomach with a pillow placed under the feet and lower legs. (See illustration on p. 191). Massage the acupoints *xinshu, geshu,* and *shenshu* on the back, using the thumb rub method. Then moving to the feet, massage the acupoint *yongquan* (or *yung chuan).*

(2) Next, have the patient roll over onto the back with a pillow under the knees,

and massage the following acupoints in order: *sanyinjiao* on the legs, *shenmen* on the wrist, *baihui* on the apex of the head, and along the occipital ridge (with gentle finger pressure) from the acupoint *fengchi* to *yifeng* and from *fengchi* to the occipital midline *fengfu*.

(3) Finally, moving to the right side of the patient, the practitioner places the left hand on the forehead area *(tianting)* with thumb touching *yintang*, and the right hand placed just below the navel on the midline of the body. (See Diagram 69.) Both hands are placed softly on the body and held there for 3 minutes or longer.

DIAGRAM 69

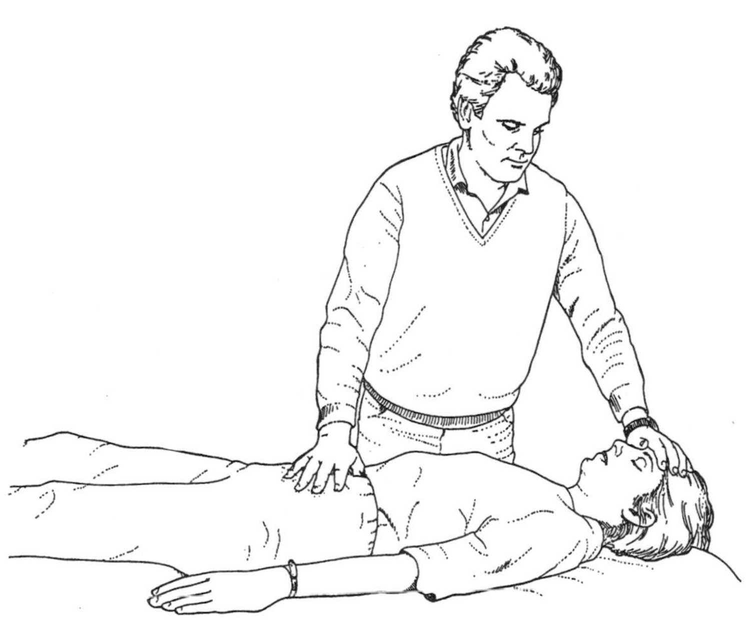

Treatment is best given in the evening before bedtime; otherwise a time of day should be chosen in which the patient can relax afterwards for 20 minutes or so. Treatment should take 15–20 minutes.

Also refer to chapter 17 of Part III for self-administered massage techniques and suggested exercises.

15. Indigestion

Indigestion is the body's outcry against an imbalanced life style; it is not a fatal outcry, but one that can be felt all too uncomfortably. Here is some relief through Chinese massage therapy.

Etiology and Symptoms

Indigestion is not a specific ailment but rather a group of related symptoms. Both Chinese and western medicine see a similar origin to this problem—mainly, overeating, hurried eating, inadequate chewing, or swallowing air while eating, as well as improperly prepared or combined foods, and lack of physical activity. These factors can cause an imbalance in the peristaltic movement of the gastrointestinal tract and in the digestive secretions, leading to indigestion. Another major factor in the cause of indigestion is emotional and mental stress, which distorts the action of the autonomic nervous system on the stomach and intestines. Not to be overlooked, however, is the possibility of a more serious problem causing the indigestion, such as tumors or growths originating in the viscera. This should be assessed by a trained medical professional.

The common symptoms of indigestion are heartburn, flatulence, constipation or diarrhea, loss of appetite (which can lead to weight loss), and nausea. Nausea can be described as a sick feeling with a desire to vomit. It is frequently associated with other symptoms such as dizziness, weakness, sweating, and headache. It is not found exclusively with indigestion and can be seen in ailments such as migraine headache and morning sickness. The following treatment gives specific acupoints that can relieve nausea accompanied by indigestion or nausea found with another ailment.

Prevention

Massage can be given during an acute attack, or as a preventive once every 1 or 2 days to strengthen the digestive system and relax the nerves. Effort must be made to correct the cause by developing proper and relaxing eating habits, reducing stress and increasing physical exercise.

Treatment

Ask the patient to lie down on his/her abdomen and chest. Place a pillow under the lower legs and feet. (See illustration on p. 191.)

(1) Begin by using the palm kneading or rub method, starting at the lower back and working up towards the shoulders; repeat 3–5 times. Then, using small circular motions, thumb rub beside the spine from the sacral area to the upper back.

(2) Next, return to the lower back and do skin pulling on the sacrum and up along the spine to the neck. The practitioner accomplishes skin pulling by placing the hands on either side of the spine (or centerline of the sacrum) with hands almost touching, and fingers bent. The skin is grasped firmly between the thumb and index finger, with the thumbnail facing towards the head. The skin being grasped is rapidly lifted away from the spine and immediately lowered. Frequently, a popping sound can be heard indicating that a release in the tissue's fascia layer has been achieved. This grasp and pull is done over each vertebra, causing a slight skin reddening afterwards. In Chinese massage therapy this is a major technique for treating gastrointestinal disorders of various kinds. During a session, it is to be done over the spine only once. (See Diagram 70)

DIAGRAM 70

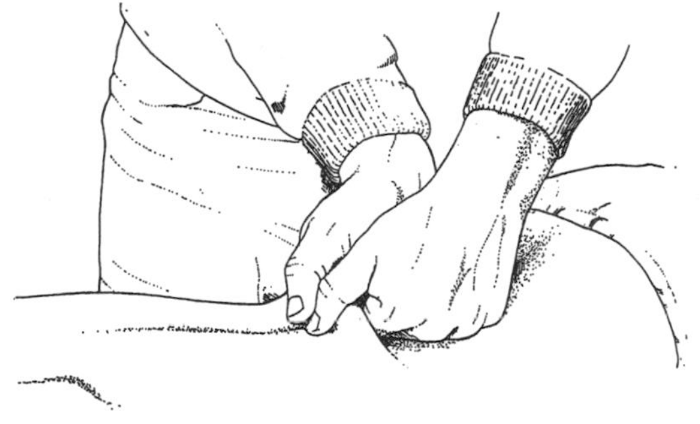

(3) After completing the skin pulling method, gently stroke the patient's back from head to lower back with relaxed fingers to ease any sensations of discomfort.

(4) Next, ask the patient to roll over onto the back, placing a pillow under the knees and head if desired. Standing on the patient's right, place your left hand on the forehead with thumb touching *yintang* and the rest of the hand covering *tianting* (this is the area of the forehead above *yintang*) and your right hand is placed in the area above the navel, *xiawan*. Slight pressure is used and the hand on *xiawan* is gently rocked. After 1 or 2 minutes of rocking with the right hand, it is moved first to the *zhongwan/shang-*

wan area on top of the stomach, repeating the rocking motion, and then to *guanyuan* below the navel, again rocking for 1 or 2 minutes. All the time the left hand is resting on *tianting.*

(v) Finally, massage the acupoints *zusanli* (or *chu san li), neiguan, quchi,* and, if diarrhea is present, *yinglingquan.*

The points *zusanli* (or *chu san li)* and *neiguan* are specific for nausea. After completing the acupoint massage, allow the patient to rest before getting up. Treatment can last for 15–20 minutes.

16. Anxiety and Nervousness

These two emotional problems are becoming more common in society as our pressures and tensions increase. Relief and balance can be restored through the simple technique of massage therapy.

Etiology and Symptoms

Anxiety and nervousness are primarily emotional reactions to pressure and stress that have lead to mental-emotional disharmony. Another cause can be hormonal imbalances, especially seen in menopause and PMS (premenstrual syndrome). Occasionally, they are symptoms of a disease process, such as the anxiety seen in intestinal obstructions, or nervousness manifesting in high blood pressure. The symptoms of anxiety are apprehension, uncertainty, and fear without cause; the symptoms of nervousness are excitability, irritability, and restlessness.

Prevention

When appropriate, counseling or psychotherapy should be urged to deal with root causes. Massage therapy is used to stabilize the mind and emotions as well as to center the physical body.

Treatment

(1) Begin with the patient lying on his/her back with pillow under knees (and head, if needed) and massage the acupoints, with thumb or finger rub method. Rub *baihui* on apex of head; *neiguan* on wrist; *zusanli* (or *chu san li), sanyinjiao* and *yongquan* (or *yung chuan)* on the legs and feet. Repeat this sequence of points 3 times or until the patient is calm and relaxed.

(2) Next, standing on the patient's right, use the thumb rub method to massage these acupoints: *yintang* on the forehead with the left hand and *guanyuan* below the navel with the right hand. Follow by resting the hands on these acupoint areas for 3 minutes.

17. Menstrual Problems and Pain

Under this heading are included irregular, prolonged, and painful menstruation, as well as premenstrual tensions.

Etiology and symptoms

A great many menstrual problems can be traced to emotional disturbances (such as anxiety and depression), causing hormonal changes that affect the reproductive organs. Other factors, such as overwork, insufficient sleep or nourishment, inadequate or excessive sexual intercourse, and menopause can also disturb the body's hormonal balance. Lastly, certain disease processes can disturb the menstrual pattern, for example, fibroid tumors, Cushing's disease, and cancer.

Symptoms associated with premenstrual tension are irritability, painful breasts, nervousness, headaches, abdominal swelling, and generalized water retention. With painful menstruation there is cramping in the lower abdomen, sometimes going down the thighs and legs, low back pain, nausea, and in some cases, increased menstrual flow. Irregular menstruation refers to a cycle abnormal either in duration or consistency.

Treatment

(1) Begin by having the patient lie face down on her abdomen and chest with a pillow under the lower legs and feet. A thin pillow placed under the abdomen will relieve the discomfort of sore breasts in this position. The pillow should be placed just below the breasts and under the abdomen. (See illustration on page 191.) Using the thumb rub or kneading method, massage the following points in order: *mingmen, shenshu,* and then the *liao* points over the sacrum (Diagram 59, p.250, points 30–33). Then, on the lower back, use the palm vibrate method for 3 min-

utes, followed by the same technique used to vibrate the sacral area. To finish the back area, gently stroke with fingers from upper to lower back/buttocks area.

(2) Next, have the patient roll over and place a pillow under the knees. Massage the following acupoints in order: *zusanli (*or *chu san li), sanyinjiao* and *taixi* on the legs and ankles.

(3) Next, massage the acupoints *guanyuan, qihai* and *qichong,* on the lower abdomen, using a gentle thumb or finger rub method.

(4) Finally, massage the acupoints *baihui* and *fengchi* on the head and base of the skull, especially if there are any symptoms of heaviness and tension in the head or upper body.

18. General Chinese Massage Treatment

The main purpose of this treatment is to promote harmony of body and mind by stabilizing the *yin yang* polarity. This is achieved by selecting and massaging acupoints that will regulate the energies of each of the main meridians. Doing so brings toning, revitalizing, strengthening, calming, and centering effects to the body and mind. This treatment is in accord with the other principles and functions of Chinese massage therapy: promoting the body's resistance to disease and increasing blood circulation. Treatment can be given on a regular basis for preventive purposes once or twice a week with good results, with each treatment lasting about 20–30 minutes.

(1) Begin by having the patient lie face down on the abdomen and chest with a pillow under the lower legs and feet. (See illustration on p. 191.) Massage the acupoint *dazhui* on the upper back, using the finger or thumb rub method. Then massage the *"shu"* points on the back (2 run lateral to each vertebra), starting at *feishu* and going down one vertebra at a time to *dachangshu.* Continue by massaging the sacral *liao* points (Diagram 59, p. 250, points 30–33), and then, in the following order, *huangtiao, chengfu, weizhong, chengshan,* and finally *kunlun,* down on the leg. The above points (except *dazhui*) are all on the bladder meridian and regulate the trunk of the body. Repeat the above sequence on the back and legs 3 times.

(2) Next, have the patient roll onto hisor her back with a pillow under the knees. Starting at the lower legs and feet, massage the following acupoints using the finger/thumb rub or the kneading method: *zusanli (*or *chu san li), yanglingquan, yinlingquan, sanyinjiao, taixi,* and *taichong,* in order. Then single-palm rub the bottom of the feet around *yongquan (*or *yung chuan).* (The free hand supports the top of the feet during palm rubbing.)

(3) Next, moving to the upper extremities, massage the acupoints *quchi, shousanli, hegu,* and the points *taiyuan, daling, shenmen, waiguan,* and *yanggu,* around the wrist.

(4) Next, using both hands, apply the push massage or drag method to the forehead, going from *yintang* and *zanzhu* acupoints between the eyebrows to *taiyang* on the temples. At *taiyang,* use a gentle vibrate method. Follow by massaging the acupoint *fengchi* at the back of the head and then, using the three-finger grasp method, pinch *jianjing* on the shoulders.

(5) Finish by applying a gentle palm press to *taiyang* on either side of the temples and then, using the three middle fingers, apply pressure to *yintang* between the eyebrows coupled with *fengchi* at the base of the skull. As *fengchi* is a bilateral point, alternate hands to effect first right then left sides. (See Diagram 71.) The pressure is gentle in both directions, or it can simply be held for 1 to 3 minutes.

DIAGRAM 71

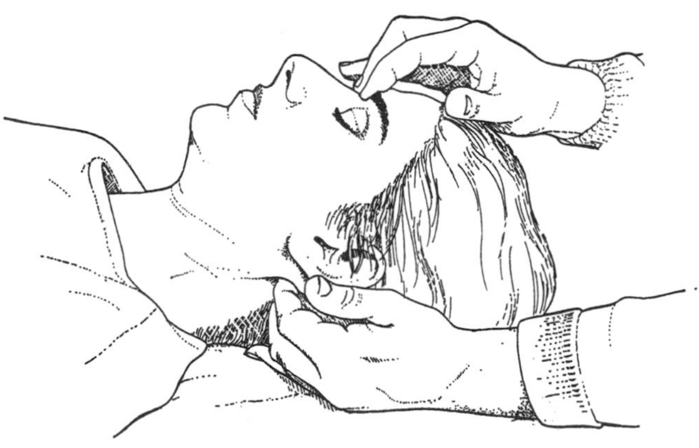

APPENDICES

Appendix 1

Self-Massage for Strengthening the Body and Preventing Disease

1. Knock on the teeth: With the lips gently closed, use the tips of the fingers to knock rhythmically against the lower and the upper teeth 30–40 times each.

2. Clean the mouth: With the lips gently closed, use the tongue to forcefully wipe out around the space between the teeth and the lips. Wipe around to the left and to the right 30 times each.

3. Rub the hands: Rub the palms together 30–40 times, with increasing speed, until they become warm.

4. Rub the face: Rub the face with the warmed palms, first going from the left side of the face across the forehead to the right side 7–8 times.

5. Knead the eyes: With the knuckles of the index, middle, and ring fingers of both hands, knead with a circular motion around the eye sockets, first going from the inside corner to the outside, then from the outside corner to the inside, 7–8 times each.

6. Knead *taiyang*: With the tips of the middle fingers of the left and right hands, press on the *taiyang* acupoints in the left and right temples and knead with a circular motion, first clockwise and then counterclockwise, 7–8 times each.

7. Wipe the forehead: With the tips of the middle finger of both hands, wipe from between the eyebrows out toward both sides, gradually reaching the hairline.

8. Push on the head: With the sides or bases of the palms of both hands, press against the sides of the head, then push from the front hairline to the back hairline. Do this 30–40 times.

9. Dig at *baihui*, *fengfu*, and *dazhui*: Dig and then knead at each of these 3 acupoints, spending about 1 minute at each.

10. Vibrate the ears: With the fingers of both hands against the back of the head, cover the ear canals with the palms and make a quick, rhythmic drumming motion, about 30–40 times.

11. Knock behind the ears: With the fingers of both hands against the back of the head, and the palms tightly covering the ear canals, tap against the back of the head with the index and middle fingers, so that a "dong" sound is heard. Do this about 20 times.

12. Pat the chest: Spread the fingers of both hands and tap against the chest with the flats of the fingers, inhaling with each tap. Do this about 7–8 times.

13. Chafe the ribs: Use the outside edges of the hands to chafe the two sides of the ribcage quickly 30–40 times.

14. Knead the abdomen: Press on the umbilical area with the left hand and press down on the back of the left hand with the right. Then deeply and forcefully knead the abdomen, going clockwise 30–80 times.

15. Chafe the lumbar area: With the hands in fists, use the thumb end of the fists (the "eye" of the fist) to chafe up and down quickly and forcefully on both sides of the lumbar region about 30–40 times.

16. Hammer the spine and the sacrum: With the hands in fists, hammer along both sides of the spine, starting from as high you can reach and going down as far as the coccyx. Do this 3–4 times.

17. Rub-roll the thighs: Sit with legs folded and rub-roll each thigh with the palms of both hands, 30–40 times.

18. Pinch the calves: Sitting with legs folded, apply a pinch massage to the gastrocnemius muscle of the back of the calf, going from the top of the muscle down to the Achilles tendon. Do the left leg first, then the right.

19. Chafe *yongquan* (or *yung chuan*): Quickly and forcefully chafe the *yongquan* acupoints of the sole of the foot with the outside edge of the hand. Chafe 30–40 times, until the center of the foot is warm. Do the left foot first.

20. Breathing exercise: Stand with the legs shoulder width apart. Lift the hands from the abdominal region upward to the throat, simultaneously lifting the

head, bending backward at the waist and breathing in. Then draw the hands downward from the throat back to the abdomen, lower the head, bend forward at the waist and breathe out. As you breathe out, make the sounds "ha-ho-hee-hoo." Repeat the exercise twice.

Self-massage is not only used to strengthen the body and prevent disease, but it can also be useful in actually treating disease and in consolidating the effect of other therapies. The 20 massage methods outlined above can be used as a group or certain of them can be selected, according to specific circumstances. When used preventively, they can be done in the morning after rising, or at night just before going to bed. When used during recuperation from illness, certain of them can be selected, according to one's condition. In disease that affects the senses, massage of the head area may be emphasized. In those that affect the lower limbs, massage of the legs is even more important. And so on.

Appendix 2

Eye-Care Massage

1. Knead the upper corners of the eye sockets: With the flats of the thumbs, press against the upper inside corners of the eye sockets, below the eyebrows (at the *tianying* point). The fingers should be slightly bent and propped against the forehead. Gently knead at the *tianying* point.

2. Squeeze and press the base of the nose: With the thumb and index finger of one hand, squeeze the base of the nose (at the *jingming* acupoint). First press down, then squeeze upward, alternating these motions.

3. Knead the cheeks: With the flats of the index fingers, press on the center of each cheek (at about the *sibai* acupoint). Hook the thumbs into the depression under the lower jaw and clench the rest of the fingers. Knead the centers of the cheeks with the index fingers.

4. Scrape the eye sockets: Slightly bend the index fingers and press the side of the second knuckle against the top of the eye socket. Press the thumbs against the *taiyang* acupoints in the temples and clench the other three fingers. Scrape down-

ward around the eye sockets with the index fingers while kneading hard on the *taiyang* points with the thumbs.

These massages should be done 20 times each, both in the morning and at night. They can also be done after looking at something for a long time, for instance after prolonged reading.

Appendix 3

Table of Weights and Measures

HEIGHT:

1 catty *(jin)* = 10 *liang* = 500 grams = 1.1 pounds
1 *liang* = 10 *fen* = 50 grams = 1¾ ounces
1 *qian* = 1⁄10 liang

DISTANCE:

1 *li* = ½ kilometer = ⅓ mile

APPROXIMATE LIQUID MEASURE:

2 catties of water = 1 liter = 1.1 quarts = 1 kilogram

Appendix 4

Table of Acupoints

I = Heart meridian; II = Small intestine meridian; III = Bladder meridian; IV = Kidney meridian; V = Pericardium meridian; VI = Three heater meridian; VII = Gall bladder meridian; VIII = Liver meridian; IX = Lung meridian; X = Large intestine meridian; XI = Stomach meridian; XII = Spleen meridian.

CHINESE NAME	TRANSLATION OF CHINESE NAME	NUMERICAL POINT
Baihui	hundred meetings	Governor Vessel 20
Chengfu	support and hold up	III-50
Chengjin	supporting muscle	
Chengshan	supporting mountain	III-57
Chize	foot marsh	IX-5
Chongyang	rushing *yang*	XI-42
Ciliao	second *liao* point	III-32
Dachangshu	large intestine correspondence	III-25
Daling	great mound	V-7
Danshu	gall bladder correspondence	III-19
Dazhui	great hammer	GV-14
Feishu	lungs correspondence	III-13
Fengchi	wind pond	VII-20
Fengfu	wind palace	GV (Governor Vessel) 16
Fengmen	wind gate	III-12
Ganshu	liver correspondence	III-18
Gaohuang	richness for the vitals	III-38
Geshu	diaphragm correspondence	III-17
Guanyan	origin of the passes	CVU-4
Hegu	joining of the valleys	X-4
Huantiao	jumping circle	VII-30
Jianjing	shoulder well	VII-21

Jianliao	shoulder *liao* point	VI-15
Jianyu	shoulder *yu* point	X-15
Jianzhen	upright shoulder	II-9
Jiexi	released stream	XI-41
Jingming	eyes bright	III-1
Juegu	bone separation	VII-39
Kunlun	*kunlun* mountains	III-60
Lieque	narrow defile	IX-7
Mingmen	gate of life	GV-4
Neiguan	inner pass	V-6
Pishu	spleen correspondence	III-20
Pucan	servants aide	III-61
Qichong	*qi* rushing	XI-30
Qihai	sea of *qi* (energy)	CV-6
Quchi	crooked pond	X-11
Quepen	broken basin	XI-12
Renzhong	person-middle	Governor Vessel 26
Rugen	breast root	XI-18
Sanyinjiao	three *yin* crossing	XII-6
Shangliao	upper *liao* point	III-31
Shangwan	upper stomach cavity	CV (Conception Vessel) 13
Shaohai	little sea	I-3
Shenmen	spirit gate	I-7
Shenque	spirit deficiency	CV-8
Shenshu	kidney correspondence	III-23
Shousanli	hand three miles	X-10
Sibai	four-white	XI-2
Taichong	supreme rushing	VIII-3
Taixi	great stream	IV-3
Taiyang	highest *yang*	an extra point
Taiyuan	great abyss	IX-9
Ten xuan	ten *xuan* points	
Tianshu	heavenly pivot	XI-25
Tianting	heaven's hall	an extra point

Tianzong	heavenly ancestor	II-11
Tinggong	listening palace	II-19
Tinghui	hearing meeting	VII-2
Waiguan	outer pass	VI-5
Weishu	stomach correspondence	III-21
Weizhong	accepting middle	III-54
Xialiao	lower *liao* point	
Xiawan	lower stomach cavity	CV-10
Xinshu	heart correspondence	III-15
Xiyan	knee-eye	
Xuehai	sea of blood	XII-10
Yamen	gate of dumbness	GV-15
Yangchi	*yang* pond	VI-4
Yanggu	*yang* valley	II-5
Yangguan	*yang* pass	GV-3
Yanglingquan	*yang* mound spring	VII-34
Yangxi	*yang* stream	X-5
Yifeng	screens the wind	VI-17
Yingxiang	welcomes fragrance	X-20
Yinlingquan	*yin* mound spring	XII-9
Yintang	hall of the imprint	an extra point
Yongquan or *Yung Chuan*	bubbling spring	IV-1
Zanzhu	collecting bamboo	III-2
Zhongfu	middle palace	IX-1
Zhongliao	middle *liao* point	
Zhongwan	middle stomach cavity	CV-12
Zusanli or *Chu San Li*	foot three miles	XI-36

INDEX

A

Abdomen
flaccid abdominal wall, 165
massage methods for, 63, 102, 163, 196, 203
relief from pain in, 63, 164, 168
strengthening and developing, 115, 160–62, 164, 165
swelling, in premenstrual tension, 297
Abdominal breathing. *See* Breathing, abdominal
Abdominal pain, massage methods for, 192
Absent-mindedness, relief from, 173. *See also* Mental concentration
Aconitum carmichaeli Debx., 261
Aconitum chinese, 262
Acupoints. *See also* individual points
for adults, 245–54
anterior view, 248d
of arms, 255
for children, 254–55
defined, 186n
lateral view, 246d
location of, 245–55
of lower limbs, 252d
names translated, 304–6
posterior view, 250
Acupressure. *See* Acupuncture points , massage of
Acupuncture for paralysis, 174
Acupuncture points, massage of, 103, 104, 129, 172
dan tian, 63
feng chi, 60
shen shu, 63
yung chuan, 64
Agility, developing, 85, 176. *See also* Flexibility
Anal fissure, 291
Anal prolapse, 291
Angelica anomala, 262
Angelica pubescens Maxim., 262
Angelica sinensis, 262
Anger, relief from, 54. *See also* Emotional State; Relaxation
Angina pectoris, 121, 135, 136, 139
Ankle joint, sprain of, 269
Ankles
flexibility, 95
Ankles, strengthening and developing, 88, 118
Anxiety, 296–97
Anxiety and depression, 167–70. *See also* Emotional state; Mental concentration; Relaxation; Well-being,
promoting
exercises for
Chi Kung, 168–69
games for, 167, 168, 169–70
Tai Chi Chuan, 168
massage for, 168, 169
mental and physical relaxation, 167–68
relief from, 54, 66, 139, 167, 173
Appetite
loss of, 264, 294
restoring, 168
Apprehension, relief from, 54. *See also* Emotional State; Mental concentration; Relaxation
Archer's position, 226n
Arms
massage methods for, 117, 203, 208, 214
strengthening and developing, 39, 41, 44, 45, 49, 53, 57, 84, 92, 101, 114, 177
Arteriosclerosis, 131–34. *See also* Circulation; Coronary heart disease
defined, 131
diabetes and, 131
emotional state and, 131
exercises for, 131–33
benefits, 131–32
Tai Chi Chuan, 132
massage for, 134
physical activity and, 131
prevention, 131
Arthritis, 20, 61, 186
Atherosclerosis, 20, 131, 137. *See also* Arteriosclerosis
Athletes
exercises for, 111–18
benefits, 111
Forward thrust, 114
Hanging and swinging, 116
massaging the shoulders, 118
Relaxing the waist and tapping the body, 116–17
Riding a horse, 112
Swallow flying, 115
Tiger walking, 113
Wall pushing, 115
massage for, 111, 117–18
Autogenic healing. *See* Mental concentration; Relaxation; Visualization
Autonomic nervous system. *See* Nervous system

B

Back. *See also* Backache; Posture; Spine
injuries, 86, 113
massage methods for, 163, 194, 196, 219, 220, 221, 1976
pain, 165, 186–91
prevention of, 93, 114, 116
problems, 56, 62, 92, 162, 165
sprains, massage methods for, 199
strengthening and developing, 41, 53, 62, 87, 111, 115, 177, 179, 185
Backache. *See also* Back; Posture
massage methods for, 197, 209
prevention, 56, 97, 98, 99, 100, 103, 115
treatment, 63, 106
Backward extension, 267
Ba Duan Jin (Eight fine exercises), 49–58
for the chronically ill, 49
Curing the five troubles and seven disorders by turning the head backward and gazing sternly, 54
for the elderly, 49
exercises, 51–58
how to practice, 49
Increasing the vital energy by tightening the fists and gazing sternly, 57
Keeping all diseases away by raising the heels seven times, 58
Regulating the internal organs by raising both hands to the sky, 50
Regulating the spleen and stomach by raising the hand upward, 53
Shooting the eagle by drawing the bow with the hands, 51–52
Strengthening the loins and kidneys by bending forward, with hands touching the feet, 56

Tranquilizing the fiery heart by turning the head around, and swinging the hips, 55
Baihui acupoint, 245, 246d, 291, 293, 296
Baixiampi, 262
Baizhi, 262
Balance, improving, 21, 123, 124, 181
Bathing, 162
BEATING THE "DRUM OF HEAVEN", 60
Bedsores, 284–86
BENDING FORWARD, 47
BENDING FORWARD WITH HANDS TOUCHING THE FEET, 56
BENDING THE TRUNK WITH THE HANDS TOUCHING THE FEET, 62
Bend method, 223–25
Bent-finger dig method, 206–7
Bingpian, 263
BITING THE TEETH, 60
Blood. *See* Arteriosclerosis; Circulation; Coronary heart disease; Hypertension
Blood pressure, high. *See* Hypertension
Borneol, 261, 263
Boswellia glabra, 261, 262, 263
Bowel illness, prevention of, 159, 163. *See also* Gastrointestinal problems
BOWING, 46
Brain concussion, exercises following, 173
Breathing
  abdominal, 21, 41, 72–73, 106, 155, 165
  in *Chi Kung,* 65, 66–67, 68, 69–70, 72, 73, 74, 75
  in anxiety and depression, 163
  in brain concussion, 173
  in coronary heart disease, 155
  counting the breaths, 72
  difficulty, 68
  exercise, traditional Chinese, 78
  following the breath, 72
  in gastrointestinal problems, 163, 165
  in hypertension, 78, 122, 123, 125, 128
  improving, 20, 36, 50, 75, 78, 94, 165
  in insomnia, 172
  in pregnancy, 108
  in *Tai Chi Chuan,* 20, 21, 165
  in *Yi Jin Jing,* 36
Bruise, 273–75
  in muscle laceration, 275–76
  swelling in, 273
Buttocks
  massage methods for, 194
  strengthening and developing, 184–85

C

Calcific arteriosclerosis, 131. *See also* Arteriosclerosis
Calisthenics, 35, 49, 78
Calves
  massage methods for, 223–25
  strengthening and developing, 58, 87
Camphor, 261, 263
Caowu, 262
Cardiorespiratory fitness, 83, 94. *See also* Breathing; Heart; Lungs
Carthamus tinctorious, 261, 263
Chafe method, 212–13
Changshan acupoint, 245
Chengfu acupoint, 245, 250d, 266, 298
Chengjin acupoint, 252d
Chengshan acupoint, 252d, 266, 292, 298
Chest
  massage, 154
  massage methods for, 196
  pain, 68, 121, 135, 136, 139, 164
  strengthening and developing, 36, 37, 38, 49, 51, 61, 62, 94
Chi Kung for Fitness, 12, 65, 70–73, 72–73, 172
  benefits of, 70
  breathing in, 70
  exercises, 71
  frequency and length of training, 73
  for hypertension, 70, 122
  principles of, 70
  program for the practice of, 73
  for psychoneuroses, 70
  quietness training, 73
Chi Kung for Relaxation, 13, 65, 69–70, 172
  benefits of, 69
  for brain concussion, 173
  breathing in, 69
  in chronic illness, 69
  frequency and length of training, 70
  for hypertension, 122
  principles of, 69–70
  quietness training, 69–70, 122
Chi Kung for Sleep, 172
Chi Kung for the Internal Organs, 65, 74–75
  benefits of, 74
  breathing in, 74–75
  for constipation, 74, 163
  for gastroptosis, 74, 164
  for peptic ulcer, 74
  principles of, 74–75
  quietness training, 75
  for viral hepatitis, 74
Chi Kung (Invigorating exercises), 65–67, 65–75, 66
  for anxiety and depression, 168–69
  breathing in, 65, 66–67, 68, 69, 72
  for constipation, 160
  defined, 65
  as "energy,saving" exercise, 65
  for gastrointestinal problems, 159–64, 165
  how to practice, 66–67
  for hypertension, 121, 122–24
  for insomnia, 172
  longevity and, 65
  meditation in, 65
  for mental and physical relaxation, 65
  mental concentration in, 65, 66, 67, 69, 70, 72
  for peptic ulcer, 159
  possible side effects, 67–69
  principles of, 65–67
Children
  amount of massage, 257
  exercises for, 83–88
  benefits, 83
  Edge walking, 88
  Eye massage, 88
  Hitting the bean bag, 84
  Monkey play, 85
  Rope jumping, 84
  Tiger walking, 86
  Tip-toe walking, 87
  Worm wriggling, 87
  indigestion, 196
  massage methods for, 196, 206, 216, 218
Chilliness, relief from, 54
Chinese exercise therapy. *See* Chinese fitness exercises; Chinese therapeutic exercises; Traditional Chinese exercises
Chinese fitness exercises, 81–118
  for athletes, 111–18

for children, 83–88
for the elderly, 97–104
for pregnant women, 105–10
for the sedentary, 89–95
Chinese therapeutic exercises, 119–91
for anxiety and depression, 167–70
for arteriosclerosis, 131–34
for coronary heart disease, 135–57
following brain concussion, 173
for gastrointestinal problems, 159–65
for hypertension, 121–29
for insomnia, 171–72
for paralysis, 174–81
for sciatica and lumbar disk problems, 180–84
Chi (Qi), defined, 200n
Chize acupoint, 245, 246d, 248d
Chongyang acupoint, 245, 252d
Chronic constipation. *See* Constipation
Chronic illness, 49, 59, 69, 78, 79
Chuandaoyou, 263
Chuanwu, 261, 262
Chu san li acupoint, 103, 187, 206n, 210n, 252d, 254, 287, 289, 291, 296, 299
Cilao acupoint, 249, 250d
Cinnamon oil, 263
CIRCLING AT A RESTING POSITION, 79
CIRCLING WHILE MOVING THE LEGS UP AND DOWN, 79
CIRCLING WHILE WALKING, 80
Circulation
in abdomen, *Tai Chi Chuan* and, 20
fibrinolysis, 137
flaccid abdominal wall and, 165
improving, 20, 60, 64, 90, 95, 98, 101, 102, 109, 131–32, 136–37
ischemia, 132, 136, 177
and massage therapy, 188
in paraplegia, 177
Club foot, 279
Commiphora myrrha Engler, 261, 262, 263
Common cold, 187
herbs for, 263
massage methods for, 213, 216
Concentration. *See* Mental concentration
Connamomum cassia, 262
Constipation, 294
causes of, 159–60
diet for, 164
exercises for, 159, 160–62
Chi Kung for the Internal Organs, 74, 163
flaccid abdominal wall, 165
massage for, 163
relief from, 164, 168
therapeutic activities, 162–63
treatment, 159
Contusion, 273–75
Coordination, improving, 21, 85, 124, 176
Coronary artery disease. *See* Coronary heart disease
Coronary heart disease, 141–54, 155–57. *See also* Arteriosclerosis; Circulation
135-57
age and, 136
angina and, 135, 136, 139
blood pressure and, 139
circulation and, 135, 136, 137, 138
defined, 136
diet and, 135, 136
emotional state and, 139
exercises for, 135–57, 139
benefits, 137–38
Chi Kung, 135
games for, 139
heart attack, 135, 136–37, 140
exercise program for recovering patients, 155–57
massage for, 154
mental and physical relaxation, 135, 137
and metabolism, 137
precautions, 135
preventive exercises, 135–38
and the sedentary, 89
symptoms, 135–37
Tai Chi Chuan, 135, 139
therapeutic exercise, 139–40
Costusroot, 261
COW LOOKING AT THE MOON, THE, 99
Cun (measurement), 247n
CURING THE FIVE TROUBLES AND SEVEN DISORDERS BY TURNING THE HEAD
CURING THE FIVE TROUBLES AND SEVEN DISORDERS BY TURNING THE HEAD BACKWARD AND GAZING STERNLY, 54
CURING THE FIVE TROUBLES AND SEVEN DISORDERS BY TURNING THE HEAD BACKWARD AND GAZING STERNLY, 54
CYCLING, 161

D

Dachangshu acupoint, 245, 250d, 298
Daemonorops draco Blume, 261
Dahengwen acupoint, 255d
Daling acupoint, 245, 246d, 248d, 289, 299
Danshu acupoint, 245, 250d
Dan tian acupoint, 63
Dazhui acupoint, 199n, 245, 250d, 291, 298
Decubitus ulcer, 284–86
Depression. *See* Anxiety and depression
Diaphragmatic breathing. *See* Breathing, abdominal
Diaphragm, strengthening, 50, 53, 163
Diarrhea, 294
Dictamnus dsycarpus, 262
Diet
and coronary heart disease, 135, 136
and gastrointestinal problems, 159, 160, 164
importance of, 136, 159
Digestion, improving, 20, 53, 90, 92, 98, 102, 109, 164. *See also* Gastrointestinal problems
Dig method, 205–7, 258
Disease, and massage therapy, 188
Disk problems. *See also* Back; Backache; Posture; Spine
chiropractic manipulation for, 190
exercises for, 186–91
massage methods for, 189, 225, 236
physiotherapy, 190
surgical intervention, 190
Divergent push method, 198
Dizziness. *See also* Vertigo
prevention, 46
relief from, 20, 54, 60, 121, 129, 139, 169, 173
Drag method, 211–12
Dragon's Blood, 261, 263
DRAGON STAMPING ON THE EARTH, THE, 100
DRAWING A BOW, 62
DRAWING THE BOW WITH THE HANDS, 51–52
Dried silkwork, 262
Drowsiness, as side effect of Chi Kung, 68
"Dry bath," 172
Dryobalanops camphora Coleb., 261
Dryobalanops draco Blume, 263
Duanzirantong, 262

Duhuo, 262
Dujiao acupoint, 254
Dyspepsia, relief from, 132

E

Edema, relief from, 110
EDGE WALKING, 88
Egg white, 260
Elbow-extension method, 222
Elbow press method, 194
Elderly, the
 Ba Duan Jin and, 49
 coronary heart disease and, 136
 exercises for, 97–104
 benefits, 97
 THE COW LOOKING AT THE MOON, 99
 THE DRAGON STAMPING ON THE EARTH, 100
 Half,squatting, 101
 Handling two chestnuts with one hand, 101
 Rowing, 100
 Swinging the arms, 98
 Walking and massaging the abdomen, 102
 massage for, 102–4
 Shier Duan Jin and, 59
Electric vibrate method, 210
Electrocardiogram, 136
Emotional state, 19, 55, 69, 121, 137, 168–69. *See also* Anxiety and depression; Mental concentration; Relaxation
 arteriosclerosis and, 131
 coronary heart disease and, 139
 gastrointestinal problems and, 163
 insomnia and, 171
Emphysema, 70
Energy-system pluck method, 208
Ephedra vulgaris, 262
Errenshangma acupoint, 254, 255d
Ershanmen acupoint, 255d
Essential hypertension. *See* Hypertension
Exercise. *See also* Calisthenics; Chinese therapeutic exercises
 for massage techniques, 237–40
 medical, 268d
Extension method, 221–22
Extreme climate, relief from, 54
Eye-care massage, 302–3
Eyesight
 improving, 88
 poor, massage methods for, 195

F

Face massage, 60, 129, 154
Faintness, 177
 as side effect of *Chi Kung,* 69
Fangfeng, 262
Fanmen acupoint, 254, 255d
Fatigue, 288–90
 relief from, 21, 164, 173 (*See also* Chi Kung)
Feet
 massage, 64, 104, 129
 numbness, 132
 strengthening and developing, 64, 87, 88, 97, 100, 104
Feishu acupoint, 246, 250d, 298
Fengchi acupoint, 60, 195n, 205n, 211, 246d, 250d, 287, 291, 293, 299
Fengfu acupoint, 247, 250d, 293
Fengmen acupoint, 247, 250d
Fen (measurement), 247n
Fibrinolysis (anti,clotting effect) in blood, 137
"Fiery heart," tranquilizing the, 55
Finger chafe method, 212
Finger-cut method, 207
Finger dig method, 265, 267
Finger-needle method, 205
Finger pat method, 218
Fingers
 flexibility of, 101
 massage methods for, 215
Finger vibrate method, 209–210, 243, 265, 267
Fitness Exercises. *See* Chinese fitness exercises; Flexibility
Five-finger grasp method, 203
Five-finger knock method, 218
Five-finger pinch method, 215
"Five troubles," the, 54
Flaccid abdominal wall, 165
Flatfoot and foot strain, 277–79
Flat-palm push method, 201
Flat-thumb push method, 197–98, 199
Flatulence, 294
 relief from, 164, 168 (*See also* Digestion, improving)
Flexibility, 46, 47, 49, 56, 86, 93, 95, 101, 113. *See also* Relaxation
 ankles, 95
 in athletes, 111
 in children, 83
 fingers, 101
 hips, 45
 increasing, 20
 knees, 45, 95, 101
 neck, 99
 shoulders, 39, 42
 spine, 39, 42, 46, 47, 49, 55, 56, 62, 86, 91, 92, 93, 99, 100, 113, 116
Flick method, 217
Flu. *See* Influenza
Food build-up, 260
Foot arch, 277
Foot strain, 277–79
Forearm, massage methods for, 215
Forehead pain. *See* Headache
FORWARD THRUST, 114
Frankincense, 261, 263
Frozen shoulder, 279–82

G

Games and sports, therapeutic
 for anxiety and depression, 167, 169–70
 for coronary heart disease, 139
 following brain concussion, 173
 for hypertension, 121, 124, 128
 injuries, preventing, 111, 117
 for paraplegia, 179–81
Gancao, 262
Ganshu acupoint, 207n, 247, 250d
Gaohuang acupoint, 247, 250d
Gaoliang, 262
Gastric activity, and massage therapy, 187–88
Gastroenteritis, massage methods for, 213
Gastrointestinal problems, 159–65. *See also* Digestion, improving; Indigestion; Peptic ulcer; Stomach
 bowel illness, 159, 163
 Chi Kung for, 159, 160, 163
 Chi Kung for the Internal Organs, 74
 constipation, 159–64, 165
 diet and, 159, 164
 emotional state and, 163
 gastroptosis, 164–65
 indigestion, 159
 massage therapy for, 159, 160, 163, 216
 obesity, 159
 peptic ulcer, 159
 psychological state and, 163
 stomach illness, 159
Geshu acupoint, 207n, 247, 250d, 292
Ginger, 263
 juice, 260
Ginger-root, 262
Grasp method, 202–4
Greater *hengwen,* 255d
Green onion, 263
Guangmuxiang, 261

Guanyuan acupoint, 247, 248d, 289
Guiwei, 262
Guiwei acupoint, 254
Guizhi, 262
Gums. *See* Periodontitis

H

HALF-SITTING AND RELAXING, 108
HALF-SQUATTING, 101
Hammer method, 219–21, 243
Hamstrings, developing, 62
HANDLING TWO CHESTNUTS WITH ONE HAND, 101
Hands
  numbness, 132
  strengthening and developing, 45, 176
HANGING AND SWINGING, 116
Head
  exercise for hypertension, 126
  massage, 60, 129, 154
Headache, 286–88
  massage methods for, 194, 195, 211, 216
  relief from, 20, 60, 121, 129, 164, 169, 173
  as side effect of Chi Kung, 69
  as side effect of Yi Jin Jing, 35
Heart. *See also* Angina pectoris; Cardiorespiratory fitness; Coronary heart disease; Palpitation
  attack
  exercises for, 155–57
  prevention, 135
  Tai Chi Chuan and, 135
  treatment, 136-37, 140
  disease, 135–57
  Chi Kung for Fitness and, 70
  lack of activity and, 89
  strengthening, 54, 84, 121, 122
Heartburn, relief from, 164, 294
HEAVING, 37
Hegu acupoint, 186, 206n, 210n, 246d, 247, 250d, 287, 289, 299
Hemiplegia, exercises for, 174, 175–77
Hemorrhoids, 291–92
Hengwen acupoint, 254, 255d
Hiking and hill climbing, 127, 128, 138
Hip-bend method, 223–24
Hip rotation method, 227, 228d
Hips
  flexibility, 45, 46, 47, 49, 56, 86, 93, 95, 101, 113
  massage methods for, 223–25
  strengthening and developing, 114
HIPS, THE, 55
HITTING THE BEAN BAG, 84
Honghua, 261, 262
Honghua (Tibetan), 263
Huangtiao acupoint, 298
Huantiao acupoint, 194n, 207n, 247, 250d
HUNGRY TIGER JUMPING TOWARDS THE FOOD, THE, 45
Hypertension, 8, 35, 45, 46, 47, 54, 121–29. *See also* Circulation
  arteriosclerosis and, 131, 132, 134
  balance and, 124
  coordination and, 124
  coronary heart disease and, 139
  exercises for, 121–29
  benefits, 121–24
  Breathing exercise, 78, 125
  Chi Kung, 121, 122–24
  Chi Kung for Fitness, 70
  Chi Kung for Relaxation, 122
  Head exercise, 126
  Relaxation exercise, 125
  Sideward stretch, 126
  Tai Chi Chuan, 19, 20, 121, 124
  Upward stretch, 127
  Walking, 127
  games and, 121, 128
  liver, 187
  massage for, 104, 121, 124, 129, 187
  and the nervous system, 123–24
  principle of descent, 123
  treatment, 19, 20, 104, 121–29
  Yi Jin Jing and, 35
Hyperventilation, 68

I

Iliac crest, pain in, 264
Imagination, in exercises. *See* Mental concentration; Visualization
INCREASING THE VITAL ENERGY BY TIGHTENING THE FISTS AND GAZING STERNLY, 57
Indigestion, 294–96. *See also* Digestion, improving
  in children, 196
  flaccid abdominal wall and, 165
  massage methods for, 196
  relief from, 63, 164
  treatment, 159
Influenza, massage methods for, 197
Insomnia, 171–72, 264, 292–93. *See also* Relaxation
  arteriosclerosis and, 132
  breathing for, 172
  Chi Kung for Sleep, 172
  emotional state and, 171
  exercises for, 55, 171–72
  massage for, 104, 172
  Tai Chi Chuan for, 171
  treatment, 20, 64, 121, 132, 171
Internal organs, massage of, 65
Intervertebral disk problems. *See* Disk problems
Ischemia (deficient blood supply), 132, 136, 177

J

Jiang, 262
Jianging acupoint, 202n, 203d, 247, 299
Jianjing acupoint, 250d, 287, 290
Jianliao acupoint, 247, 250d
Jianyu acupoint, 246d, 247, 266
Jianzhen acupoint, 247, 250d
Jiexi acupoint, 247, 252d
Jingmang acupoint, 246d, 247, 248d
Jogging, 20
  for anxiety and depression, 167, 168, 169–70
  for coronary heart disease, 135, 138, 139
  for gastrointestinal problems, 159, 160, 162, 163
  for hypertension, 128
Joints, massage methods for, 217, 225–29
Juegu acupoint, 249, 252d

K

KEEPING ALL DISEASES AWAY BY RAISING THE HEELS SEVEN TIMES, 58
KICKING, 95
Kidneys, 54
Kneading method, 208–9, 267
KNEE BENDING, 160
KNEE BENDING AND RELAXING, 107
Knees
  degeneration of cartilage, 43
  flexibility, 45, 95, 101
  massage, 118, 129
  strengthening and developing, 35, 43, 92, 104, 111, 112, 115, 177
Knock method, 217–18

Kunlun acupoint, 249, 252d

L

LEG RAISING, 161
Legs. *See also* Ankles; Calves; Feet; Knees; Thighs
  circulation, 64, 95
  massage methods for, 214, 215, 235
  numbness as a side effect of *Chi Kung*, 68
  reducing of swelling in, 105, 110
  relief from pain in, 186
  strengthening and developing, 49, 62, 101, 103, 115, 122, 123
Liao acupoint, 265, 266, 292, 298
Licorice-root, 262
Lieguan acupoint, 246d, 248d, 249
LIFTING THE PLATES, 43
Lipid levels
  and arteriosclerosis, 131
  and coronary heart disease, 137
Liquor, medicinal, 261
Liufu acupoint, 254, 255d
Liver, 54, 187
Loin sprains, massage methods for, 199
Longevity, 65
Lower-limb shake method, 230
Lower-limb stretch method, 235
Lumbago, massage methods for, 192
Lumbar disk problems. *See* Disk problems
Lumbar pain, 265, 271. *See also* Disk problems
  chronic, 266–69
  massage methods for, 196
  from sciatica, 181
Lumbar rotation method, 228–29
Lumbar sprain, 271–72
Lumbar strain, 264–66
Lumbar stretch, 230–33, 268d
Lumbar suspension, 268d
Lungs. *See also* Breathing
  developing, 54, 84, 121
  emphysema, 70
Lymphatic vessels, 273

M

Mahuang, 262
MAKING A GESTURE OF RESPECT WITH BOTH HANDS FACING THE CHEST, 36
Mallets, for exercise, 221
Maqianzi, 262
Massage, 17–18, 59, 102–4. *See also* Acupuncture points: massage of; Yi Jin Jing
  abdomen, 63, 102, 163
  for anxiety and depression, 168, 169
  arms, 117
  for arteriosclerosis, 132, 134
  for athletes, 111, 117–18
  back, 63
  for constipation, 160, 163
  for coronary heart disease, 154
  for the elderly, 102–4
  eyes, 88
  face, 60, 129, 154
  feet, 64, 104, 129
  following brain concussion, 173
  for gastrointestinal problems, 159
  head, 129, 154
  for hypertension, 121, 124, 129
  for insomnia, 172
  internal organs, 65
  knees, 118, 129
  neck, 60, 129, 154
  for paralysis, 174, 175
  for sciatica and lumbar disk problems, 180
  shoulders, 118
  stomach, 50
  thighs, 117
  touch, 190
Massage techniques
  physical training for, 237–44
  practicing, 237–44
Massage therapy
  amount of massage, 257
  applications of, 265–66
  considerations during, 259–60
  degree of force, 257–58
  for disk problems, 189
  effect on disease, 186, 188
  general, 298–99
  and hypertension, 187
  individual needs, 259
  media used in, 260–63
  sequence of, 258, 259
  and skin temperature, 188
  strength of, 258
Medications, 261
  bone injuries, 262
  cartilage injuries, 262
  for hypertension, 122
  for massage of children, 260
  medicinal liquor, 261
  for perspiration, 261
  pneumonia, 262
  wound massage, 263
Meditation. *See* Mental concentration; Visualization
Megalo-spondylitis, 266
Meibingpian, 261
Menstrual problems, 296, 297–98
Mental concentration, 19, 167. *See also* Visualization
  for anxiety and depression, 167, 168
  in *Chi Kung*, 65, 66, 67, 68, 69–70, 72–73, 75
  for hypertension, 122, 124
  for insomnia, 172
  in *Tai Chi Chuan*, 20, 21
  Yi Jin Jing for, 35, 36, 37, 38, 39, 40–41, 42, 43
Mental relaxation. *See* Relaxation
Mental stress. *See* Anxiety and depression; Emotional state; Relaxation
Metabolism. *See also* Digestion, improving
  diseases, 159
  improving, 137
Middle-finger knock method, 217–18
Migraine, 286–88
Mingmen acupoint, 249, 250d, 265, 266, 291
MONKEY PLAY, 85
Morus alba L., 262
Motion sickness, 290–91
MOVING THE TONGUE AROUND, 60
Moyao, 261, 262, 263
Mulberry twigs, 262
Muscle dividing method, 199
Muscle laceration, 275–77
Muscles. *See also* Flexibility; Massage
  flaccid, 174
  massage methods for, 212, 230–35
  relaxation, massage methods for, 212
  spastic, 174
  strains, massage methods for, 204
  tone, 35
  weakness, 132, 173
Muscle-snapping method, 203–4
Muscle-straigthening method, 211–12
Muscle strengthening exercises, See *Yi Jin Jing*
Musculoskeletal problems
  in the elderly, 97–104
  in the sedentary, 89–95
Musk, 263
Myofasciitis, 283
Myrrh, 261, 262, 263

N

Native copper, 262
Nausea, 290, 294
Neck
flexibility of, 99
massage, 60, 129, 154
pain, 283
preventing stiffness, 39, 42, 91, 99
relief from pain, 35, 39, 42
stiff, 282–84
strengthening and developing, 45, 54, 97
Neck rotation method, 225
Neiguan acupoint, 206n, 210n, 246d, 248d, 249, 287, 296
Neilaogong acupoint, 206n, 254, 255d
Neixiyan acupoint, 252d
Nerve function
and disease, 186–87
effect of massage on, 186
Nervousness, 296–97
Nervous system, 123–24. *See also* Emotional state; Relaxation
Neuromuscular tension, reducing, 169
Nocturnal emissions, relief from, 63
Notopterygium incisum Ting., 262

O

Obesity, 159. *See also* Diet
Occupational strain, 264
Occupational therapy for paralysis, 176
Old form *Tai Chi Chuan*. *See Tai Chi Chuan*
Overeating, 159
relief from, 54

P

Pain
ankle, 270
foot, 277–78
lower back, 264
lumbar, 267, 271
menstrual, 297–98
muscular, 275
neck, 283
relief, massage methods for, 210
shoulder, 279
Pain shifting method, 186–87
Palm, massage methods for, 215
Palm chafe method, 213
Palm-edge chafe method, 213
Palm-edge hammer method, 220
Palm-edge rub-roll method, 214
Palm-heel kneading method, 265
Palm-heel push method, 201–2
Palm-heel rub method, 196–97
Palm kneading method, 209
Palm pat method, 219
Palm press method, 192–93
Palm rub method, 196, 265
Palm rub-roll method, 213–14
Palm-vibrate method, 210
Palpitation, 121
relief from, 64
side effect of Chi Kung, 68–69
Paralysis. *See also* Hemiplegia; Paraplegia
acupuncture for, 174
benefits of exercises for, 174
duration of exercises, 174
functional training exercises, 174
massage for, 174, 175, 200
spinal cord injury, 174
stroke, 174
walking, 174
Paraplegia
causes of, 176
circulation and, 177
defined, 176
exercises for, 174, 176–80
benefits, 176–78
faintness and, 177
games for, 179–81
ischemia and, 177
surgical intervention, 177
therapeutic sports, 179
treatment, 176
Pat method, 218, 243
Peach kernel, 262
Peck method, 218
PELVIC ROCKING, 106
Pelvis
relaxation of, 107, 108, 109
relief from pressure on, 105
Peptic ulcer. *See also* Gastrointestinal problems; Relaxation; Stomach
Chi Kung for the Internal Organs, 74
exercise with *Tai Chi* stick for, 79
treatment, 159
Periarthritis, 61. *See also* Arthritis
Periodontitis, 60
Peripheral ischemia. *See* Ischemia
Perspiration, 187
Phobias, relief from, 167. *See also* Anxiety and depression; Emotional state; Relaxation
Physical Fitness. *See Ba Duan Jin;* Chinese fitness exercises; Flexibility; *Yi Jin Jing*
Physical relaxation. *See* Relaxation
Physical training, for massage, 237–40
PICKING UP BEANS, 92
Pillows, in massage therapy, 191
Pinch method, 215–16, 243
Pishu acupoint, 187, 207n, 249, 250d
Pitu acupoint, 255d
Pitu line, 200
Pluck method, 207–8
Pneumonia, herbs for, 262
Popliteal fossa, massage of, 129
Posture. *See also* Back; Spine
in *Chi Kung*, 65
for children, 83
faulty, 165
improving, 35, 36, 37, 38, 49, 50, 58, 87
Pregnant women, exercises for, 105–10
Abdominal breathing, 106
benefits, 105
Half-sitting and relaxing, 108
Knee bending and relaxing, 107
Pelvic rocking, 106
Squatting and relaxing, 109
Stretching and relaxing, 110
Tailor sitting (sitting cross-legged) and rhythmic breathing, 108
Walking, 109
Premenstrual syndrome, 296
Press method, 192, 193d, 194
Prone-fist hammer method, 220
Prunus perspica, 262
Psychological state. *See* Anxiety and depression; Emotional state; Mental concentration
Psychoneuroses. *See also* Anxiety and depression; Emotional state; Relaxation
Chi Kung for Fitness for, 70
exercise with *Tai Chi* stick for, 79
Psychosomatic illness. *See* Anxiety and depression; *Chi Kung;* Emotional state
Pucan acupoint, 249, 252d
PULLING THE EAR, 42
PULLING THE TAILS OF NINE OXEN, 40–41
PUSHING THE MOUNTAIN, 41
PUSHING TOWARDS THE SKY
(Shier Duan Jin), 61
(Yi Jin Jing), 38
PUSHING WITH THE HANDS WHILE RIDING A HORSE, 92
Push method, 197–202

Q

Qianghuo, 262
Qi (chi), defined, 200n
Qichong acupoint, 248d, 249
Qihai acupoint, 248d, 249
Quadriceps, 112
Quchi acupoint, 246d, 249, 255, 296, 299
Quepen acupoint, 248d, 249
Quietness training in *Chi Kung*, 66, 72–73, 75. *See also* Relaxation

R

REACHING THE STARS, 39
Red blood cells, 188
REGULATING THE INTERNAL ORGANS BY RAISING BOTH HANDS TO THE SKY, 50
REGULATING THE SPLEEN AND STOMACH BY RAISING THE HAND UPWARD, 53
Relaxation, 20, 116. *See also* Breathing; Emotional state; Mental concentration
- for anxiety and depression, 167–68
- *Ba Duan Jin* for, 54, 55
- *Chi Kung* for, 64, 65, 66, 69–70, 72–73, 75
- in coronary heart disease, 135, 137
- exercise with the Tai Chi stick for, 79
- following brain concussion, 173
- in hypertension, 121, 122, 123–24, 125
- in insomnia, 171–72
- in pregnancy, 106, 107, 108, 109
- *Tai Chi Chuan* for, 19, 20
- *Yi Jin Jing* for, 36

RELAXING THE WAIST AND TAPPING THE BODY, 116–17
Renzhong acupoint, 246d, 248d, 249, 291
Respiration. *See* Breathing
Respiratory system, massage methods for, 201
Restlessness, 55. *See also* Relaxation
Rheumatic disorders, massage methods for, 204, 213
Rheumatism, treatment of, 20, 54
Rhus verniciflua Stokes, 261
Rhythm, in massage therapy, 190
Rib pain, as side effect of Chi Kung, 68
RIDING A HORSE, 112
Roll method, 204–5, 242, 265, 267
ROPE JUMPING, 84
Rotation method, 225–29
Rowing, 162
ROWING, 100
Rub method, 195–96, 267
Rub-roll method, 213–14
Rugen acupoint, 248d, 249
Running. *See* Jogging
Ruxiang, 261, 262, 263

S

Safflower, 261, 262, 263
Saliva, secretion of, 60
Sandbags, for massage practice, 240
Sanguan acupoint, 254, 255d
Sanguan line, 200n
Sangzhi, 262
Sanyinjiao acupoint, 249, 252d, 287, 296, 299
Saussurea lappa Clarke, 261
Scalp, massage methods for, 217
Sciatica, 186–91, 267. *See also* Back; Backache; Posture; Spine
- causes, 180, 186
- defined, 180, 186
- disk problems and, 184, 190
- exercises for, 180–84, 187–91
  - benefits, 186
  - inflammation of nerves, 186
  - lumbar pain, 181
  - lumbosacral arthritis, 186
  - massage, 180
- massage for, 180, 186
- sacroiliac arthritis, 186
- sciatic neuritis, 186
- symptoms, 180, 190
- treatment, 180, 190

Scoliosis, 87
Sedentary, the, 89–95
- arteriosclerosis and, 131
- coronary heart disease and, 89
- exercises for, 90–95
  - benefits, 89
  - Kicking, 95
  - Picking up beans, 92
  - Pushing with the hands while riding a horse, 92
  - Spreading the "wings," 94
  - Swaying from the waist and hips, 93
  - Swinging the arms, 90
  - Twisting the trunk and looking backward, 91
  - Walking like the wind, 94

Self-administered massage. *See* Acupuncture points, massage of; Massage; Self-massage
Self-control, increasing, 19
Self-esteem and confidence, enhancing, 19, 169. *See also* Well-being, promoting
Self-massage, 288, 300–301
Sesame oil, 263
"Seven disorders," the, 54
Shake method, 229–30
Shaking grasp method, 203
Shangliao acupoint, 249, 250d
Shangwan acupoint, 248d, 251, 295
Shanmen acupoint, 255, 255d
Shaohai acupoint, 246d, 248d, 251
Shaoshang acupoint, 200n
Shaoshang method, 200
Shenmen acupoint, 246d, 248d, 251, 289, 299
Shenque acupoint, 248d, 251
Shenshanqi, 261
Shenshu acupoint, 63, 103, 250d, 251, 265, 292
Shexiang, 263
Shier Duan Jin (Twelve fine exercises), 59–64
- for the chronically ill, 59
- for the elderly, 59
- exercises, 60–64
  - Beating the "drum of heaven," 60
  - Bending the trunk with the hands touching the feet, 62
  - benefits, 59
  - Biting the teeth, 60
  - Drawing a bow, 62
  - Moving the tongue around, 60
  - Pushing towards the sky, 60
  - Stretching the legs, 64
  - Stroking the *dan tian* (field of pills), 63
  - Stroking the *shen shu* (kidney point), 63
  - Stroking the *yung chuan*
  - "Washing" the face, 60
  - Winding the pulley, 61

SHOOTING THE EAGLE BY DRAWING THE BOW WITH THE HANDS, 51–52
Shoulder-extension method, 221
Shoulder rotation method, 226, 227
Shoulders
- flexibility, 39, 42
- frozen, 279–82
- massage, 118
- massage methods for, 215, 234
- medical exercise, 281d
- pain in, 279
- pariarthritis, 279–82
- strengthening and developing, 51, 53, 61, 62, 90, 98, 114, 177, 179

Shousanli acupoint, 246d, 251, 299
Sibai acupoint, 246d, 248d, 251
Side-of-the-thumb push method, 200
Siegesbeckie, orientalis var. pubescens, 262
Sihengwen acupoint, 255d
Silkworm, dried, 262
Simplified *Tai Chi Chuan. See Tai Chi Chuan*
Single-finger dig method, 205–6
Sit ups, 162
Skin
  circulation in, 60
  temperature, and massage therapy, 188
Sleep, lack of. *See* Insomnia
Soft tissue injuries, 204, 269, 273
Songhua powder, 261
Sorghum liquor, 262
Spinal pinch method, 216
Spinchter spasm, 291
Spine. *See also* Back; Backache; Posture
  compressive fracture of, 266, 267
  curvature of, 87, 165
  flexibility of, 39, 42, 46, 47, 49, 55, 56, 62, 86, 91, 92, 93, 99, 100, 113, 116
  injury to, 174, 176
  and surgical intervention, 177
"Spiritual exercise," 167
Spleen, 53, 54
Sports. *see* Athletes; Games and sports, therapeutic
Sprain, 269–75
  of ankle joint, 269
SPREADING THE "WINGS", 94
SQUATTING AND RELAXING, 109
Stamina, increasing. *See* Chinese therapeutic exercises
Standing *Chi Kung* and hypertension, 122–23
Stiff neck, 282–84
Stomach. *See also* Digestion, improving; Indigestion; Peptic ulcer
  illness, prevention of, 159
  massage, 50
  strengthening and developing, 164
Strengthening and developing
Stress, relief from. *See* Anxiety and depression; Mental concentration; Relaxation
STRETCHING AND RELAXING, 110
Stretching exercises, 44, 62, 64, 110, 116, 126–27, 141, 142, 148–49. *See also Yi Jin Jing;* individual exercises
STRETCHING THE ARMS, 44
STRETCHING THE LEGS, 64
Stretch method, 230–35
Stroke, exercises following, 174
Strychnos nux vomica, 262
SWALLOW FLYING, 115
SWAYING FROM THE WAIST AND HIPS, 93
Swelling
  in bruises, 273
  reduction of, massage methods for, 211–12
Swimming
  and coronary heart disease, 139
  and hypertension, 121, 124, 127
SWINGING THE ARMS, 90, 98
Symbolism in Chinese exercises. *See* Visualization
Sympathetic nervous system. *See* Nervous system
Syncope. *See* Faintness
Szechuan *honghua,* 261

T

Tai Chi, 191
Tai Chi Chuan, 19–34
  for anxiety and depression, 168
  for arteriosclerosis, 132
  benefits of, 19–21
  breathing and, 20, 21, 165
  circulation and, 20
  for coronary heart disease, 135, 139
  defined, 19
  digestion and, 20
  how to practice, 20–22
  for hypertension, 121, 124
  for insomnia, 171
  intensity of, 20–21
  mental concentration and, 20, 21
  need for a teacher, 22
  Old form, 124
  physical relaxation and, 21
  popularity of, 21
  principles of, 21–22
  Simplified
  21, 124
  illustrated, 23–34
Tai Chi stick, exercise with
  benefits, 79
  exercises, 79–80
  Circling at a resting position, 79
  Circling while moving the legs up and down, 79
  Circling while walking, 80
  possible side effects of, 80
Taichong acupoint, 251, 252d, 299
TAILOR SITTING AND RHYTHMIC BREATHING, 108
Taixi acupoint, 251, 266, 299
Taiyang acupoint, 194n, 211, 246d, 251
Taiyuan acupoint, 246d, 248d, 251, 289, 299
Talcum powder, 261
Taoren, 262
Tao yin, 20, 59
Teeth. *See* Periodontitis
Tension, relief from, 168. *See also* Anxiety and depression; Emotional state; Flexibility; Mental concentration; Relaxation
Ten xuan acupoint, 251
Terrain cure, 138
Therapeutic exercise. *See* Chinese therapeutic exercises
Thighs
  massage methods for, 117, 215, 220
  strengthening and developing, 35, 43, 51, 55, 114
Three-finger grasp method, 202, 203d
Three-finger pinch method, 215
Thumb kneading method, 209, 265
Thumb press method, 194
Thumb push method, 241–42, 267
Thumb rub method, 195–96
Thumb-tip push method, 200n
Tianchong, 262
Tianheshui acupoint, 255, 255d
Tianshu acupoint, 248d, 251
Tianting acupoint, 246d, 248d, 251, 293, 295, 296
Tianzong acupoint, 250d, 251
Tibetan *honghua,* 261
TIGER WALKING, 86, 113
Tinggong acupoint, 211, 246d, 251
Tinghui acupoint, 246d, 253
TIP-TOE WALKING, 87
Torticollis, 282–84
Touch, importance of, 190
Traditional Chinese exercises
  Ba Duan Jin (Eight fine exercises), 49–58
  benefits of, 167–68
  Breathing exercise, 78
  Chi Kung (Invigorating exercises), 65–75, 122, 123, 139, 163, 164–65, 168–69, 172
  Shier Duan Jin (Twelve fine exercises), 59–64

Tai Chi Chuan, 19–34, 124, 135, 139, 168, 171
Tai Chi stick, exercise with, 79–80
Yi Jin Jing, 35–47
TRANQUILIZING THE FIERY HEART BY TURNING THE HEAD AROUND AND SWINGING, 55
Tread method, 236
Tweak method, 216–17
TWISTING THE TRUNK AND LOOKING BACKWARD, 91
Twist method, 216–17
Two-hip bend method, 224–25
Typing-up method, 200

U

Ulcer, necrotic, 284–86
Upper-limb shake method, 229–30
Upper-limb stretch method, 234
Upright-fist hammer method, 220
Urine retention, 187

V

Vertigo, 133, 164, 169, 173
Vibrate method, 209–10
Viral hepatitis, 74
Vision, improving, 88
Visualization. *See also* Mental concentration
for athletes, 112, 113, 115
in *Ba Duan Jin*, 51–52, 54, 57
for children, 85, 86, 87
for the elderly, 99, 100
for the sedentary, 92, 94
in *Shier Duan Jin*, 60, 61, 62
in *Tai Chi Chuan*, 21, 22
Vitality, enhancing, 103. *See also Chi Kung;* Chinese fitness exercises; Well-being, promoting
Vomiting, 290

W

Waiguan acupoinjt, 250d, 253, 299
Waijianshi acupoint, 255, 255d
Waixiyian acupoint, 252d
Walking, 94, 102. *See also* specific ailments and individual parts of the body
for anxiety and depression, 169
for arteriosclerosis, 132
for constipation, 162
for coronary heart disease, 138, 139, 141, 152, 156
for heart attack, 156
for hypertension, 121, 124, 127, 128
for insomnia, 171
for paralysis, 174, 175, 176, 178–80
for pregnant women, 109
WALKING AND MASSAGING THE ABDOMEN, 102
WALKING LIKE THE WIND, 94
WALL PUSHING, 115
"WASHING" THE FACE, 60
Water, use in massage, 260
Weight control. *See* Diet; Obesity; Overeating
Weishu acupoint, 187, 250d, 253
Weizhong acupoint, 202n, 252d, 253, 266, 298
Well-being, promoting, 54, 59–64, 78, 90, 98, 103. *See also* Mental concentration; Relaxation; Self-esteem and confidence
WINDING THE PULLEY, 61
WORM WRIGGLING, 87
Wushaoshe, 262
Wuzhjie acupoint, 255d

X

*Xialiao a*cupoint, 249, 250d, 251
Xiaohengwen acupoint, 255d
Xiawan acupoint, 248d, 253, 295
Xinshu acupoint, 250d, 292
Xixiancao acupoint, 262
Xiyan acupoint, 252d, 253
Xuehai acupoint, 252d, 253
Xuejie acupoint, 261, 263

Y

Yamen acupoint, 250d, 253
Yangchi acupoint, 250d, 253
Yanggu acupoint, 250d, 253, 299
Yangguan acupoint, 250d, 253, 291
Yanglingquan acupoint, 252d, 253, 299
Yangxi acupoint, 246d, 250d, 253
Yifeng acupoint, 246d, 250d, 253, 291, 293
Yi Jin Jing (Muscle strengthening exercises), 35–47
as body/mind exercises, 36–47
exercises, 36–47
Bending forward, 47
Bowing, 46
Heaving, 37
Lifting the plates, 43
Making a gesture of respect with both hands facing the chest, 36
Pulling the ear, 42
Pulling the tails of nine oxen, 40–41
Pushing the mountain, 41
Pushing towards the sky, 38
Reaching the stars, 39
Stretching the arms, 44
hungry tiger jumping towards the food, 45
mental concentration in, 35, 36
principles of, 35
as stretching exercise, 36–38
Yin and *Yang*, 19, 186
defined, 186n
Yinglingquan acupoint, 296
Yingxiang acupoint, 246d, 248d, 253
Yinlingquan acupoint, 252d, 253, 299
Yintang acupoint, 199n, 211, 248d, 254, 289, 295, 297, 299
Yin Yang, 298
Yiwofeng acupoint, 206n, 255
Yongquan acupoint, 252d, 254, 292, 296, 299
Yung chuan acupoint, 64, 104, 129, 172, 252d, 254, 292, 296, 299
Yushushenyou, 263
Ywofeng acupoint, 255d

Z

Zanzhu acupoint, 246d, 248d, 254, 299
Zaocys dhumnades, 262
Zhangnao, 261, 263
Zhanjindan, 263
Zhijie acupoint, 254, 255d
Zhongfu acupoint, 248d, 254
Zhongliao acupoint, 249, 250d, 251
Zhongwan acupoint, 248d, 254, 295
Zuanzhu acupoint, 199n
Zusanli acupoint, 187
Zusanli acupoint, 206n, 210n, 252d, 254, 287, 289, 291, 296
Zuzanli acupoint, 252d, 299